T0257247

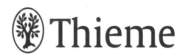

The Business of Dermatology

Jeffrey S. Dover, MD, FRCPC
Co-director
SkinCare Physicians
Chestnut Hill, Massachusetts
Associate Professor of Clinical Dermatology
Yale University School of Medicine
New Haven, Connecticut
Associate Professor of Dermatology
Brown Medical School
Providence, Rhode Island

Kavita Mariwalla, MD, FAAD
Director
Mariwalla Dermatology
New York, New York

50 illustrations

Thieme
Stuttgart • New York • Delhi • Rio de Janeiro

Library of Congress Cataloging-in-Publication Data is available from the publisher

Important note: Medicine is an ever-changing science undergoing continual development. Research and clinical experience are continually expanding our knowledge, in particular our knowledge of proper treatment and drug therapy. Insofar as this book mentions any dosage or application, readers may rest assured that the authors, editors, and publishers have made every effort to ensure that such references are in accordance with the state of knowledge at the time of production **of the book.**

Nevertheless, this does not involve, imply, or express any guarantee or responsibility on the part of the publishers in respect to any dosage instructions and forms of applications stated in the book. **Every user is requested to examine carefully** the manufacturers' leaflets accompanying each drug and to check, if necessary, in consultation with a physician or specialist,whether the dosage schedules mentioned therein or the contraindications stated by the manufacturers differ from the statements made in the present book. Such examination is particularly important with drugs that are either rarely used or have been newly released on the market. Every dosage schedule or every form of application used is entirely at the user's own risk and responsibility. The authors and publishers request every user to report to the publishers any discrepancies or inaccuracies noticed. If errors in this work are found after publication, errata will be posted at www.thieme.com on the product description page.

Some of the product names, patents, and registered designs referred to in this book are in fact registered trademarks or proprietary names even though specific reference to this fact is not always made in the text. Therefore, the appearance of a name without designation as proprietary is not to be construed as a representation by the publisher that it is in the public domain.

Georg Thieme Verlag KG
Rüdigerstrasse 14, 70469 Stuttgart, Germany
+49 [0]711 8931 421, customerservice@thieme.de

Thieme Publishers New York
333 Seventh Avenue, New York, NY 10001 USA
+1 800 782 3488, customerservice@thieme.com

Thieme Publishers Delhi
A-12, Second Floor, Sector-2, Noida-201301
Uttar Pradesh, India
+91 120 45 566 00, customerservice@thieme.in

Thieme Publishers Rio, Thieme Publicações Ltda.
Edifício Rodolpho de Paoli, 25º andar
Av. Nilo Peçanha, 50 - Sala 2508
Rio de Janeiro 20020-906 Brasil
+55 21 3172 2297 / +55 21 3172 1896

Cover design: Thieme Publishing Group
Typesetting by DiTech Process Solutions, India

Printed in Germany by CPI Books   5 4 3 2 1

ISBN 978-3-13-242779-2

Also available as an e-book:
eISBN 978-3-13-242780-8

Experience has taught us that the practice of dermatology is not just an art and science but also involves a bit of pluck and determination. Bringing this project together was a labor of love. Thank you to our colleagues and friends who selflessly gave their time and were bold enough to be truly honest in their written words.

Jeffrey S. Dover, MD, FRCPC
Kavita Mariwalla, MD, FAAD

To my mentor Kenneth Arndt, a true scholar whose enthusiasm, inquisitiveness, support, and friendship have guided me through my career.
To Michael Kaminer, who has taught me much of what I know of the business of medicine.
To my colleagues at SkinCare Physicians and to my support team of Chris Foley, Maureen Teahan, Beth Hartigan, Joanne Shortell, Andrea Digiulio, and Joan Buchanan.
And, most importantly, to Tania Phillips, my constant companion, guide, and moral compass.

—Jeffrey

To Jeff Dover whose grace and friendship through the years has been a blessing.
To create a successful practice, you need a few key ingredients. For me they have been:
My teachers who gave me the skills to create a successful life—Jean Bolognia, David Leffell, and Lisa Donofrio.
My cheerleaders who are always there with words of wisdom—Raju and Rajesh Mariwalla.
My friends who answer calls at any time of day—Mona Gohara and Allison Hanlon.
My practice family to whom I am indebted—Lori Ulrich and the staff at Mariwalla Dermatology.
And, of course, none of it is worthwhile without Kabir, Shyer, Ashar, and Ayan—the writer, poet, verses, and muse of life.

—Kavita

Contents

Contents

50 Marketing and Advertising Your Dermatology Practice 320

Michelle Henry

Section VII Miscellaneous 327

51 Growing Your Practice 328

Vince Bertucci and Alessia C. Bertucci

52 Mohs: Outsource or Keep In-House 335

Allison Hanlon

53 The Ground Rules of Teaching in a Private Practice 338

Lauren Taglia

Preface

Though it may seem strange to put the word "Business" next to a field of medicine, whether you are in private practice or part of an institution, there exists this component of our specialty which was not taught in residency but is vital to understand. Unfortunately, as a group, we do not talk about it enough. New residents graduate, pass the Boards each year, and feel like they have to reinvent the wheel before they join a group or decide to hang their own shingle. Owning your own practice can feel like you are on an island with insurmountable questions; this is where *The Business of Dermatology* can help. There is no doubt that joining an established practice can make you feel like there must be better ways to do things than the model you are inheriting; this is also where *The Business of Dermatology* can help. And, finally, there are those of us who feel like we made it work so far but wish that we had an inside look into how a colleague did it; this is also a place where *The Business of Dermatology* can add value.

For us, having the conversation is where this book started. In putting the table of contents together, we thought of questions from the perspective of a doctor starting out in practice but also asked ourselves what we wish we knew back then and the advice we wish we had. We have broken it down into sections specific to different parts of practicing dermatology. We asked for contributions from authors with whom we have worked, whose practices are flourishing, but most importantly, those who were willing to give honest advice. For this reason, the book is written in an informal tone. It is meant to be a quick read to give you insight but also to stimulate conversation and questions for yourself. To our surprise, the submissions we received made us rethink some of what we already do in our practices now. And ultimately, that is what we are most proud of—that *The Business of Dermatology* is not just for beginners, it is like a 40-way group chat with the people we trust.

We hope that you will find it helpful and informative whether you are 2 months out or 20 years.

Jeffrey S. Dover, MD, FRCPC
Kavita Mariwalla, MD, FAAD

Contributors

Murad Alam, MD, MSCI, MBA
Professor and Vice-chair
Department of Dermatology
Northwestern University, Feinberg School
   of Medicine
Chicago, Illinois

Jusleen Ahluwalia, MD
Resident Physician
Department of Dermatology
University of California
San Diego, California

Kenneth A. Arndt, MD
Adjunct Professor
Department of Dermatology
Brown University
Providence, Rhode Island
President
SkinCare Physicians
Chestnut Hill, Massachusetts

Curtis Asbury, MD, FAAD
Owner
Delmarva Skin Specialists
Selbyville, Delaware

Jessica Awerman, MD
Dermatology Resident
Department of Dermatology
Tufts Medical Center
Boston, Massachusetts

Eileen L. Axibal, MD
Fellow, Micrographic Surgery & Dermatologic
   Oncology
Department of Dermatology
University of Colorado
Aurora, Colorado

Alessia C. Bertucci, BComm
Business Operations Analyst
Digital Marketing and Analytics
EHN Canada
Toronto, Ontario, Canada

Vince Bertucci, MD, FRCPC
Instructor
Division of Dermatology
University of Toronto
Toronto, Ontario, Canada

Neal Bhatia, MD
Director
Clinical Dermatology
Therapeutics Clinical Research
San Diego, California

Mariah R. Brown, MD
Associate Professor
Department of Dermatology
University of Colorado School of Medicine
Aurora, Colorado

Kim Campbell, MA
Founder
Dermatology Authority
New York, New York

David B. Chaffin, JD
Partner
White and Williams LLP
Boston, Massachusetts

Annie Chiu, MD
Founder and Director
The Derm Institute
Hermosa Beach, California

Doris Day, MD
Clinical Associate Professor
Department of Dermatology
NYU Langone Health
New York, New York

Amy Derick, MD
Academic Associate Member
Section of Dermatology
University of Chicago
Chicago, Illinois;
Clinical Instructor
Department of Dermatology
Northwestern University
Evanston, Illinois

Jeffrey S. Dover, MD, FRCPC
Co-director
SkinCare Physicians
Chestnut Hill, Massachusetts
Associate Professor of Clinical Dermatology
Yale University School of Medicine
New Haven, Connecticut
Associate Professor of Dermatology
Brown Medical School
Providence, Rhode Island

Matthew J. Elias, DO, FAAD
Clinical Assistant Professor
Nova Southeastern University;
Private Practice
Elias Dermatology, LLC
Fort Lauderdale, Florida

Merrick D. Elias, DO, FAAD
Clinical Assistant Professor
Nova Southeastern University
Fort Lauderdale, Florida
Private Practice
Elias Dermatology, LLC
Pembroke Pines, Florida

Aleksandra G. Florek, MD
Resident Physician
Department of Dermatology
University of Colorado School of Medicine
   Anschutz Medical Campus
Denver, Colorado

Christine E. Foley, BA
Chief Operating Officer
SkinCare Physicians
Chestnut Hill, Massachusetts

Cynthia Forbush, BA, SPHR
Human Resources Business Partner
SkinCare Physicians
Chestnut Hill, Massachusetts

Joseph K. Francis, MD
Adjunct Clinical Assistant Professor
Department of Dermatology
University of Florida College of Medicine
Gainesville, Florida

Chloe Gianatasio, MS
Project Specialist
Miami Dermatology and Laser Institute
Miami, Florida

Mona A. Gohara, MD
Associate Clinical Professor
Department of Dermatology
Yale School of Medicine
New Haven, Connecticut

David J. Goldberg, MD, JD
Director
Skin Laser & Surgery Specialists of NY/NJ;
Clinical Professor of Dermatology
Past Director of Mohs Surgery and Laser Research
Icahn School of Medicine at Mount Sinai;
Clinical Professor of Dermatology
Chief, Dermatology Surgery
UMDNJ–Rutgers Medical School
Adjunct Professor of Law
Fordham Law School
New York, New York

Michael T. Goldfarb, MD
Lecturer
Department of Dermatology
University of Michigan
Ann Arbor, Michigan

Elizabeth K. Hale, MD
Clinical Associate Professor
Department of Dermatology
NYU Langone Health;
Co-founder
CompleteSkinMD
New York, New York

Allison Hanlon, MD, PhD
Assistant Professor
Department of Dermatology
Vanderbilt University Medical Center
Nashville, Tennessee

Heather Hamilton, MD
Dermatologist
Dermatology Physicians of Connecticut
Shelton, Connecticut

Michelle Henry, MD
Clinical Instructor of Dermatology
Department of Dermatology
Weill Cornell Medical College
New York, New York

Byron K. Ho, MD
Resident Physician
Department of Dermatology
Johns Hopkins Medicine
Baltimore, Maryland

Sara Hogan, MD
Health Sciences Clinical Instructor
Division of Dermatology
University of California
Los Angeles, California

Deirdre Hooper, MD
Co-founder
Audubon Dermatology;
Assistant Clinical Professor
Department of Dermatology
Louisiana State University School of Medicine;
Assistant Clinical Professor
Department of Dermatology
Tulane University School of Medicine
New Orleans, Louisiana

George J. Hruza, MD, MBA
Adjunct Professor
Departments of Dermatology and Otolaryngology
St. Louis University School of Medicine
St. Louis, Missouri

Omer Ibrahim, MD
Dermatologist
Chicago Cosmetic Surgery and Dermatology
Chicago, Illinois

Brooke A. Jackson, MD
Medical Director
Skin Wellness Dermatology Associates
Durham, North Carolina

Sarah Jackson, MD
Co-founder
Audubon Dermatology;
Assistant Clinical Professor
Department of Dermatology
Louisiana State University School of Medicine
New Orleans, Louisiana

Reena Jogi, MD
Dermatologist
Village Dermatology
Houston, Texas

Michael S. Kaminer, MD
Associate Clinical Professor
Department of Dermatology
Yale School of Medicine
New Haven, Connecticut
Adjunct Assistant Professor
Department Dermatology
Brown Medical School
Providence, Rhode Island
Co-founder
SkinCare Physicians, Inc.
Chestnut Hill, Massachusetts

James D. Kelso, JD, LLM (Health)
Managing Partner
The Law Office of James D. Kelso, PC
San Antonio, Texas

Kyle Kieffer, BA
Student
Department of Neurobiology
Northwestern University
Evanston, Illinois

Sailesh Konda, MD, FAAD, FACMS
Assistant Clinical Professor of Dermatology
Department of Dermatology
University of Florida College of Medicine
Gainesville, Florida

Laura Kruter, MD
Dermatologist
Skin Associates of South Florida
Coral Gables, Florida

Edward (Ted) Lain, MD, MBA
Chief Medical Officer
Sanova Dermatology
Austin, Texas

Keith LeBlanc, Jr., MD, FAAD, FACMS
Assistant Clinical Professor
Department of Dermatology
LSU Health Sciences Center
New Orleans, Louisiana

Wendy Lewis, BA
President
Wendy Lewis & Co Ltd, Global Aesthetics
  Consultancy
New York, New York

Aleksandra Lindgren, BA, MS3
Medical student
University of Queensland Ochsner Clinical School
New Orleans, Louisiana

Peter A. Lio, MD
Clinical Assistant Professor
Dermatology and Pediatrics
Northwestern University, Feinberg School
  of Medicine
Chicago, Illinois

Kavita Mariwalla, MD, FAAD
Director
Mariwalla Dermatology
New York, New York

Ellen Marmur, MD
President/Founder
Marmur Medical, & MMSkincare
New York, New York

Gabriel J. Martinez-Diaz, MD, FAAD
CEO, Owner, and Medical Director
M D Aesthetics and Dermatology, LLC
Chicago, Illinois

Girish S. Munavalli, MD, MHS, FACMS
Medical Director
Dermatology, Laser, and Vein Specialists of the
  Carolinas
Charlotte, North Carolina

Colton Nielson, MD
Chief Resident
Department of Dermatology
University of Florida
Gainesville, Florida

Rajiv Nijhawan, MD
Assistant Professor
Department of Dermatology
University of Texas Southwestern Medical Center
Dallas, Texas

Jeffrey S. Orringer, MD
Professor, Service Chief, and Division Chief
Department of Dermatology
University of Michigan
Ann Arbor, Michigan

Briana Paiewonsky, BS, MS2
Medical Student
Charles E. Schmidt College of Medicine
Florida Atlantic University
Boca Raton, Florida

Chad L. Prather, MD
Clinical Assistant Professor
Department of Dermatology
Louisiana State University School of Medicine;
Private Practice
Sanova Dermatology
Baton Rouge, Louisiana

Heather D. Rogers, MD
Co-owner of Modern Dermatology;
Founder and CEO of Doctor Rogers RESTORE
  Skin Care;
Clinical Professor of Dermatology
University of Washington School of Washington
Seattle, Washington

E. Victor Ross, MD
Director
Laser and Cosmetic Dermatology
Scripps Clinic
San Diego, California

Anthony M. Rossi, MD, FAAD
Assistant Attending
Memorial Sloan Kettering Cancer Center;
Assistant Professor of Dermatology
Weill Cornell Medical College
Memorial Sloan Kettering Cancer Center
New York, New York

David A. Rubin, BBA, MPA
Partner
Telecom Consulting Group
Pompano Beach, Florida;
Vice President
KB Technologies
Deerfield Beach, Florida

Nazanin Saedi, MD
Associate Professor
Department of Dermatology and Cutaneous Biology
Thomas Jefferson University
Philadelphia, Pennsylvania

Sarah Sawyer, MD
President
Dermatology & Laser of Alabama
Birmingham, Alabama

Daniel I. Schlessinger, MD
Resident Physician
Department of Medicine
Massachusetts General Hospital
Boston, Massachusetts

Contributors

Joel Schlessinger, MD, FAAD
Director
Advanced Skin Research Center
Omaha, Nebraska

Camile A. Silva, AIA, LEED AP
Owner
C.SILVA Architect, LLC
Baton Rouge, Louisiana

Lauren Taglia, MD, PhD
Dermatologist
Department of Dermatology
Northwestern Regional Medicine Group
Naperville, Illinois

Nikki D.Y. Tang, MD, FAAD, FACMS
Mohs Surgeon
The Clinic for Dermatology and Wellness
Medford, Oregon

Elizabeth L. Tanzi, MD
Associate Clinical Professor
Department of Dermatology
George Washington University School of Medicine
Washington, District of Columbia

Abel Torres, MD, JD, MBA
Professor and Chairman
Department of Dermatology
University of Florida College of Medicine
Gainesville, Florida

Robin Travers, MD
Dermatologist
SkinCare Physicians
Chestnut Hill, Massachusetts

Jill Waibel, MD
Medical Director and Owner
Miami Dermatology & Laser Institute;
Assistant Voluntary Professor
Miller School of Medicine
University of Miami
Miami, Florida

Jordan V. Wang, MD, MBE, MBA
Dermatologist
Department of Dermatology and
  Cutaneous Biology
Thomas Jefferson University Hospital
Philadelphia, Pennsylvania

Daniel I. Wasserman, MD
Dermatologist
Skin Wellness Physicians
Naples, Florida

Susan H. Weinkle, MD
Associate Clinical Professor
Department of Dermatology
University of South Florida
Tampa, Florida

Kathleen M. Welsh, MD, FAAD
Founder and Principal
Bay Area Cosmetic Dermatology
San Francisco, California

Misha Zarbafian, MD
Resident
Department of Dermatology & Skin Science
University of British Columbia
Vancouver, British Columbia, Canada

Section I

Bricks and Mortar

I

1 To Rent or to Buy: That Is the Question

Jill Waibel MD, Jusleen Ahluwalia MD, Chloe Gianatasio MS

Abstract

When opening a practice in dermatology, a doctor has a multitude of factors to consider beyond mere knowledge of dermatological care. Patients may be the most important focus, but one also requires a functional place to treat them. Buying versus renting an office space is a high-capital, high-maintenance, important decision that lays the groundwork of a developing office. Both alternatives have advantages and disadvantages, but the ultimate decision must coincide with overall practice goals and qualities appropriately. This chapter reviews the principles of buying or leasing an office space, and discusses key considerations that are involved in the decision-making of buying or leasing a practice.

Keywords: office space, location, equity, operating expenses

Top 10 Things You Need to Know

1. Before anything else, establish your practice qualities and goals. What does your patient population look like? What are you most passionate about treating? How do you want the environment to feel?
2. Location determines your clientele, expenses, and resources. Make sure it matches your needs and your goals prior to setting up your office.
3. It is important to involve your business consultants, lawyers, and accountants early to formulate a game plan for your practice.
4. Owning a building is a long-term investment but involves greater upfront expenses and reduces flexibility if you plan to move in the future.
5. Owning a building entails all maintenance and repair costs but enables complete customization of the space.
6. The size of a space that your budget allows you to buy versus lease is likely to be two very different stories. Consider your current size, growth goals, and their respective needs when choosing an office space.
7. Leasing allows greatest flexibility if you wish to change location but it involves relinquishing a substantial amount of control.
8. Leasing often has hidden costs. You can better protect yourself by setting terms in advance.
9. Changing locations can lead to the loss of a significant amount of clientele. Be mindful of your future plans when setting up your first practice.
10. Be cognizant of the similar practices in your desired area. Overabundance will diminish your ability to thrive.

1.1 Twelve Years of Education and Yet...

Twelve years of education went by and now you have fulfilled your dream of becoming a dermatologist! You know every minute detail about psoriasis, graft-vs-host disease (GVHD), acne vulgaris, and rhytid treatments. Yet, none of the high-powered, Nobel Prize-winning, medical scientists mentioned anything about business acumen. It feels as though someone taught you the most beautiful peanut butter and jelly-spreading technique but neglected to mention that you need bread. Most well-trained dermatologists successfully graduate from residency but are completely devoid of the knowledge required to open a practice.

Alternatively, you may be an established dermatologist who is in the process of adding new physician partners, or a professional who opened a practice sometime back that has been so wildly successful that your patient base and business offerings have outgrown the space that was sufficient for a young budding dermatologist. If you are to continue to grow, you need a larger location, a relocation, or an expansion. With real estate prices skyrocketing and the multitude of leasing options rising correspondingly, making the right decision has become an increasingly muddled proposition. Any self-made entrepreneur will tell you that you learn business dynamics on the go. However, there exists an opportunity to educate practitioners a little bit in advance about the nitty-gritty of the business of dermatology. This resource aims to carry out a discussion about the bricks and mortar of your practice.

1.2 Location, Location, Location

The location of your practice not only sets the tone but also defines many of the qualities of your practice; after all, it serves to be your stage, where your actors perform in front of your audience. Differences exist with regard to establishing a practice in a medical center, university town, urban mecca, or strip mall. Location determines the patient population to which you should cater. For example, if you are passionate about treating melasma, an ideal location would house a significant population with darker skin. Alternatively, a practice primarily focused on lasers and energy-based devices may benefit from an urban city environment to effectively fulfill practice demand. Neighborhood competitors should also influence decision-making. If every surrounding office performs the same procedures, then that market is likely to be saturated and will be less fruitful in terms of the growth of your practice.

While not impossible, relocating a practice requires time, money, and a potential loss of patient volume. On average, it costs thousands of dollars to move one clinic room to another state. These costs sequentially rise when considering the expenses required to move hefty lasers and other devices which form an integral part of the practice (see also Chapter 2). When you add in zoning for medical facilities or the pursuit of class A office space, these costs climb even further.

1.3 Buying versus Leasing 101

It is important to analyze the two forms of financing: buying or leasing. The eventual choice will instill different dynamics in your practice. Buying real estate can be very complex on account of the sizeable time, research, and planning required. However, it offers the opportunity to build equity, make your expenses more predictable, customize your business as it evolves, and even gain tax advantages. Owning a building is also a long-term investment that can one day be sold separately from the medical business or passed on to a prodigy. In some situations, it is also possible to become a partial owner of a building if you have relationships with international property companies. Alternatively, leasing allows flexibility, greater liquid assets over capital to divert to other areas of the practice, and fewer maintenance tasks for a busy dermatologist.

The decision to buy or to lease a property can be difficult for even the most business-savvy dermatologist because there is no one-size-fits-all formula. There are several key concepts to survey prior to pursuing any business decision, such as costs, risks, and specific practice needs. Although it may sound excessive, a team of experts may be the best choice to help in making an educated and informed decision. These experts include commercial brokers, mortgage brokers, accountants, and lawyers.[1] Their firms may be local, regional or national. It is also advisable to choose firms that are experts in the medical field due to the unique laws surrounding medicine and medical practices that can impact endeavors such as renovation (i.e. there must be a sink in every room). Commercial brokers help to locate potential properties in your price range that meet your needs. Mortgage brokers can aid in financing needs and arm you with knowledge about down payment requirements, mortgage rates, commercial real estate loans, and so on. Accountants can assess practice revenue, help create an appropriate budget, provide insight on tax benefits, and forecast your operating budget. A legal representative can negotiate terms before you sign that contract and help complete the entire transaction. Overall, when considering the alternatives of buying versus leasing, it is important to keep the primary goal in mind: higher revenue, lower costs.

1.4 Are You Ready for Commitment? The Pros and Cons of Purchasing Office Space

Purchasing is a long-term commitment that requires a hefty down payment.[1,2] The cash upfront can range from 20 to 25% of the property value. In urban cities, estimated property value can be around $15 million without even considering Class A highly sought locations. For this reason alone, many early career dermatologists elect to lease their office space, as resident salaries have not quite adjusted for this. However, those electing to pursue their practices in suburban or lower traffic areas, this overhead is less prohibitive as the property values entail a lower cost per square foot. The cost of down payment in an urban city may equal the cost of an entire office space in the Midwest. In these places, purchasing may be a viable option but it may also cater to a different clientele. As such, practice goals and expertise are extremely relevant and intertwined.

Office real estate value is also subject to fluctuation and appreciation like any other real estate, in accordance with the general economic situation of the area. For example, during the financial crisis in 2008, consultants more frequently recommended purchasing property as values were significantly lower than in previous years. Typically, the office value will appreciate over a career lifetime and the appreciated value of the property can then be passed to subsequent generations.[3] However, due to the time factor, this asset should not be incorporated into a practice's overall revenue. Times of financial crisis also increase the difficulty of obtaining loans if required which should also be taken into account.

A primary advantage of purchasing an office space is an increased understanding and control of total costs. Typically, commercial mortgage payments are locked-in for long-term periods.[2] Moreover, you are provided with the property of flexibility in your space. You can also modify your office as the need arises rather than engaging in long-term wrestling with a property manager. Besides, you have the freedom of choosing any maintenance contract and insurance company without fear of violating a leasing contract. However, even though base costs are fixed, an owner is liable for all extraneous building-associated expenses. This includes operating, maintenance, capital improvement, real estate, alterations, insurance, landscaping costs, and other costs.[2,3,4] Luckily, these costs can incur benefits as well in the form of tax deductions.[2,4]

Another important factor to consider is the projected geographical future of your practice. Purchasing an office space becomes impractical if, for example, your family is in, or considering relocating to, a different state. Purchasing effectively grounds you to your office space unless a buyer or renter is easily accessible, making it an arduous task to then try to relocate again.

In summary, purchasing your office space is a big investment that requires a lot of capital upfront; however, the primary advantage involves the ability to establish your practice in your own way. You can create a business from the ground up, building, decorating, and operating without restraint. However, it is important to understand that the cash paid upfront is completely removed from the cash flow of your practice. If you do not possess the resources to fully invest both in acquiring an office space and in operating the said office space (staff, lasers, devices, etc.), and it is advisable to consider leasing options.

1.5 Constant Vigilance: The Pros and Cons of Leasing Office Space

Leasing is a relatively short-term commitment that can provide locational flexibility and the opportunity to build working capital to allocate across other practice requirements (e.g., energy-based devices, staff, and equipment).[2,5] Typically, a refundable deposit is the only upfront cash requirement associated with leasing.

Many advisors accurately claim that leasing office space allows your practice to be more agile, flexible, and scalable.[6] However, moving your practice from one location to another is not ideal, unless in mandatory circumstances, because you may lose a portion of your patient base. Another advantage to leasing is that monthly lease payments are typically tax deductible as business expenses.

When you negotiate an office lease, your rent becomes another business expense. Currently, at our practice, the lease payment is the second highest monthly expense following payroll. Property managers are highly motivated to obtain the maximum profit while leasing space, and thus, learning to spot hidden costs and restrictions helps in protecting a lessee's interests. There can be hidden costs in the actual building structure of the office space. Lessees are charged per rentable square foot and this includes any space that is considered unusable (stairways, closets, lobbies, etc.). Usable rented area is typically only 75 to 90% of what is actually paid for.[2] In addition, there can be added charges for factors such as common space and hurricane readiness that can be reassessed at various times throughout the year. New assessments often imply rent increases when you go to renew your lease.

Operating expenses can be a tricky area for practitioners to figure out and thus an opportune area for lessors to exploit. Property managers occasionally use the operating expense clause as an opportunity for a blank check from your practice, so out-of-pocket costs of running a building need to be defined within a leasing contract for maximum protection of your assets. Certain costs should be excluded from operating expenses, such as electricity, maintenance contracts, advertising costs, landscaping costs, structural repairs, and legal fees to resolve disputes.[2] Property management can impose these expenses on the lessee in order to obtain profit. Properly negotiating terms in your contract can save you from signing your life away on the dotted line.

Leasing renewals also require a discussion because the price can be raised at the lessor's discretion. In some cases, leases will have yearly increases already built-in prior to reassessment that you have to watch for. Contracts may include an extension option to ensure uninterrupted operation in your office space for more than the short-leased time frame without full lease renewal. This not only allows for the assurance that the practice will not be subject to opportunistic eviction but also avoids the legal process of renewal which would essentially invalidate the original lease and open the new lease to potentially new negotiation terms. Frequently, the process involves a formula that is linked to the fair market rate in order to determine lease payments during the extended term. Fair market rates are subject to the lessee's credit rating, operating expenses, and lease term. Renewals are also not guaranteed. A colleague of mine was in the situation where, at the time of her next lease renewal, the lessors, without warning, declined to renew because they had other plans for the space. She had no choice but to comply and lose her office. Unfortunately, in the world of leasing, this is a risk.

Lessees payments typically reflect increasing real estate taxes and building expenses following the base point, which are determined initially with the property manager. These rising costs may, in extreme circumstances, climb insurmountably and force the practice to consider leasing elsewhere. Knowledge of escalation formulas within your contract and awareness about the definitions of base year versus expense stops can help avoid this dramatic predicament. Rent escalation formulas that are linked to direct operating expenses are dependent on either the building's "rented" or "rentable" area as the denominator in the fraction.[2] These definitions will need to be clearly spelled out within the leasing contract.

Real estate taxes should be the landlord's legal responsibility. However, without proper scrutiny, increasing real estate taxes can fall in either camp depending on the contract terms. A good contract should protect you from paying the property manager's income tax, inheritance tax, and payroll tax. Should the property tax of your office space decrease, ensure your lease entitles you to participate in the benefits of devaluing the property.[2]

Flexibility can be defined in many ways. Leasing has the aforementioned flexibility of movement and impermanence but often reduces the flexibility to alter your office space. Typically, lessees may make nonstructural changes (mirrors, paintings, etc.) to the office with the landlord's permission but structural changes (lighting fixtures, landscape settings) are not guaranteed to be approved by a landlord.[2] So, you may not be able to redesign a space in your desired way. On the other hand, by purchasing, you may be able to fully design your own space but you may have to sacrifice size. When I was searching for a property, I had the option of buying two beautiful rooms to design in my own way or leasing 15 rooms to make work. For my specific needs, two rooms would not have been sufficient.

Maintenance costs of the office building such as structural elements, the exterior, and building common areas, are usually at the expense of the property manager.[2,3,5] Yet, those that are within your office space such as repairs may fall under your purview. When something breaks, leaks, or needs to be fixed to operate your practice, there is often a back and forth with the leasing company; in other words, the owner and you. This can serve to add legal expenses to the already expensive repairs. In the event of casualties affecting the building, property managers have the right to force you out of your office space, although this is very rare.[2]

Finally, insuring your office space may be your liability if you have leased an office space. In many cases, property managers are bound to specific insurance companies and/or policies based on prior agreements. Insurance is also variable, based on what you choose to place in your office such as energy-based devices and other high-liability equipment.

In summary, while there are several upfront and hidden costs associated with leasing office space, negotiating a contract and involving a legal representative can help in protecting the practice. It is important to clearly define who is responsible for extraneous costs and clarify the long-term plan of your office space with property management. In court, contracts behave just like medical notes; if it was not documented, it was never said.

1.6 City Mouse, Country Mouse

As the nursery rhyme goes, a city mouse may practice in a lavish area. However, there is very little real estate left to buy[7] in overcrowded cities like New York City, Los Angeles, or Miami. There may be a surplus of demand to supply but a deficit of space. Whereas a country mouse may be able to afford a large space, he or she may not have sufficient demand to fill it. You need to find your happy medium which satisfies your practice's goals in order to maximize revenue and minimize costs.

Building your practice from the ground up can be daunting. Sometimes, older established practices can provide a lower cost and lower stress option than starting anew. Of course, older practices risk dragging along "old home issues," such as outdated plumbing systems, surface stains, and malfunctioning outlets. However, the costs to repair these issues should be lower than doing all of the work from scratch unless the former owners were truly careless. Moreover, an existing practice may have more space, allowing you accommodate more patients and can result in greater patient capacity than a smaller, newer practice.

1.7 There's a Perfect Match for Everyone

Matching your practice size to your practice space is of critical importance in the business of dermatology. A larger space with more clinic rooms may cost more when buying or leasing than a smaller space with less clinic rooms. Yet, revenue can be generated more easily in the larger alternative. It is important at some point in your business life to look at returns on investment per room per hour to help find this optimal point. This becomes especially important in aesthetic practices where laser machines occupy a significant space in clinic rooms and require more space. So, make sure your eyes are not bigger than your stomach when choosing a building size and layout. Analyze growth projection accordingly, so as not to miss the mark in either direction.

1.8 Office Configuration

Another important aspect to consider in office success is that you are not the only person in it. Patients and staff must travel to your office for it to function, making their ease of access a relevant factor. Parking for patients and staff can be an exorbitant overlooked expense that ultimately will factor into your costs of providing care and payroll expenses, respectively.

Personal Anecdote from Jill Waibel

When seeking my office space, I wanted to ensure that my patients and my staff could reach the office in a reasonable amount of time. I had been looking at city areas with high-rise buildings, and realized that it would take my patients and staff an extra 20 minutes just to park their cars and ride an elevator to the office. Since I also treat celebrities who want to be able to come and go with discretion, it was important for me to have a ground floor with an alternative back route into the clinic to make this feasible. Moreover, I also recognized that a large amount of my clinic space would have to be devoted to stationary patients waiting for topical analgesia to take effect. Therefore, I needed an office space with a large enough space (40 × 40 sq ft) for a "patient care center," so that multiple patients can be accommodated comfortably out of the major flow of clinic while still being divided visually for privacy. Finally, the new office space I was considering had two rooms versus an older office space with 15 rooms for the same price. I am passionate about laser treatments and personally own a wide variety of devices which takes up multiple rooms. So, for me, it made the most sense to take over the older practice at the time. Now that I have had time to build my business in this space for many years, I am looking into the option of partially owning a newer building. But back when I was starting, this option would not have been feasible.

To-Do Checklist

- [ ] If you're lucky enough to have picked up this book before graduating from school, I strongly recommend taking a financial minor. This will save you a great deal of stress.
- [ ] It is important to involve your financial consultants, lawyers, and accountants early to formulate a game plan for your practice.
- [ ] Before anything else, establish your practice qualities and goals. What does your patient population look like? What are you most passionate about treating? How do you want the environment to feel?
- [ ] Carefully weigh the pros and cons of buying versus leasing office space in the context of your experience, finances, and goals.
- [ ] Seek advice from your mentors to help guide your decision-making.

References

[1] Introduction to Buying Commercial Property for Your Business. Bank of America. Available at: https://www.bankofamerica.com/smallbusiness/business-financing/learn/intro-to-buying-commercial-propertyPublished 2019. Accessed January 16, 2019

[2] Manley M. Before you sign that lease.... Harvard Business Review. Available at: https://hbr.org/1988/05/before-you-sign-that-lease. Published 1988. Accessed January 16, 2019

[3] Pretorius F, Ho M. Real estate and capital structure decisions–lease-versus-buy analysis. Hbr.org. Available at: https://hbr.org/product/real-estate-and-capital-structure-decisions-lease-versus-buy-analysis/HKU253-PDF-ENG. Published 2019. Accessed January 16, 2019

[4] Fabian K. Leasing vs. buying office space. business.com. Available at: https://www.business.com/articles/leasing-vs-buying-office-space/. Published 2018. Accessed January 16, 2019

[5] Zahorsky D. The pros and cons of leasing vs. buying office space. The Balance Small Business. Available at: https://www.thebalancesmb.com/the-pros-and-cons-of-leasing-vs-buying-office-space-2951249. Published 2018. Accessed January 16, 2019

[6] David C, Sperry V. Should you buy or lease space for your business? Business News Daily. Available at: https://www.businessnewsdaily.com/4424-buy-lease-office-space-business.html. Published 2013. Accessed January 16, 2019

[7] Rudy M. City Mouse, Country Mouse. 1st ed. New York, New York: Henry Holt and Co.; 2017

2 Location

Keith LeBlanc Jr., MD, FAAD, FACMS

Abstract

The location in which we practice is a vital decision not only for the success of the practice but also for our own happiness and well-being. A variety of other factors play significant roles in this decision. Family preferences, proximity to training programs, population and demographic makeup, market saturation, and mobility are just some of the topics to consider when debating about where to practice. Your desired practice type (e.g., solo private vs. multispecialty group vs. academic, general dermatology vs. Mohs vs. dermatopathology) and job availability at each possible location also factor into this decision. This chapter will aim at reviewing all relevant topics regarding the location of your practice, including a rough chronology of the order in which these decisions should be made in order to set up yourself and your practice for long-term success.

Keywords: location, family, population, demographics, market mobility, market saturation, market share, long-term goals

Top 10 Things You Need to Know

1. Macro decisions versus micro decisions.
2. Family first (spouse preference, cost of living, access to schools, social life, proximity to extended family, etc.).
3. Proximity to residency/fellowship program.
4. Population of chosen location.
5. Understand the specific demographic of the patient population you are attempting to attract or will most likely make up the bulk of your desired patient base (age, income level, ethnicity, etc.)
6. Competition—other BCD/non-BCD practices in area.
7. Proximity to hospitals, medical office buildings, and medical resources.
8. Is patient population in chosen area mobile or would you need to establish multiple locations within the region to capture the market?
9. What is your long-term goal in establishing the practice? (Is this the practice you plan to be in until retirement, or does the goal involve building a multiprovider practice vs. potential sale to a hospital or private equity group?)
10. Solid, evidence-based medicine and exceptional customer service will succeed in any location, regardless of the factors working against it. But never forget the adage: Location, Location, Location!

The location in which you choose to practice is of vital significance, and one of the decisions you should be making early on, as you contemplate your future career. Before we begin our discussion, I would like to outline the structure of my thought process. I will be (admittedly, somewhat arbitrarily) referring to decisions regarding the placement of your practice as macro-level (e.g., in what region, state, city do I want to practice?) versus micro-level (e.g., what neighborhood, and typically medical vs. commercial/nonmedical real estate, etc.). As you would expect, most of the decisions you should be making early on in the process are macro-level, while those you make later will be more consistently micro-level.

Most would tell you that there are two main decisions to be made in concert with one another: what type of practice would I like to have (e.g., solo private, group private, academic, or multispecialty)? And what availability exists for this chosen practice type in my desired location?

These questions are certainly macro-level, practical queries you need to address as you plan your career. I would posit that another, more important macro-level question must be asked when first thinking about the location of your practice: What location will place me, as well as my immediate and extended family, in a setting where I will be emotionally and spiritually most secure *outside* of the office to better serve my patients and build a successful practice?

On its face, this seems illogical. Why think about spheres outside the office setting when deciding where to practice? The answer lies in my firm belief that the best version of me—as a physician, dermatologist, husband, father, son, etc.—exists in an environment where my whole self, not just my professional self, is satisfied. Furthermore, this best version of me is the greatest gift that I can give not only to my patients in practice, but also to my immediate and extended family and friends.

These coexisting versions of yourself are so obviously dependent on one another, and yet are so often overlooked. I see so many graduating residents and colleagues settling into jobs in locations not because they desired the location but rather because it was the best financial deal that was offered to them. While it may be the best monetary decision at the time (due to other common factors early in your career such as student loans, the costs of starting a family, etc.), these decisions are often short-sighted and contribute to early burnout and job turnover.

To successfully choose a location in which to practice, the first questions I believe anyone should ask himself or herself are as follows: Where do I want to live? What about my spouse, partner, or significant other? Are there any locations where they would be particularly happy or unhappy? If children are part of the equation, what is the day care availability and what are the school systems like in potential locations? What about the cost of living? What are the restaurants, public parks, and facilities available with regard to night life and outdoor activities? All of these are important questions that need to be answered when it comes to location.

Once these questions are answered, my guess is that 1 to 2 and perhaps as many as 4 to 5 locations will be considered as possible landing spots. Then, and only then, do I feel it best to evaluate another macro-level topic: What opportunities exist for your desired type of practice setting?

What type of practice do you feel most comfortable in: private solo practice, private group practice, multispecialty practice, or academics? Furthermore, what opportunities exist in relation to your selected practice type in the locations where you and your family would be satisfied? If you plan to go into solo private practice, you may be more inclined to look for a rural area or one

that is underserved by dermatologists in order to ensure that your schedule is not empty starting out. If so, do you see yourself comfortable professionally being the sole decision maker for the practice immediately after finishing residency or fellowship with minimal input or assistance from partners or nearby colleagues? If not, perhaps a location where a group-practice setting exists may be more suitable. Conversely, if one chooses to practice in a seemingly saturated area, a multispecialty group, or perhaps academics, would prove to be a better choice. When tackling the notion of practice setting, be aware that many graduating residents begin their post-training careers by playing a hybrid-type role, engaging in part-time practice in a private or multispecialty setting and part-time practice in an academic setting.

If you are planning to start a solo private practice, another factor to consider that is intricately tied to location involves framing a business plan and securing a corporate loan. The use of a consulting firm can be particularly helpful in this circumstance. With regard to existing group practices, multispecialty groups, and academics, these concerns are not applicable. Hopefully, once these first couple of questions, family preference and practice setting, are answered, you would find yourself with 1 to 2 possible locations to begin your practice.

Another consideration when choosing the location of your practice is the proximity to the location of your residency or fellowship program. This is the point where two main macro-level decisions have been made, and most of the remaining decisions to be made fall under the micro-level category. This decision in particular is somewhat of a segue between the two. The reason that this is considered most important is because data shows that a majority of residents and fellows typically settle into practice within a limited radius from their training program.

This outcome is the result of a variety of factors. Residents are typically in their late 20s to early 30s upon completion of residency or fellowship, coinciding with a time at which many are getting married and/or having children. This family "anchor" can limit the mobility of a resident and his or her family in the immediate post-training phase and while seeking a job post-residency. In addition, information regarding available job opportunities near training programs is commonly disseminated among residents who may be interested and these positions are often filled quickly by local graduating residents and fellows.

This data point can lead a trainee in one of two directions. If the resident has matched into a training program in or near the location of his or her desired post-residency job opportunity, then he or she is quite likely to stay nearby if a good job offer presents itself. Conversely, if the resident matched into a program a considerable distance from his or her desired landing spot (e.g., the resident or his or her spouse wants to return to his or her hometown after traveling for training), then they are still more likely to settle within the radius of their training program than someone who trained elsewhere, but these various outlying factors may cause them to buck the trend and move back to their desired location in order to settle post-training if an offer is available there.

This becomes important from the perspective of collegiality and camaraderie. We can all agree that residencies often function like family units, with all the complexities and dynamics of interpersonal relationships in play between the trainees. Fellowships are akin to marriages, as the fellows spend countless hours working alongside their fellowship director. We less frequently take note of the fact that professional life immediately post-training can be lonely, especially in a solo private practice setting. Taking a position near the residency or fellowship program in which you trained, where co-trainees are also more likely to settle, sets one up for a future in which the relationships developed during training are more likely to continue into future careers, even if starting a solo private practice.

For many residents and fellows, particularly those who develop strong relationships with their colleagues in training, the possibility of continuing such a collaboration into future careers is enticing. While less likely, there are those who view their experiences with colleagues during the course of training as toxic, and for these individuals a change of scenery post-training is more than welcome. Regardless, an honest assessment of the relationships developed during residency or fellowship and the want to continue (or discontinue) them should be undertaken when thinking about where to locate your practice.

The population of the location (including all relevant suburbs) is another important factor to consider when examining potential locations for your practice. In 2015, the average clinically active per capita workforce in dermatology was 36 dermatologists per 1 million patients (which averages out to 1 dermatologist per 27,000–28,000 patients).[1] This means that, ideally, the population of the location you choose would currently have less than 1 dermatologist per 27,000 patients. If the location in question has equal to or more than this per capita figure, it would suggest that the market is at or near saturation, as compared to the national average. This does not, however, mean that the location is necessarily a poor choice. If you offer a service currently not provided by the dermatologists at that location (e.g., you could be the only fellowship-trained Mohs surgeon or pediatric dermatologist), then a seemingly saturated market may, in fact, be a great site for your practice.

This segues into another factor to consider when looking at possible locations: the makeup of the current dermatology landscape in the area. You need to not only consider the number of board-certified dermatologists in the area, but also non-board-certified physicians and midlevels who may be providing dermatologic care and would therefore prove to be possible competition for your practice. If you plan to start a practice with a bent toward cosmetics, consideration of medispas, laser centers, and similar sites also need to be factored in as potential competitors. When analyzing the current landscape in your possible practice locations, even if the market seems saturated, I would urge you each to determine if there is a particular niche within the market that you can fill. As an example, if multiple successful practices which incorporate cosmetics exist within a seemingly saturated market, it could turn out to be an ideal landing spot if you intend to practice complex medical dermatology, or vice versa.

For Mohs surgeons, much is dependent upon your ideal weekly case load, but a typical Mohs surgeon, on average, needs between 5 to 7 full-time practicing general dermatologists referring the majority of their Appropriate Use Criteria worthy cases to maintain a busy schedule.

The number of dermatologists in the area is not the only aspect that needs to be weighed when considering a location. I would argue that the demographic data regarding each of these possible competitors is just as important. How old are the existing dermatologists and their practices? If the practices employ midlevels, how many midlevel providers does each dermatologist oversee, and at how many locations? Is the supervising physician always on site or are the midlevels allowed to practice independently with only remote support and supervision? How loyal is their patient population? What is their reputation among patients in the community?

If you are looking to move into an area that seems saturated when looking at the number of dermatologists in a vacuum, but on further inspection realize that many of the providers in the area are later in their careers with loyal patient populations, then perhaps this is an ideal scenario to approach an older physician with a mature practice to gauge his or her interest in bringing you on as an employee physician with a potential for future ownership of their practice. If, however, many of the practices in a given area are young (< 3–5 years old), it would be a poor choice in which to locate another new practice. On the other hand, this is conceivably a scenario where the immaturity of the practices in existence may suggest a lack of patient loyalty and a possibility for growth of your own practice.

Similar demographic data on your potential patients is just as important. What is the average age of the patient in a given location? What is the average income level? What is the average level of education? What is the typical insurance coverage and/or payer mix? All of these factors may or may not be important to your particular practice structure but should nevertheless be considered when evaluating each possible location. If you are looking to start in a private practice setting with a cosmetic arm, it would be wise to choose a location where a sizeable portion of the population is over 35 years with a somewhat high education level and a mid-to-high income level, as these patients are more likely to possess the disposable income needed to support such a practice (with cosmetic procedures becoming more mainstream, however, these age and income figures may actually be skewing slightly lower). If, however, you are interested in academics or complex medical dermatology, the payer mix, income level, and education level of the patient become less important to a certain extent. Rather, you should consider a location with a large population, typically in an urban setting, and ideally, access to a large hospital system that will draw in such cases from the surrounding regions.

Market mobility is also important when assessing a potential location. Situating your practice in a convenient location for your patients will set you up for success. How far is the average patient you plan to serve willing to travel for the services you provide them? There are a number of ways to assess this. Average workplace commute in a given area is a good place to begin to evaluate how willing to travel patients within that area may be. Why, you may ask. Most patients when questioned would readily tell you that barring unusual circumstances, they would prefer services to be provided at a location that is close to either their home or their workplace, as these are the two locations in which the average patient spends the bulk of their time. This is human nature, which especially pertains to medical services: We would all prefer to have such services performed at a location in which we feel comfortable, and most people by nature are most comfortable in attending such sessions in the areas in which they spend the most time. As such, the locations of the home and workplace of your desired patient demographic, and their willingness to travel, become important in the placement of your practice.

Furthermore, does your particular desired patient demographic alter this average willingness to travel in any way? As an example, a Mohs surgeon's expected patient demographic will likely limit expected market mobility. Think about it, would your grandmother choose to see a good Mohs surgeon who is located 5 minutes away or would she go visit the best surgeon in the state whose nearest location is over an hour away? My grandmother, and I expect most patients over the age of 65, would be more likely to visit a good surgeon who is 5 minutes away as opposed to an excellent one an hour's drive further. In such a situation, you would perhaps be required to travel on a weekly basis to multiple locations in order to truly capture the market share in a particular area.

Conversely, if you are the only fellowship-trained dermatopathologist for 200 miles in every direction, or the only pediatric dermatologist specializing in rare genodermatoses, then you should expect the market mobility in your case to be increased, as you provide a service to the area not previously offered by any of your competitors.

Finally, as you consider all your options regarding the location of your practice, the final question I would urge you to answer is this: What is my long-term goal in establishing this practice at this location? You may not have an answer to this question at first. If so, that is acceptable because, at least, it will have you asking the right questions of yourself when you consider where to place your practice.

Is my goal just to test the waters and build some experience before moving on to another location? Perhaps I will be taking up a position that I assume to be temporary as I await a spouse or partner to finish his or her training, and so on. Are you joining a practice to perhaps be under the tutelage of a particular mentor, unknowing of whether or not you have a long-term future in that locale? Alternatively, are you planning to return to your hometown after a time away in training, and start and build a practice that will be yours until retirement?

These questions do not all require answers as you begin your search for a practice location. Nevertheless, asking these questions over the course of the process, as your search evolves, will aid you in finally settling down in a location that will set both you and your practice up for long-term success.

I wish you all the luck in the future and urge you each to believe in yourself and your abilities as board-certified dermatologists. We are all well-trained and capable to serve our patients on a daily basis. If our focus is consistently on the best patient care and evidence-based medical decision-making, then no changes in location, market saturation, new governmental regulations, invasion of outside corporate entities, etc. can stop us from what should be our primary focus: to always combine sound medical practice and exceptional patient/customer service in an environment that promotes the health and well-being of not only our patients but also ourselves. If we succeed in this goal, then we will be on the right path no matter our location.

Reference

[1] Sargen MR, Shi L, Hooker RS, Chen SC. Future growth of physicians and non-physician providers within the U.S. Dermatology workforce. Dermatol Online J 2017;23(9):13030/qt840223q6

3 How Much Space Do I Need?

Camile A. Silva AIA, LEED AP; Chad L. Prather MD

Abstract

How much space do I need? The amount of space needed for a dermatology clinic is inherently dependent on the program, and determined by the number of providers and staff, types of services offered, the anticipated productivity, and other special requirements. Various configurations of clinical and support areas may be used depending on physician preferences and desired workflow. The program matrix presented in this chapter is an interactive tool that can assist in figuring the number of rooms recommended in the clinical area, and reception desks in the reception area based on the number of staff and patients attended to per hour. The spatial matrix then follows, using assumptions from the program matrix to help determine the square footages for every room and for the dermatology clinic in total. These areas are often required by building code or have been calculated by recent trends in health care design. Engaging the appropriate professional can be instrumental in identifying these trends and evaluating the specific needs for each type of dermatology practice.

Keywords: dermatology clinic, configuration, program, square footage, area calculation

---

Top 10 Things You Need to Know

1. An ideal dermatology clinic design delivers a patient-focused experience without compromising functionality or operational efficiency.
2. Flexibility and adaptability are key design considerations when planning for multiple lines of service or multiple providers.
3. The initial step in space planning involves determining the number of providers, support staff, and the anticipated productivity (patients per hour) of the clinical team.
4. The general rule of thumb for medical and surgical dermatology practices is three to four examination/procedure rooms per provider.
5. Planning for nonclinical support space such as reception areas, restrooms, break rooms, and storage areas will follow.
6. Identifying the necessary number of rooms and support spaces without regard for room size is known as building a program. This is the starting point for working with your architect.
7. The amount of space necessary may also vary depending on the organizational pattern chosen. The ideal configuration varies based on your workflow priorities.
8. Spatial planning guidelines can assist in converting the program into a range of square footage, which will assist the dermatologist and architect in quantifying the necessary space.
9. Federal, state, and local regulations, as well as the American with Disability Act (ADA) regulations, will dictate some requirements of the medical office.
10. Engaging an architect experienced with outpatient health care can be instrumental in identifying the specific needs for each type of dermatology practice.

3.1 Introduction

An ideal dermatology clinic design delivers a patient-focused experience without compromising functionality or operational efficiency. Whether 2,000 square feet (sf) or 20,000 sf in size, layout and workflow have a direct impact on productivity and patient experience. Flexibility and adaptability of spatial configuration are key design considerations when planning for multiple lines of service or multiple providers. Defining the number of providers (physicians and extenders) and types of services are the first steps in determining how much space is necessary. Planning for nonclinical support space and choosing the ideal configuration will follow. Spatial planning guidelines can then assist in converting these considerations into a range of square footage, which will assist the dermatologist and architect in quantifying the necessary space.[a]

3.2 Number of Providers and Workflow

The initial step in space planning involves determining the number of providers, support staff, and anticipated productivity (patients per hour) of the clinical team. How many physicians and physician extenders will use the space? Will the providers work full-time and be present in clinic at the same time, or part-time with varying schedules such that the clinic rooms may be shared? Once built, the clinic design and size become limiting factors in the revenue potential of a particular site. Thus, determining how many providers the space needs to accommodate, and whether there is any room in the site and budget to build additional space for potential future growth, become considerations of utmost importance.

The number of providers and their anticipated schedules determine the planned workflow for the practice and the relationships between clinical areas and support spaces, such as laboratories, storage rooms, offices, restrooms, and administrative areas. The general rule of thumb for medical and surgical dermatology practices is three to four examination/procedure rooms per provider. Nurses' stations and restrooms (staff and patient) will vary in number and size according to the number of staff and anticipated number of patients, which affect the occupancy of the building.[1] The following two scenarios illustrate the relationship between efficiency and spatial needs:

In scenario 1, two full-time providers work simultaneously. The typical clinical program would require six to eight examination rooms, two nurses' stations, and two offices or dictation rooms to be shared by both providers.[b] The nonclinical program would consist of a waiting room, restrooms, and support spaces, which are generally determined by the number of patients and staff, and have no direct relationship to the number of examination rooms provided. Federal, state, and local codes are used to help in determining the minimum spatial requirements for these nonclinical spaces, and adequate space must be allotted to pass necessary inspections and obtain a license for occupancy.

In scenario 2, two providers work on a part-time basis and are never in the practice at the same time. While the number of examination rooms, nurses' stations, and dictation rooms can be cut in half, waiting spaces, restrooms, and general support spaces typically cannot due to building codes and federal standards such as ADA standards for accessible design. Regulatory codes will dictate clearances and minimum room sizes, and sometimes vary little even if the number of patients attended to in the practice is doubled. For example, the area requirement for a toilet room is the same whether 40 or 80 patients will use it on any given day.

Spatial calculations take into account the throughput (number of patients per hour) of the staff and providers as well as their schedules.[2] Since space is typically at a premium with regard to practice costs, every effort should be made to utilize space efficiently across the work week. Anticipating the day-to-day workflow of a medical practice is critical to establish the spatial configuration and planning of the new medical office.

3.3 Service Type

In dermatology space planning, there are generally four areas of focus: medical (including pediatric), surgical, cosmetic, and dermatopathology (often occurs in a separate space and will not be considered here). A practice may have a particular focus in one area, or may need space for multiple lines of service within the same clinic. The amount of space needed for clinical and support areas is directly related to and varies with the services rendered. In multiple-provider practices that provide a mix of services, the best layout for clinical areas may be grouped pods of standard-sized examination rooms with fewer, shared procedure rooms, whereas in surgical or procedural-heavy practices, larger procedure rooms that also suffice as examination rooms constitute the bulk of clinical space. In cosmetic-heavy practices, waiting rooms become more spacious, equipment storage space with direct

---

[a] Building occupancy is the classification provided to structures primarily for building and fire code enforcements. Building and fire codes vary by location, and typically result from a combination of federal, state, and local ordinances. The International Building Code (IBC) is the most commonly used building code in the United States of America. According to IBC, a doctor's office is classified as a Business Occupancy.

[b] In recent years, many physicians have replaced nonrevenue generating office space with revenue generating spaces, such as examination or procedure rooms. Rather than a dedicated office, some providers prefer smaller, more centralized spaces where they can process clinical notes between patient visits to improve efficiency.

access to the treatment rooms improves workflow and flexibility, and a retail space is usually incorporated into the spatial program. Consequently, when considering a combination of any of these subspecialties of dermatology, flexibility, and adaptability become key design considerations as they directly impact efficiency and workflow.

3.4 Spatial Configurations and Design Organizational Patterns

It often helps to think of zones or groups of areas with similar functions when laying out the plan for a new practice. The four different spatial configurations presented (▶Fig. 3.1, ▶Fig. 3.2, ▶Fig. 3.3, ▶Fig. 3.4) are examples of how the clinical and

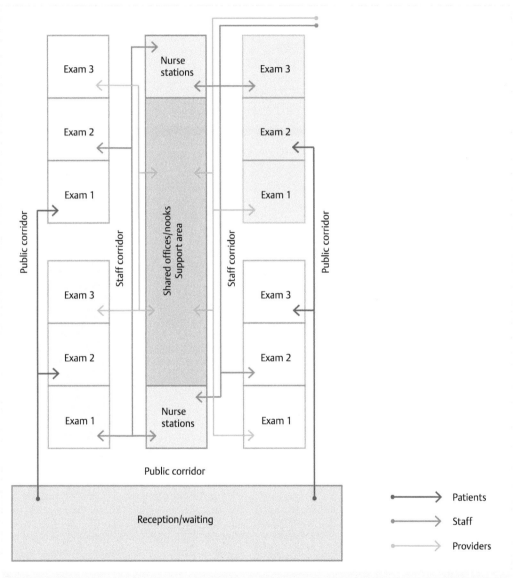

Fig. 3.1 Axial pattern. Spaces are connected through a well-defined axis and organized so that staff and public don't mix outside of examination rooms. Examination rooms have two doors: one for providers and one for patients. Provider offices can take the place of examination rooms or be remote. Nurses' stations and support spaces are internal and separate from public access. Each provider uses a cluster of examination rooms, but may utilize other rooms if available. Most typically used in general dermatology.

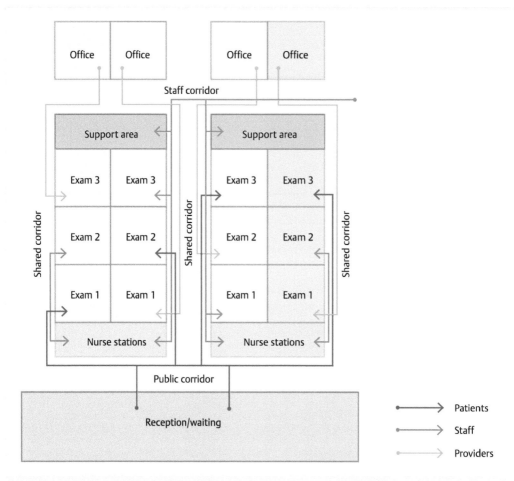

Fig. 3.2 Grid pattern. Staff and public originate from opposite ends and separate corridors. Examination rooms are placed along shared corridors. Providers' offices and support spaces are close to clinical areas, but opposite from the nurses' stations, which are closest to the public waiting area.

nonclinical functions of a dermatology practice may be arranged in ways that best serve the type of service and workflow anticipated, typically predetermined before the planning phase begins. Patient flow is shown in red, staff flow is shown in orange, and provider flow is in green.

Areas for examinations and procedures are shown grouped according to providers, while workspaces such as physicians' nooks or dictation rooms, instrument processing rooms, supply storage, restrooms, and laboratory spaces are assigned as support areas. The nurses' stations are zoned separately, as they often function as a bridge between the public/waiting areas and the examination/procedure rooms. Both support areas and nurses'

stations should be designed with regard to the fewest number of steps necessary between the most frequently used spaces to optimize efficiency.[3]

Visualizing different flow patterns between patients, staff, and providers at this stage will help make adjustments to better accommodate the workflow desired within the amount of space available. Each configuration has advantages and disadvantages, and your priorities may steer you toward a particular configuration. For example, is there flexibility in the number of examination rooms per provider? How important is it for the examination rooms to have access to natural light? Or is it important to separate patients from staff and providers?

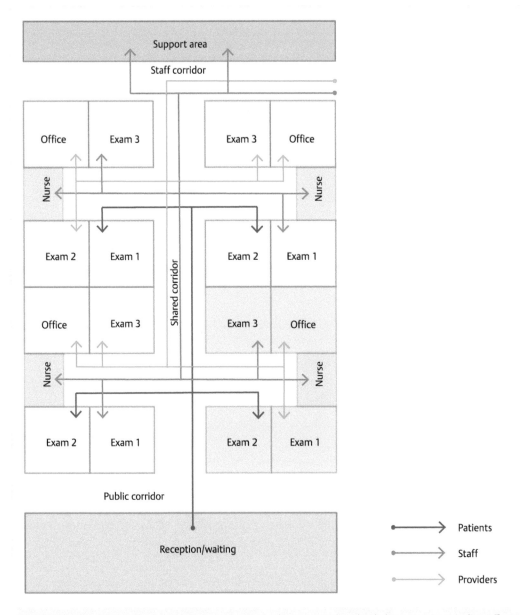

Fig. 3.3 Cluster pattern. More commonly known as the "pod system." Each pod includes a separate provider's office or consultation room and a separate nurse station. The support area, separated by a staff corridor, is shared by all "pods." This pattern is efficient and best utilized when multiple providers have similar schedules and require a set number of examination rooms.

The amount of space necessary may vary depending on the organizational pattern used.[4] Axial and cluster configurations take the most area, as a result of the number of corridors, but allow for a more controlled circulation and a clear separation of provider/staff areas from the patient/public areas. This contrasts with the radial configuration, where the less restrictive circulation allows for more flexibility of use, better visual connection between patients and staff, and a smaller footprint.

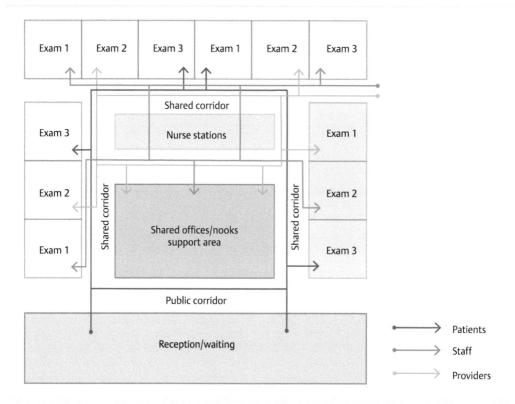

Fig. 3.4 Radial pattern. All functions radiate from a central point. This is the most compact and flexible of the organizational patterns, and thus used for mixed (medical, surgical, cosmetic) lines of service practices. As in the axial configuration, provider offices can replace examination rooms or be remote, while nurses' stations and support spaces are internal, including dictation rooms, laboratory, storage, restrooms, etc. Nurses' stations are centralized and function as a hub, allowing for maximum interaction between spaces with fewer distances to travel in between rooms. Public and staff share corridors.

Consider which rooms you would prefer to have window access. In the grid pattern, providers' offices are prioritized for exterior views and natural light intake. In the axial and cluster arrangements, the examination rooms tend to be placed internally, thus they are without windows. This layout compromises exterior views but improves patient privacy. The radial pattern, on the other hand, prioritizes patient views by placing the majority of the examination rooms on the perimeter and support rooms centrally.

3.5 Clinical and Support Areas Needed

Becoming familiar with the spaces required in a medical office prior to meeting with your architect will expedite the planning process. According to the guidelines of hospitals and outpatient facilities, the following clinical and support areas shall be provided regardless of the spatial configuration chosen: (1) examination, treatment, or procedure rooms, or a combination of these; (2) support areas for these clinical rooms, such as nurse station, clean supply storage, soiled holding room, equipment and supply storage, clean linen and soiled linen holding area, and laboratory spaces when applicable; (3) support areas for patients such as toilet rooms; (4) support facilities such as janitorial closets, and engineering and maintenance service rooms such as electrical closets, mechanical rooms, and telecommunications equipment room; (5) public and administrative areas such as vehicular drop-off and pedestrian entrances, reception, waiting space, public toilet rooms, interview space, or an area where private communications with patients shall be situated away from public areas; (6) equipment and supply storage; (7) staff lounge and toilet room(s); (8) space for business or nonclinical work; and (9) medical record storage when applicable.

Examination rooms should be accessible to the nurses' station and patient toilet room(s), and have a minimum clear floor area of 90 sf.[c] When centrally located, examination tables should have a 2 feet 8 inches clearance around the entire table. A documentation area (written or electronic) should be provided in each examination room, and at least one hand washing station should be provided for each of the four examination rooms.

With regard to support spaces for examination rooms, the recommendations are as follows: (1) the nurse station shall include a work counter, communication system, space for supplies, and accommodation for written or electronic documentation; (2) when applicable, work areas for preparing, dispensing, and administering medications, including work counter, handwashing station, lockable refrigerator, lockable storage for controlled drugs, and sharps containers; (3) a space for clean supply storage[d]; (4) a space for medical/hazard waste holding room[e]; (5) equipment and supply storage, including wheelchair and emergency equipment storage; (6) clean linen storage and soiled linen holding area[f]; and (7) when applicable, a space for soiled instruments and/or instruments processing room.[5]

[c] The typical examination room has become larger in order to accommodate a computer station, in addition to accompanying family members or interpreters. The optimal examination room size is 10 ft x 10 ft (approx. 100 sf), although slight variations can occur without affecting the function of the room. For procedure rooms, especially in Mohs surgery suites, the optimal size is 12 ft x 12 ft (approx. 144 sf), where the examination table is centered in the room. Smaller rooms such as 8 ft x 10 ft or 9 ft x 9 ft, which used to be the common examination room size, are optimal for quick examinations such as surgical follow-up visits. In these configurations, the examination tables are placed at an angle or against a wall.

[d] Such space can be in a room or cabinet located in or close to the nurse's station.

[e] Medical waste shall be disposed in clearly labeled containers, preferably separate from patient areas with direct access to the exterior, where it can be picked up by third-party vendors.

[f] For clean linens, the storage area can be in a dedicated room or cabinet located in or close to the nurse's station. For soiled linens, the holding area can be separate or shared with hazard/medical waste, where it can be picked up by third-party vendors.

Although these guidelines provide the general criteria for design of a medical facility, it is important to note that federal, state, and local regulations, as well as ADA regulations, will dictate some requirements of the medical office. Other aspects enforced by the regulatory codes are as follows: height and location of counters; size and location of toilet rooms; width of hallways; accessibility and clear floor space (wheelchair turnaround diameter) in examination/procedure rooms, workspaces, toilet rooms, etc.; width of door openings (32 inches minimum); and wall mounting heights, among other requirements.

3.6 Program and Area Requirements Calculations

When engaging an architect or designer for the new space, one of the first questions you will be asked is "What is your program"? Although the architect can assist with providing a program, this program planning phase is usually separate from the design phase. Determining your program prior to engaging an architect will expedite the process and save money. To create a spatial program and determine how much space you need, follow this process:

Step 1: Determine number of providers and staff and also determine anticipated productivity or patients per hour and approximate time each patient takes to check-in and check-out.

Step 2: Using your answers from Step 1, complete the matrices in ▶ Table 3.1 and ▶ Table 3.2 to determine the total area needed for the new practice. The program matrix is used to determine the program requirements, such as number of examination rooms and waiting area based on number of providers and staff in your planned practice. The spatial matrix is used to convert the program requirements into area needs for clinical, administrative, and support spaces, such as waiting, reception, and building services. A hallway factor is also added to the formula in order to account for necessary circulation between spaces. The accumulation of these areas will generate the overall area, in square footage, needed for the practice.

In the program matrix (▶ Table 3.1):
- Determine number of providers for each specialty (a, b, c, d) before totaling the number of providers (P).
- Determine the number of rooms per provider by multiplying the number of providers in each

Table 3.1 Program matrix

Providers	Number of providers
General dermatology medical doctors (MD)	a
Mohs surgeon	b
Physicians' assistants (PA)	c
Aesthetician	d
Total providers (a + b + c + d)	**P**
Clinical space	**Number of rooms**
3 examination rooms per MD	3a
4 treatment rooms per Mohs surgeon	4b
2 rooms per PA	2c
1 room per aesthetician	d
2 rooms per MD for clinical research	2a
Total rooms* (3a + 4b + 2c + d + 2a)	**R**
Anticipated productivity	**Patients per hour**
8 patients per day per Mohs surgeon + follow-up patients[1]	2b
5–6 patients per hour per MD	6a
4 patients per hour per PA	4c
½ patient per hour per aesthetician	0.5d
Total patients per hour (2b + 6a + 4c + .5d)	**PT**
Reception area	**Number of front staff**
Total number of patients x check-in time[2]/60 minutes (PT x 4/60)	x
Total number of patients x check-out time[3]/60 minutes (PT x 4/60)	y
Total number of staff/desks (x + y)	**D**
Waiting room area	**Number of people**
Number of patients per hour	PT
1 family member accompanying each patient per hour	PT
Minus number of examination/treatment rooms	–R
Total number of waiting room seats (PT + PT – R)	**S**

[1] Assume 8-hour days, with a productivity of one surgical patient plus one follow-up patient per hour. This number varies greatly depending on Mohs surgeon efficiency.
[2] Assume check-in average time = 4 minutes
[3] Assume check-out average time = 4 minutes

specialty and the average number of rooms listed per provider. For example, in a practice with two general dermatologists, the number of examination rooms required is six. The sizes of each room type will be assigned in the spatial matrix. Find the total number of rooms needed by adding the number of rooms assigned to each subspecialty (R).

- Determine the anticipated productivity by calculating the number of patients each subspecialty is expected to care for per hour. This number is also based on number of providers. The result of the addition of all patients per hour (PT) will help in determining the amount of waiting space based on the number of seats needed.

Table 3.2 Spatial matrix

Waiting room			
Number of rooms	**Type of room**	**Area per room**	**Total area**
S	Waiting chairs/seats	25 sf/per	S x 25 sf
	Public toilet room	60 sf/per	
	Coffee area	60 sf/per	
Reception			
Number of rooms	**Type of room**	**Area per room**	**Total area**
D	Receptionists' desks	65 sf/per	D x 65 sf
	Administration office	120 sf/per	
	Medical records cabinets[1]	15 sf/perp	
	Product display	50 sf/per	
	Work area for front (copier, etc.)	50 sf/per	
Clinical areas			
Number of rooms	**Type of room**	**Area per room**	**Total area**
3a	Examination room for MD	120 sf/per	3a x 120 sf
4b	Procedure room for Mohs	144 sf/per	4b x 144 sf
2c	Exam room for PA	100 sf/per	2c x 100 sf
P = 1 per provider	Nurse station	50 sf/per	P x 50 sf
P = 1 per provider	Dictation room	65 sf/per	P x 65 sf
	Mohs lab (area per cryostat)	120 sf/per	
	Soiled room	60 sf/per	
	Clean room	80 sf/per	
	Instrument processing room[2]	75 sf/per	
	Patient toilet room	60 sf/per	
	Clinical storage	100 sf/per	
	Equipment room	50 sf/per	
	Waste room	50 sf/per	
Administrative areas			
Number of rooms	**Type of room**	**Area per room**	**Total area**
	Provider offices	140 sf/per	
	Dictation room	65 sf/per	
	Staff cubicles	48 sf/per	
	Staff toilet room	60 sf/per	
	Workroom area	80 sf/per	
	Breakroom	40 sf/per	
	Storage	150 sf/per	
	Locker room	5 sf/per	
	IT room	120 sf/per	

(continued)

21

Table 3.2 (*continued*) Spatial matrix

Building services			
Number of rooms	**Type of room**	**Area per room**	**Total area**
	Electrical room	60 sf/per	
	Mechanical room	100 sf/per	100 sf
	Janitorial closet	30 sf/per	30 sf
	Elevator	80 sf/per	80 sf
Subtotal			**ST**
Hallway factor	30%	ST + (ST x .3)	
Total			**T**

[1] Consider each cabinet to take up 6 ft x 2.5 ft of floor area. Medical records cabinet lengths can vary, but depth is typically 12 inches.
[2] A single instrument processing room is an alternative to a soiled and clean room.

- The number of staff needed at the reception area is related to the number of patients per hour, which is determined by the anticipated productivity and the average time spent checking them in and out. The result will inform the number of reception desks or check-in/check-out stations (D).
- To calculate the waiting room area, it is important not only to consider the number of patients per hour, but also the number of examination rooms and accompanying family members. This calculation will result in the number of seats to be provided (S).

In the spatial matrix (▶ Table 3.2):

- Determine spaces needed as per function. Functions are listed as waiting room, reception, clinical areas, administrative areas, and building services. These spaces can vary depending upon suite location within an existing building.
- Refer to program matrix for number of rooms or spaces needed per function, for example, number of seats in waiting area (S), reception desks (D), exam rooms (R), etc.
- Determine individual area requirement per line item. When spaces are deemed not needed, the total area for that line item shall be computed as zero.
- Use the following rule of thumb for business occupancy code calculations:
  - *Occupancy* 100 sf per occupant;
  - *Plumbing*
    - One toilet per 25 occupants for the first 50 occupants;
    - One lavatory (sink) per 40 occupants for first 80 occupants;
    - One drinking fountain per 100 occupants;
    - One service sink.
  - *Parking* One space per examination room + 1 space for every 300 sf of administrative space (or use number of staff for a more accurate count)
- The code requirement for toilet rooms is often exceeded by the convenience and comfort of providing separate restrooms for public, patients, and staff. The spatial matrix below accounts for this convenience, and thus can be adapted to take into consideration existing facilities and area availabilities.
- Soiled and clean rooms are generally requirements pertaining to surgical suites. For general or cosmetic dermatology, instruments can be processed in the same room, which is identified below as instruments processing room. Depending on the type of practice, either instruments room or soiled and clean rooms would be computed as 0 sf.
- Clinical and equipment storages vary per size and type of practice. Cosmetic dermatology practices usually require an equipment room, whereas medical dermatology practices do not require more than a clinical storage area, although an equipment storage room would be an added bonus. It is important to note that clinical storage space does not require a dedicated room, and cabinet spaces within the nurse station can be utilized to fulfill this need.
- Patient and staff toilet rooms shall be unisex in nature.
- Building service spaces such as electrical, mechanical, and IT rooms will vary according

to engineering design and recommendations. These spaces are usually provided in buildings when a suite renovation occurs. Nonetheless, the location of these areas is important and should be taken into consideration when planning a new medical office.

- The hallway factor can vary between 30 to 40% depending on how spacious the corridors are. The minimal corridor width for business occupancies is 4 feet, but 5- to 6-foot wide corridors are more comfortable, especially when shared between providers, staff, and patients.

In the following examples, both program and spatial matrices were used to help the owner/client build a program and determine the area needed for the new dermatology office.

▶ Fig. 3.5 shows a renovation of a shell space within an existing building. The office is primarily used for two medical and cosmetic providers, but also allows for a part-time Mohs surgeon to utilize the entirety of the suite once per week. The space is configured in a cluster format with a centralized support area and two pods, each composed of three procedure rooms, an office, and a nurses' station located on either end of the suite.

▶ Fig. 3.6 is a new project for construction of a medical office specialized in medical, surgical, and cosmetic dermatology. A Mohs surgeon utilizes this space three times per week and had desired all rooms to be built as procedure rooms. The space is configured in a radial format where the support area and nurses' stations are centrally located and

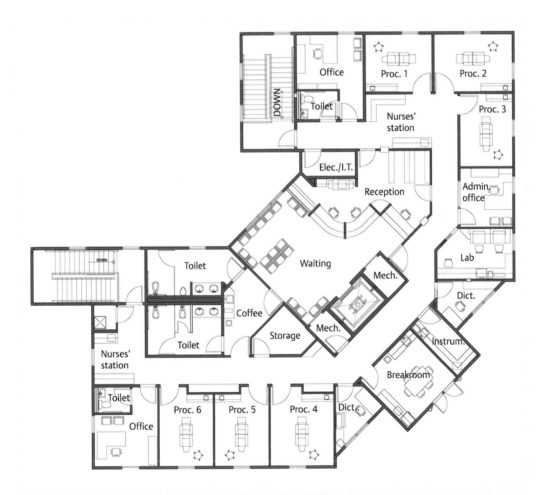

Fig. 3.5 Dermasurgery center. Lafayette, LA. Total floor area = 4,690 sf.

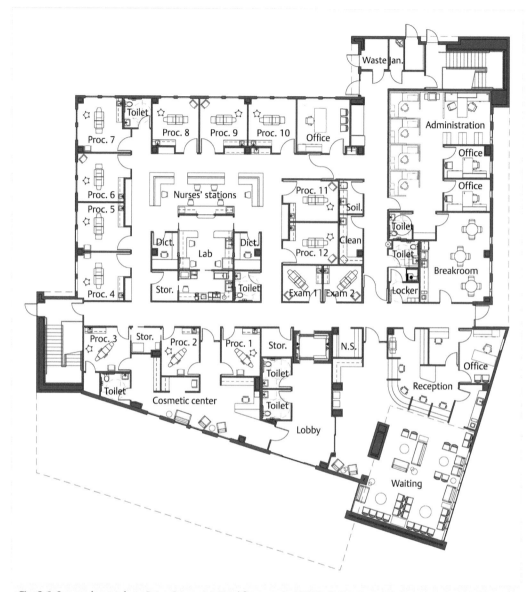

Fig. 3.6 Sanova dermatology. Baton Rouge, LA. Total floor area = 10,570 sf.

the procedure rooms are organized on the perimeter of the building to allow for maximized efficiency and adaptability to different providers on different days.

In summary, the size and layout of the practice should support the planned delivery of care based on the particular type of service, number of providers and rooms per provider, number of staff, spatial configuration desired, and priorities regarding the patient experience. Efficiency of space contributes to the success of the practice it serves. It is important to note that both matrices are meant to help guide the creation of a spatial program, so the area per room listed is for reference only and may vary. Final areas and plans can be customized and modified according to each individual style of practice, spatial needs, and budget.

References

[1] Malkin J. Medical and Dental Space Planning: A Comprehensive Guide to Design, Equipment, and Clinical Procedures. New York, NY: John Wiley & Sons; 2002: 198–208

[2] Brooks L. Practice Flow Concepts Every Doctor Should Know. Available at: http://practiceflowsolutions.com/wp-content/uploads/2015/09/09–12-Allergan-Access-Practice-Flow-Concepts-Every-Doctor-Should-Know.pdf. Accessed March 30, 2018

[3] Brooks L. Understanding the four S's that govern physician productivity. Pract Dermatol 2004(July):21–22

[4] Ching FDK. Architecture: Form, Space, and Order. Hoboken, NJ: John Wiley & Sons; 2015: 196–197

[5] Facility Guidelines Institute (FGI). Guidelines of Hospitals and Outpatient Facilities. Chicago, IL: American Society for Healthcare Engineering of the American Hospital Association; 2014

4 Creating a Business Plan

Deirdre Hooper MD, Sarah Jackson MD

Abstract

This chapter will outline how to create a business plan for your dermatology practice. In the banking world, a business plan is a document you present to lenders in order to access the capital you require. You need money to not only start your practice but also get to the point in time when you cover your overhead expenses and become profitable. Lenders want to be assured that they will be paid back, and your business plan will explain exactly how this payback will materialize. In our opinion, the process of creating a business plan is especially important for physicians. We are incredibly well trained to provide care, but often incredibly poorly trained with regard to running a business. Creating a business plan requires you to take a very real look at your market, competition, the risks you are facing, and the work you will have to do to become profitable. Once you have framed your plan, you have your roadmap to success.

Keywords: business plan, executive summary, business description, pro forma income statement, pro forma balance sheet, pro forma cash flows, break-even analysis

Top 10 Things You Need to Know

1. A business plan's primary objective is to get someone to lend you capital.
2. A business plan needs to be based on facts.
3. A business plan needs to clearly review the reality of the pros and cons of your business.
4. Your plan should include an executive summary that someone with no medical background can understand.
5. The term "pro forma" means projected and you will use the projected financial outcomes of your company to engage the help of lenders or investors.
6. An income statement explains how your business will make profit or loss.
7. A balance sheet will show a business's assets, liabilities, and equity.
8. A cash flow analysis shows the money moving in and out of your business.
9. A break-even analysis predicts the income level required to cover the cost of conducting business.
10. You can seek advice and business plan preparation from a professional, but you should possess in-depth knowledge of your own business plan and financials in order to meet with lenders or investors.

4.1 Introduction

In August 2005, we were living in two different worlds of private practice and residency, when our worlds were turned upside down by Hurricane Katrina. One of us was in the third year of being an employee, without a thought in the world about a business plan, while the other was thinking of Mohs fellowship, and not entrepreneurship. Our career paths and lives were forever changed by the flight of many dermatologists out of the city, including one of our employers and the other's Mohs directors. By December, we decided to take a chance and start a practice in the city.

Knowing what you want to do is one thing, but honestly evaluating how you are going to go about it is crucial. Starting a business not only involves risk to but also requires funds. Unless you are independently wealthy, you are going to need to borrow and then pay back. Whoever lends you money is going to ask for a business plan. A business plan is used primarily by the lender to decide on whether he or she would help you access capital you require to start your business. Your plan should focus on interesting lenders in providing the funds you need to operate your practice until you start covering your overhead expenses and begin making profit. Lenders want to be assured that they will be paid back.

The best business plans tell a clear story about how and why your business will be a success. It is important to be realistic about financial estimates and projections, and to be able to back up those claims with data. The good thing happens to be that doctors understand reality and worst-case scenarios. The challenge we face is that we do not possess much business training to even know how to create financial estimates. You may need to hire a consultant to help you with the parts you find confusing, but you should understand the process behind the numbers. Taking the time and effort to ensure your plan is realistic will payoff for you in the beginning, as you secure funding and enter the real world of private practice. We actually suffered a net loss in year one of practice (our K-1 was −$60,000), but we expected that, planned for that, and have achieved great success year over year since!

The rest of this chapter is devoted to breaking down the components of a business plan. Keep the primary objective in mind through the process of creating a plan. You are framing the plan to gain access to money which is required to manage your practice. Most business plans include several sections. They begin with an executive summary that explains the fundamentals of your business. The following sections serve to educate a lender, who may know absolutely nothing about dermatology practice, about the financial implications of running your practice, including your market, competition, and plans to operate and manage your practice. There is no single correct way to write a plan and you may modify the sections, expanding some and limiting others based on your particular practice, but the overarching context involves the use of the data to make your business a success. Good luck!

4.2 Creating Your Business Plan

Start with a clean, attractive cover page. Open with an executive summary (see below) and then proceed to narrate the story of your business. You do not have to include every step below, as there is no specific format that every lender uses. The following sections should serve as a guideline of what your plan should contain.

4.2.1 Executive Summary

The executive summary explains the fundamentals of your business. It should provide a short and clear synopsis of your business plan, describing your business concept, financial features and requirements, company's current business position, and any major facts that are relevant to the practice's success.

Ideally, composed across one page, the summary should include the following points:
- **Overview:** Describe the services your practice will provide.
- **Strategic logic:** Explain why opening your practice makes sense, based on the demand for your services in your market.
- **Business organization:** Describe the legal form of business your practice will take and where you plan to locate.
- **Business development:** Describe where you are situated in the start-up stage and what you have done to get ready to open your practice. Review when the company was formed, who the principals are, and identify key personnel.
- **Financial objectives:** Be clear about the amount of money you are seeking and how you will use the lender funding. Mention cash flow and sales projections as well as capital required.

Remember to keep your summary short and uncomplicated. Do not attempt to summarize every element of the plan. Focus on the elements that will prove to be the most interesting to the lender.

4.2.2 Business Description

This is a clear explanation of your business strategy. It is not a definition of the business or a summary of the market, but rather a summary of the one or two key factors that set your practice apart from the competition which is explained as follows:
- **Specialty description:** A precise, substantial description of your focus. For example, will you be engaged in medical/general dermatology, Mohs, or cosmetics? Discuss what makes your practice stand out from similar ones. Is your training more specialized or prestigious?
- **Impact factors:** Other aspects of your practice that are fundamental to your strategy. Do you have an alliance with a hospital or university? Do you have community ties that will aid in your success?
- **Product features and benefits:** Describe any other distinguishing features of your practice (your services and products) and delineate any strong health care consumer benefits. For example, you may be skilled in certain

procedures that other physicians in your area are not trained to perform.

- **Current situation:** Present basic information about demographics, competition, staffing, and marketing plan. List specific milestones that you have achieved.

4.2.3 Review of the Market

This is where you define your target market (who you will be treating) and how you plan to reach out to it. Market analysis requires research and familiarity with the market, so that you can clearly make out your specific targets and structure your practice to reach them.

- **Market segmentation:** Analyze your market (your potential patients) in terms of size, trends, and growth potential. Almost every market possesses some distinctive segments. For a dermatology practice, the market is segmented according to payers, age, income, nationalities, language, and race. You will need to discuss how you plan to cope with any positive or negative effects these segments may have on your practice.

  How large is the potential market? What is the physician to population ratio for dermatologists? How many dermatologists are practicing in your area? Overall, is the market growing, flattening, or shrinking?
- **Consumer analysis:** Describe your consumers and focus on factors that best determine how viable your practice will be in your market. Explain how you will attract patients in order to fulfill your plan. Look at the following points:
  - **Services:** What procedures, services, and products will appeal to your patient base?
  - **Choices:** Who are your competitors?
  - **Marketing:** What marketing approach is best suited to reach out to the patient base? How do you plan to align yourself to capture and maintain referrals from other physicians?

4.2.4 Competitive Analysis

What is the competitive advantage that your practice will offer? What are the possible weaknesses of your practice? This section should be a detailed analysis of the competitive advantages and weaknesses of your practice.

Overview other physicians who specialize in dermatology in your area. Identify the leading practice and define what makes it successful. Emphasize what sets your practice apart. For example, if there are no other physicians who specialize in advanced cosmetic dermatology and that is your focus, explain how that will serve to differentiate your practice.

Your practice may be competing with established practices in the area, and you need to let investors know how you will stand out. How do patients choose one provider over another? Prices, image, or visibility? What services will you offer that your competition does not offer? A couple of things to consider are that word-of-mouth publicity and provider referrals are key. How will your practice target these areas?

Honestly put forth your weaknesses in this section. This will help you and lenders identify problems that may hinder your success. A few other things to consider include other practices may have established patient bases, name recognition, and financial strength.[1]

4.2.5 Positioning

Lay out your strategy for how your brand will distinguish itself and how you will portray your practice to the community. Provide details on how customers will benefit from your professional services and products. A positioning statement should be a succinct description of your target market and an explanation of how you want that market to perceive your brand.[1]

4.2.6 Advertising and Promotion

A dermatology start-up practice can utilize many different promotional and advertising means. Begin this section with a general promotional plan. Provide a summary of different media and methods you intend to use and explain why. Go into the details if you know what types of promotional programs, publicity, or advertising media you will utilize.[1]

4.2.7 Sales

Part of your business plan should include how you plan to "sell" yourself and your skills. Physicians will not refer to you unless they know about you. Focus on introducing yourself and any skills that you possess that set you apart. Describe how you are an essential part of the marketing and business strategy.[1]

4.2.8 Operations

This section should first overview the practice as a business. Discuss all the critical elements of a dermatology practice. Explain how your practice will include management, front-office employees, and back-office employees. Detail how copays and insurance payments will be collected. If you plan on selling products, provide an overview of your retail plan. Break down insurance payments, patient responsibility, cash procedures, and products, so the lender can understand your dermatology practice. Summarize how your major business functions will be carried out. "Operations" should include any important aspect of your business that is not described elsewhere in your business plan.[1]

4.2.9 People

Describe your organizational culture, including your mission, vision, and core values. First, focus on any professionals in the practice. A curriculum vitae for each professional should be included. Explain the focus of each professional, their past experiences and successes, and how they will contribute to the practice. Then, highlight any mid-level or physician extenders. If you will employ extenders, explain how they will be used. Point out that extenders can allow a dermatologist to attend to more patients and increase the availability of dermatology services. Also, consider including any other key people who have committed to joining your practice. You can also include any outside services or contracting firms that you intend to use to help run your practice. Explain their expertise and how you will utilize them.[1]

4.2.10 Payback

Paying back loans is a crucial part of your business plan. Use this section to realistically outline how you will pay back your lenders. You must first find out from investors what a comfortable payback period would be for their investment. Payback period is the number of years required for an organization to recapture the initial investment. If your practice involves using loans rather than outside investors, your loan terms will be set upon closing of the loan. Outline what time period has been established for all your loans. Do you plan on paying the minimum until a certain time period or certain income is achieved? If there is

accelerated payback plan, verify there are no pre-payment penalties. Finally, estimate when you will be debt-free.[1,2]

4.2.11 Financials

Your financial section will include projected income statements, balance sheets, and cash flow and break-even analysis. The term "pro forma" literally means "for the sake of form" and is used in business and investing interchangeably with "projected." Financial projections for three to five years should be shown. Sometimes, three scenarios are presented, which pertain to the varying courses your practice might take financially. Consider presenting a weak or underperforming scenario, a realistic average-case scenario, and also a high-achieving scenario, where revenues exceed expectations. The goal of these financial projections is not to perfectly predict exactly how many patients you will attend to, but rather convince the lenders, as well as yourself, that you will provide a return on investment.

The pro forma income statement is also known as a profit and loss statement or P&L. It involves accounting of income and expenses that indicate a practice's net profit or loss over a certain period of time. It is recommended to show asset inflows, cost of operation, and profits on both a monthly and an annual basis for three to five years. Your income statement should be able to inform a lender, at a simple glance, when your practice will be profitable. Your bottom line or net profit should be clearly listed at the end. Every income statement uses the same following formula:[1,3,4]

Net profit = Revenue – Total expenses

Annual pro forma balance sheets should be presented. A balance sheet is a statement of your practice's assets, liabilities, and capital at a particular point in time, detailing the balance of income and expenditure over the preceding period. The balance sheet is the current financial state of your company in a snapshot. It will summarize what you own (assets), what you owe (liabilities), and your investment money plus profits (equity). The formula for a balance sheet is as follows:[1,5,6]

Assets = Liabilities + Equity

Cash flow pro formas should be included in both monthly and annual form for a period of three years. Cash flow is the total amount of money being transferred into and out of your practice. Your cash flow statement shows how cash is moving in and out of your business, and your liquidity, over a given period of time. Include any information that will help potential lenders understand your projections. If you can reference benchmarking data to support your projections, it will prove to be meaningful to lenders. The cash flow formula is as follows[1,7,8]:

$$Cash\ flow = Cash\ received - Cash\ paid\ out$$

4.3 Obtaining Financing

You will require several documents for your presentation to prospective lenders. If you possess experience with preparing business plans and pro forma documents, you can do this on your own. You can also enlist a consulting firm to help you prepare these. A firm that has expertise in medical practices or has helped a dermatology practice previously is ideal. Either way, you must understand the financial data that you are presenting, and be able to answer any questions from the lenders. These documents will serve as your outline for your first few months of practice. They will serve as your budget, and help you to keep track of performance and realization of goals. If you understand the business and financials of your practice, you will be more likely to secure the funding you require, and more likely to succeed in your venture.

A bank may not be your only option for financing. Make sure to approach your hospital or local health system to assess the possibility of them cosigning a bank loan. Another option may be to approach any venture capital or private equity who pursue other practices in the community. Dermatology practices are not usually as supported by hospitals as our other colleagues, but in a rural or underserved area, there may exist options for funding.

4.3.1 Pro Forma Income Statement

This is a financial statement that goes by many different names, so do not get confused—profit and loss statement, P&L, income statement, or pro forma income statement. It provides an explanation of how your business made a profit or incurred a loss over a certain period of time. It will include a table that lists all of your asset inflows and expenses, which subsequently helps in calculating your net profit and loss. Items in the document are as follows:

Revenue

Use projected number of patients seen and estimated collected amount per patient to calculate revenue. Remember to provide three estimates for variable performance in the first year. If your practice will rely on insurance collections, remember to adjust for a 90-day collections lag.

Direct Cost

Direct cost is also referred to as the cost of goods sold. If you pay for something only when you make a sale, that is a direct cost. The main example of this type of cost in a dermatology practice will be the product inventory. This is in contrast to regular expenses such as salaries, utilities, rent, or insurance, which are the same no matter how much you sell.

Gross Profit

Gross profit or gross margin refers to the difference between the revenue and direct cost on your P&L. The gross profit can be compared with the total operating expenses to determine whether you are profitable. The formula for gross profit is as follows:

$$Gross\ profit = Revenue - Direct\ cost$$

Operating Expenses

Operating expenses are all of your regular expenses other than your cost of goods sold. These expenses are best grouped into categories than listed individually. This should include fixed and variable expenses such as the following: rent, payroll, utilities, office supplies, and advertising and marketing cost.

Operating Income

Operating income is your earnings before interest, taxes, depreciation, and amortization (EBITDA). It is calculated by subtracting your total operating expenses from your gross profit. It is a reflection of your profitability and is exactly what investors are looking for.

$$Operating\ income = Gross\ profit - Operating\ expenses$$

Total Expenses

Total expenses is the total of all your expenses including interest, taxes, depreciation, and amortization. It is calculated by adding the direct cost, operating expenses, and additional expenses mentioned above.

Total expenses

$$= Direct\ cost + Operating\ expenses$$
$$+ Interest + Taxes + Depreciation$$
$$+ Amortization$$

Net Profit

Net profit is also referred to as net income and serves as your bottom line. It is calculated by subtracting total expenses from revenue. If this number is in the negative, then you are running at a loss.

$$Net\ profit = Revenue - Total\ expenses$$

When you are starting your practice, many of these line items will be estimates based on projected income. There are several options available for finding realistic projections based on other practices. One such resource is Association of Dermatology Administrators and Managers (ADAM), and another is Medical Group Management Association (MGMA). Your financial advisor may also have resources to help you project realistic data. It is important for your investors and you, as you start your practice, to have these estimates and frequently monitor your financial operations.[1,3,4]

4.3.2 Pro Forma Balance Sheet

The balance sheet is one of the essential parts of the financial statements other than your income statement and cash flow statement. The balance sheet shows your company's assets, liabilities, and owner's equity at a specific time. This sheet, too, represents future projections. The pro forma balance sheet can be used to project the overall financial position of your practice. A balance sheet always has to balance, hence the name; liabilities and owner's equity on one side and assets on the other.

The equation for a balance sheet is as follows:

$$Assets = Liabilities + Equity$$

If you think about the equation, and the definitions, it is common sense. Assets, or what the company owns, had to be paid for by either borrowing money from lenders (liabilities) or obtaining money from investors or owners (equity).

Your practice's net worth can also be determined at any given point in time from the balance sheet. Net worth is calculated by subtracting liabilities from assets.

The equation is as follows:

$$Net\ worth = Assets - Liabilities$$

The balance sheet will include the following:

Assets

Your assets should be organized from top to bottom based on liquidity, or how easily the asset can be converted into cash. Your assets will be broken down into two major categories, current and long term or fixed. Your current assets are assets that can be converted to cash within one year.

- **Current assets:**
  - **Cash:** Pertains to the money you have on hand in the bank or checking account balance. It can also include cash equivalents that are liquid and easily converted to cash, like a money market account or treasury bill.
  - **Accounts receivable:** This is what you have billed already, but have not received from insurance companies or patients. This projection is based on average collection time taken to receive payment.
  - **Inventory:** This includes the value of all products that you have on hand but have not sold yet.
  - **Total current assets:** This includes cash, accounts receivable, and inventory.
- **Long-term or fixed assets:** These are all the assets you possess with long-standing value, such as vehicles, lasers, building and land, or other equipment. These items are ones that can typically not be converted into cash quickly.
- **Accumulated depreciation:** Depreciation occurs when your asset loses value over time. Your accountant can use this depreciation for certain tax benefits, and your insurance can be adjusted to reflect the value of your property with depreciation. It is important to understand depreciation as a business owner.
- **Total long-term or fixed assets:** This term is used to describe long-term assets plus depreciation on a balance sheet.

Liabilities

Similar to how you ordered your assets, you should order your liabilities in accordance with how quickly you need to pay them off. Current liabilities will be those liabilities due within one year. Your long-term liabilities would be those due at any point after one year.

- **Current liabilities:**
  - **Accounts payable:** The amount that your business owes at the beginning of balance sheet period is known as the accounts payable. This includes all regular bills that you will need to pay.
  - **Accrued payroll payable:** This is the amount of payroll unpaid at the beginning of the balance sheet period.
  - **Sales taxes payable:** This applies to a business that does not pay sales tax right away. Some businesses only pay sales tax each quarter. Check with your accountant in order to find out how you will be paying sales tax.
  - **Short-term debt:** This is any debt that must be paid by your business within a period of one year. This can also be referred to as notes payable or current liabilities.
- **Total current liabilities:** This is the sum total of accounts payable, accrued payroll, sales tax payable, and short-term debt.
- **Long-term liabilities:** These are the financial obligations that will take your business more than a year to pay back. It does not include the interest on the obligations. This includes your mortgage note payable minus the principal paid in the upcoming year. It also includes any long-term loan taken to buy expensive equipment. This number will decrease over time as your business makes principal payments.
- **Total liabilities:** This is the total of your business's current and long-term liabilities.

Equity

- Owner's equity refers to the money paid into the company as an investment. This is different from the market value of stock. Equity is the actual money paid into the company as equity investments by owners. This is sometimes referred to as paid-in capital.
- **Common stock:** This does not change unless new stock is issued.

- **Retained earnings:** These are earnings or losses that have been reinvested with the company and not paid out as dividends. It can be a negative or positive number. If negative, the company has accumulated losses. Not all legal entities will be the same; however, if your company is a pass-through tax entity, then your balance sheet will reflect that. This means that all losses or profits will be passed onto the owners.[1,5,6]

4.3.3 Pro Forma Cash Flows

Cash flow is the measure of actual money that is moving in and out of your bank accounts. Positive cash flow is cash that is entering your business and negative cash flow is cash that you pay out. A pro forma or projected cash flow can help you determine when or if there will be a shortage of cash. The cash flow calculation is as follows:

$$Cash\ flow = Cash\ received - Cash\ paid\ out$$

Cash will be critical to running your dermatology practice. Your cash sources will be funds you receive based on the services you provide and the products you sell. You will need cash to purchase supplies and pay fixed operating expenses. In some months, you may encounter negative cash flow. This is a very common occurrence as you grow your business. You will need money from investors to be able support negative cash flow for some time while your business is growing. Negative cash flow during the initial days is called burn rate. Burn rate is the measure of how much cash you are "burning" every month.

Your cash flow will be delayed because insurance payments are often delayed and patient responsibility can delay your collections even further. Some tips for improving your cash flow include the following:

- Try collecting payments from patients up front instead of invoicing or billing them. This will lower your accounts receivable. If you accept insurance, it is often prudent to have your front office check patient responsibility at the time of service. If the patient has a copay or has a deductible that has not been met, then that money should be due at the time of service.
- Consider paying bills a little more slowly. Many injectable companies will let you delay your payment by 90 days without interest. In your first few months of practice, try to negotiate

later payments without interest from all vendors. The longer you can hold onto your cash, the better your cash position will be.

- Get a line of credit to cover any periods of negative cash flow. This is a short-term loan that you can withdraw from as you need and repay without penalty. Many start-up dermatology practices use lines of credit to help them through periods of low cash, or to manage larger purchases on a more short-term basis than a long-term loan.
- Manage your inventory carefully. Do not make the mistake of buying too much inventory. Many companies will provide discounts for larger purchases, but in your early months of practice, you must have cash to pay the bills. Also, consider only outfitting part of your office or few examination rooms to start with, and then add as needed. It makes more sense to carry less inventory and order only when needed in your start-up practice.
- Use a collection service to outsource your problem or overdue accounts receivable. If you do not have any extra employees, at first, to track down patients for outstanding balances, consider a collection service. These services will collect a fee for successful payments and do not charge for any uncollected fees. Use this only for problem patients and if your office has not been able to collect on their own.

"Cash is king," as they say. Cash flow is extremely important to monitor, as it is necessary for the survival of your business. Having an understanding of your cash flow will be critical for the health of your practice. Use your pro forma cash flow statement to show investors the metrics of your practice, and then use that statement during the initial months to monitor cash flow.[1,7,8]

4.3.4 Break-even Analysis

A break-even analysis predicts what level of income is required to cover the cost of condcuting business. Your break-even point is achieved when all expenses due are covered by money received. The break-even analysis is different than the payback period discussed earlier. Payback period is the time it takes to recover an investment.

The break-even analysis uses all fixed expenses, including ones that are paid quarterly or yearly. It is recommended that you include all regular running fixed costs or total monthly operating expenses. Gross profit must exceed all total monthly operating expenses to reach the break-even point. These expenses include the following:
- Rent
- Payroll
- Insurance
- Utilities
- Taxes
- Interest
- Medical supplies
- Office supplies
- Telephone/Cable/Internet
- Advertising
- Any other miscellaneous expenses required to run your business

At first, your break-even analysis will be based on assumptions. Make the most educated assumptions that you can make about the number of patients you would attend to, and number of products you would sell, for your initial assessment. Later, you may be able to use more detailed forecasts and profit and loss numbers as your practice builds. Review this analysis during your first few months of practice and compare your actual financial status to your projection.[1,2]

4.4 Dos and Don'ts

- Do call on experts to help you analyze the market, competition, and report numbers.
- Do not let others do the work for you without understanding everything.
- Do understand every aspect of the business end of your practice.
- Do not let dreams and hopes outweigh reality.

4.5 Conclusion

Starting your dermatology practice can be both exciting and overwhelming. Being prepared with a sound business plan will help you navigate both obtaining funding and staying on course in your first few months of practice. As dermatologists, we are trained to operate at the highest level of expertise in our fields, but most of us possess no formal business training. You must take the time to understand the business aspects of starting a practice, and utilize experts when needed. We hope that this chapter will help you in preparing your business plan. Best of luck in your endeavor!

References

[1] Brady W, Chaudhari R, eds. Starting and Marketing a Dermatology Practice. American Academy of Dermatology, Des Plaines, Illinois, 2013

[2] Berry T. What Is a Break-Even Analysis? Available at: https://articles.bplans.com/break-even-analysis/?_ga=2.265356175.1847499318.1548611832–124031931.1544387348. Accessed October 9, 2019

[3] Parsons N. How to Read and Understand Your Profit and Loss. Available at: https://www.liveplan.com/blog/how-to-read-and-understand-your-profit-and-loss/?utm_source=liveplan&utm_medium=download&utm_campaign=income_statement&utm_content=how_to_read_an_income_statement. Accessed October 9, 2019

[4] O'Rourke A. What Is an Income Statement? Available at: https://articles.bplans.com/income-statement-2/?utm_source=liveplan&utm_medium=download&utm_campaign=income_statement&utm_content=what_is_an_income_statement. Accessed October 9, 2019

[5] Parsons N. What Is a Balance Sheet, and How Do You Read It? Available at: https://www.liveplan.com/blog/what-is-a-balance-sheet-and-how-do-you-read-it/?utm_source=liveplan&utm_medium=download&utm_campaign=balance_sheet&utm_content=how-to-read-a-balance-sheet. Accessed October 9, 2019

[6] O'Rourke A. What Is a Balance Sheet? Available at: https://articles.bplans.com/balance-sheet/?_ga=2.260010890.1236268530.1548612780–124031931.1544387348. Accessed October 9, 2019

[7] Parsons N. Understanding Your Cash Flow Statement. Available at: https://www.liveplan.com/blog/understanding-your-cash-flow-statement/?utm_source=liveplan&utm_medium=download&utm_campaign=cash_flow_statement&utm_content=understanding-cash-flow-statement. Accessed October 9, 2019

[8] Parson N. What Is Cash Flow? Available at: https://www.liveplan.com/blog/cash-flow-metrics-minute/?utm_source=liveplan&utm_medium=download&utm_campaign=cash_flow_statement&utm_content=what-is-cash-flow. Accessed October 9, 2019

5 Room Layout

Jessica Awerman MD, Rajiv Nijhawan MD

Abstract

The examination room is the primary setting of contact with a patient and, thus, has the inherent ability to either maximize your efficiency or completely hinder your progress. Creating a room design that is focused on physician efficiency without negotiating patient comfort will enable quick transitions, easy movements, increased productivity, and higher patient and team satisfaction. We believe the key to physician efficiency is standardization of the examination room to promote seamless transitions and provision of easy access to all necessary materials. This chapter will walk through the basic elements that a dermatologist should consider in their clinic room setup and provide some visual examples of design that have been successful in our high-volume clinic.

Keywords: room design, layout, workflow, efficiency, exam room, organization, standardization

Top 10 Things You Need to Know

1. All aspects of the clinic and room design should optimize physician efficiency.
2. You must understand your patient demographics in order to anticipate their needs and the aim of your practice.
3. Examination rooms should be standardized to streamline access to materials and instruments while maximizing patient safety.
4. Standardization should be based on the types of practice (i.e., medical dermatology versus surgical dermatology) or implement a universal care model.
5. A central patient examination chair that adjusts and converts to a table allows for easy transfers and transitions from consultation to procedures with access from both sides.
6. Work stations should allow you to face the patient and seamlessly transition the screen for patient viewing.
7. Rooms should be well-stocked and have the most used materials most easily accessible.
8. All access points to patient should have easy disposal of sharps and trash.
9. Communication systems that enable nonverbal cues to staff speed up retrieval of needed supplies and preparation of patients.
10. Do not underestimate the importance of patient comfort and satisfaction in improving a streamlined visit.

5.1 Introduction

The objectives of a clinic visit are to assess, diagnose, and treat a patient, all of which occur within the confines of an examination room. Thus, the room layout has the potential to help you streamline each visit and fly through your day; conversely, it can hinder your progress, frustrating you, your staff, and your patients, and make your day seem to drag on forever. Creating a room design that is focused on physician efficiency without negotiating patient comfort will enable quick transitions, easy movements, increased productivity, and higher patient satisfaction.

5.2 Where Do I Start?

In order to design a well-organized room layout, it is important to have a full grasp on the demographics you anticipate treating as well as what you will be doing within your scope of practice. Start by asking yourself: How old are my patients? Do they have mobility issues? How often do family members accompany them? What type of procedures do I anticipate performing frequently (e.g., surgical, cosmetics, lasers, etc.)? Some of these questions may be difficult to answer, as you may not know what demographic you will attract until you are open and operational. However, you need to be prepared and ready to treat this population prior to starting, while giving yourself a buffer to accommodate any future expansion.

With most aspects of clinical medicine, there is a constant learning curve and progressive improvements can be made throughout your practice. In this chapter, we will break down the basic elements needed to design an efficient room layout suitable for the general dermatologist. Given the nature of dermatology practice, ranging from medical consultation to surgical procedure and encompassing all age ranges, we recommend using a "universal care" examination room model to avoid any need for lengthy transitions of patients within the clinic to specialized rooms or delays in compiling supplies within the same room for common procedures.

5.3 Elements of the Room Layout

5.3.1 Room Dynamics

The location and the building setup or whether you are designing your own space will contribute to determining room dynamics. However, most importantly, any aspect over which you do have control should be completely standardized. Standardization decreases your cognitive load, mental memory, and overall stress to enable a smoother workflow and more efficient visit.[1] It streamlines your visit, knowing what you have within your reach versus what you need your staff to bring you.

Recent literature debates over designing mirrored rooms (i.e., standardization across a shared wall) versus handedness rooms (i.e., all rooms are truly identical). A study in an acute medical-surgical setting found that there was no clear difference in the two setups, and an overall global view of the patient care environment upon entry is the most important factor to reduce cognitive load.[2]

Some clinics are also implementing a two-door system. The overall idea is to increase patient privacy and improve flow of the visit, and it can be implemented in two different scenarios. In some cases, clinics are using separate entrances for physicians versus patients. An alternate option is to have patients enter through one door and exit through the other door, so that patients do not walk back through the waiting room to exit; further, it respects patient privacy postvisit. This approach may be especially useful for certain patients seeking the upmost privacy, such as cosmetics patients and/or in practices that often treat celebrities.

In addition, the size of rooms is an important consideration if you are designing your clinic space. Most physicians prefer at least a 10-foot by 10-foot examination room with an increase to 12-foot by 12-foot for procedure rooms. These sizes allow for easy flow in the room without feeling overcrowded if the patient, nurse, and physician need to be in the room at the same time. We recommend allocating more overall space to examination/procedure rooms than the waiting area to maximize your productivity. You likely need to only have approximately two to three waiting room chairs per examination room.

5.3.2 Exam Table

Upon entry into the room, the examination table should be visible with a clear path for the patient. The examination table is the classic symbol of a "doctor's office" and its importance stems from the fact that it is the place where the key physician–patient exchange occurs and where all the three tasks of assessment, diagnosis, and treatment are carried out. Use this to your advantage by investing in an examination table that optimizes efficiency, comfort, and safety.

That being said, the classic examination table is no longer practical, can be inconvenient, and even dangerous for both staff and patients when attempting to get a patient onto the table. The best option is an examination chair that can be easily accessible by patients of all mobility statuses and quickly converted into a flat table through a remote control and/or a foot pedal to avoid any potential injury to staff manually adjusting the chair either. One source suggests the height of 17 to 19 inches for best patient access of elderly patients.[3] This should have access from both sides for patient ease, and for later ease of treatment and assessment of all patient sides. Foot pedals are convenient for midprocedure adjustments, so that neither the dermatologist nor the staff has to unglove and reglove (▶Fig. 5.1). Procedure chairs

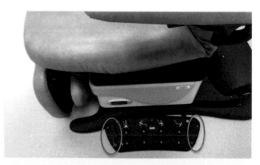

Fig. 5.1 Examination chair with foot pedal. Red circles note the automatic memory functions which when pressed will easily change the chair from a seat to a flat table or vice versa.

with some memory options (e.g., reclined position, flat table, or sitting position) help expedite proper positioning as well, instead of, for example, individually having to adjust the head, back, and legs. For dermatologists who prefer to sit while performing certain examinations/procedures, chairs that adjust height can also help with efficiency.

It is important to remember that the longer it takes a patient to get on and off an examination table, the more time it will take in reaching the goal toward maximum efficiency. Patient flow in the room depends on physicians' personal preference; patients can be directed to the examination table immediately (and not any extra seating in the room) by the assistant rooming the patient to limit an extra step in the patient's evaluation. The assistant should be able to easily access a gown in the room and direct the patient to change into it to help initiate the medical examination. However, some physicians prefer to first sit the patient on a chair beside the desk where the history can be taken and confirmed and a relationship can be established before the patient is seated on the chair for the full examination or procedure depending on the situation.

Friends or family often accompany patients to medical visits, so it is beneficial to have 1 to 2 extra chairs on the side of the examination room which are out of the way for the patients' companions. Unless absolutely necessary, it is best if any companions beyond 1 to 2 people remain in the waiting room to prevent congestion in the patient's room. The proximity of the patient to the physician should be the closest to establish that he or she is the focus of the appointment that day. In addition, seating in general should be able to accommodate patients of all sizes as at least 39% of American adults are obese.[4] Having a designated area for placement of assistive mobility devices, such as walkers and canes, out of the workflow path also helps accommodate elderly patients safely. Hooks on walls can also be helpful to have for patients' clothes if they need to disrobe or even just for their coats.

5.3.3 Technology

The dependence on digital data and charting in the electronic medical record (EMR) has become essential to the patient visit in most cases and often serves as key source of communication throughout the entire clinic visit (i.e., medication prescriptions, requesting future visit scheduling, referrals, messages to collaborative providers, etc.). Thus, it should have a permanent, easily accessible space within the examination room. There are varying opinions across specialties on whether this workstation should be placed in order to allow patient eye contact or patient viewing. It also depends if the physician is the one who enters the majority of the information into the EMR.

Given that the nature of dermatology depends less on the EMR "facts" and "data" and more on the visual inspection of the patient, we suggest the ideal option is to position the computer to enable the physician to engage with the patient while working on the computer. Yet, it is similarly important to have the option to turn the screen, usually with a moveable bracket, and engage the patient in the conversation (i.e., identifying a prior biopsy site via a clinical photograph or showing them the pathology report) without either having to change positions (▶ Fig. 5.2). In addition, fixed desktop computers in each room help mitigate any issues with the cognitive load of having to move with a laptop from one place to another and the issues that come with this option such as battery dying and even infection risk. If you do elect for a mobile workstation, remember to have a docking or charging station in each room. In ideal situations, the practice employs scribes for documentation, maybe even with tablets, and the positioning of a workstation/screen is not as relevant to the practice.

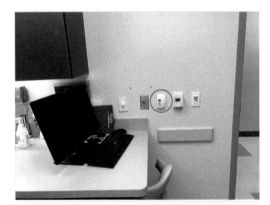

Fig. 5.2 Desktop computer with movable screen. This setup allows charting while maintaining eye contact and easy ability to turn screen to allow for patient involvement. Red circle notes the easy access to call button in order to alert clinic staff that assistance is needed.

One aspect to keep in mind is patients need to sign electronic consent. Tablets make this process very easy. Yet, if your practice elects for a fixed workstation, consider an electronic signature pad that is long enough to reach the patient's seat.

In our technologically savvy society, patients and their companions will often want to use the wireless Internet connection while waiting in your office. If you decide to offer Wi-Fi access to patients, it is important to never give out any secure network passwords. A separate guest Wi-Fi network should be setup that is separated from the main office network, with the appropriate access points and firewalls that create secure boundaries. Be extremely careful to not leave any vulnerabilities in this separation and contact your wireless provider or an information technology (IT) specialist, if needed, to ensure that your patient and office data are secure. Hospital-run IT teams often have this aspect appropriately addressed, but if there is no guest Wi-Fi available in your hospital, never give out passwords to patients, as this could allow them access into secure data. If you are in a private practice setting where you are responsible for setting up the Internet connection, your provider should be able to help you setup a guest access Wi-Fi connection separated by a firewall from the clinical Wi-Fi network.

5.3.4 Room Setup

Once the patient is in the examination chair, everything should be within arm's reach from that position and identical in each room (▶ Fig. 5.3). You

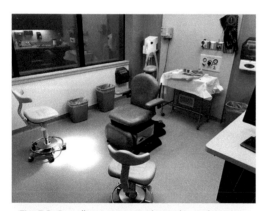

Fig. 5.3 Overall room setup is identical in each room. Examination chair is central to allow for movement on each side. Each side of room has a separate trash can and sharps container.

will need stationary lighting fixtures for each room, the exact specification may depend on the type of procedures you are performing, but we recommended a fixed overhead light to declutter the floor workspace and provide optimal viewing. Most examination rooms in dermatology benefit from at least three overhead lights. Ideally, one of the ceiling mounted lights is an adjustable operating room style light to allow for procedures and closer viewing of patients. However, given that this may be cost prohibitive, another more affordable option is LED flashlights, wall-mounted lamps, or headlamps in each room. As much natural light as possible also helps with dermatologic examinations, but this often needs to be a balance with patient privacy and your office layout. New lighting fixtures are remarkable in their ability to light a patient and his or her skin.

There should also be a horizontal stable workspace, likely a counter or movable cart/table, in close proximity to the patient. It is important to place the most used objects in your practice directly on the counter to avoid time spent searching through drawers. In our clinic, this includes: alcohol pads, gauze, hand sanitizer, bandaging materials, handheld mirrors, and gloves (▶ Fig. 5.4). Underlying and overlying this space should be ample cabinet and drawer storage that is fully stocked with the most used items to avoid any unnecessary time in having to go outside the room for more materials (▶ Fig. 5.5).

Four overhead cabinets seem to work well for practices with high-surgical volume, although three may be ample for more medical dermatology practices. Drawers below the counter can be great

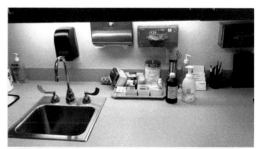

Fig. 5.4 Counter space with most used items. This includes alcohol pads, gauze, hand sanitizer, bandaging materials, handheld mirrors, and gloves.

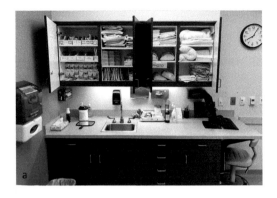

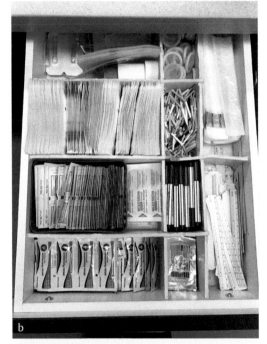

Fig. 5.5 (a) Cabinets and **(b)** drawers in each room are standardized with the most commonly required materials that are fully stocked each day.

ways to easily access commonly used items. In high-volume clinics, it seems you can never have enough storage in each room, because inevitably something runs out at the most inopportune time. A staff member should be designated to maintain accurate inventory frequently to ensure appropriate quantity of supplies. While some minimalist-type rooms may look sleeker, ample storage is critical to maximize efficiency and minimize time required to constantly restock rooms.

There are some items used in daily practice, such as needles, that ideally should be kept out of patient rooms to protect them from tampering and theft. Multi-dose vials, such as local anesthesia, should stay out of patient treatment areas and only be accessed in a dedicated clean medication preparation area. Similarly, prefilled syringes should be kept in this clean preparation area to avoid tampering and inadvertent contamination. While this approach adds an extra step to retrieve these syringes from another location, it helps in ensuring patient safety. Locking and unlocking drawers in each room can often be cumbersome, but if expensive or sharp tools are to be left in patient rooms, it may not be a bad idea.

5.3.5 Safety Elements

Keeping harm away from patients, staff, and self fulfills the Hippocratic oath and also maximizes efficiency. The most common safety hazard in the dermatology clinic settings is sharps, given our frequent injections, biopsies, and in-office procedures. Thus, sharps containers on both sides of the room help avoid travelling with a sharp object that could end in harm (▶Fig. 5.3). Apart from disposal of sharps, it is important to have easy access to general disposal of garbage. In our clinic, this is executed through stationary trash cans on either side of the room (▶Fig. 5.3). For a cleaner look, some practices prefer to keep their trash bins below the sinks.

Another option that is preferred by some surgical practices includes mobile biohazard buckets on wheels. The advantage to this option is it is easily mobile and moved with one's foot to avoid any need to unglove to move it. Yet, the mobile nature has an inherent lack of standardization that will decrease efficiency when searching for the bucket. However, a general dermatology room may not have utility for these buckets.

Safety considerations also include protecting patients from preventable infections by having a sink in the room and multiple access points to hand sanitizers within the path of the physician to avoid unnecessary movements. Some argue that with the ubiquitous use of hand sanitizers, sinks may not even be needed in each room and can be reserved for procedure rooms.

5.4 Other Important Considerations

5.4.1 Portable Items

In order to avoid clutter of the room, it is reasonable to have certain medical devices that are kept outside of the room and brought in when needed. These can be easily transported on carts/poles with wheels. One example is having a vital sign cart that is brought in to take the patient's vitals and then is removed from the room. Other potential devices include lasers and energy-based devices. If these are going to be a large component of your practice, it is very important to pay particular attention to location, patient flow, and flexibility of room use to optimize their use. Special outlets may be necessary for devices, so be sure to consider this aspect in the build-out plans.

5.4.2 Clinic Communication

Do not underestimate the efficiency gained from a functional team. Having a standardized communication system that is consistently used by all members of the team helps in reducing unnecessary trips for supplies or searching for staff. In our rooms, we have an easily accessible call button within each room that makes an audible sound within the work room and lights up over the door to allow quick and easy identification of a room where staff is needed (▶ Fig. 5.2). This allows seamless transitions for procedure preparation or supply collection.

Headsets or other electronic communication technologies can also be very helpful in improving efficiency, especially in large practices or in layouts that are not very open. Front desk staff can seamlessly communicate with back office members without having to physically track them down. Hands-free devices can even allow for physicians to request additional assistance when gloved in a sterile manner.

▶ Fig. 5.6 shows our flag system, which is immediately outside each door. This helps facilitate flow. Flags can also be used to signify who is in the room (e.g., patient, attending physician, trainees such as residents or fellows, nurse, etc.). In our clinic, each role has an assigned color flag.

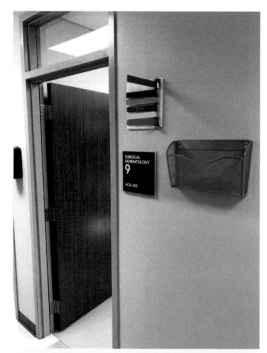

Fig. 5.6 Flag system outside every examination room door allows for nonverbal communication among staff. Each flag in our clinic represents a different role (i.e., red = patient, blue = attending 1, orange = attending 2, green = resident/fellow, and yellow = nurse).

Thus, without any discussion, everyone easily knows who is in the room with each patient. Other options for flags is as follows: (a) using them to determine which patient needs to be seen next by a physician or nurse or (b) using them to signify to team members which room needs to cleaned and turned over.

5.4.3 Privacy

Optimizing patient's privacy both visually and acoustically should be incorporated into the room layout. Visual privacy can be controlled by the use of privacy curtains; however, these also increase the potential for cross-contamination, laundry costs, and need for physician recall to pull these closed.[5] The cost-benefit analysis will be specific to your practice and whether you are consistently having total body skin checks, in which patients are at their most vulnerable, changing fully into a gown. Training your staff and yourself to be mindful of the door being closed can also ensure more privacy. Studies have shown that nurses and doctors tend to leave the door open at the beginning and end of visits, right when patients are changing, even though the door is closed during the visit.[5] Traditional doors that open inward are often less noisy than sliding doors, but sliding doors may be a better fit for smaller examination rooms. It is imperative to train your staff to not slam the door shut to ensure an optimal experience. Curtains for doors do provide an extra level of privacy, especially if a staff member inadvertently enters without knocking during a full body skin examination, but they are often bulky and unnecessary if team members are conscious when to enter a specific room. Flags can be used as a cue in instances when not to enter.

In addition, you must consider privacy to the outside through windows and the need for window curtains. Attaining a balance between optimizing natural light to improve visibility for your examination/procedure while ensuring that patients' privacy is protected is essential.

Of note is the fact that acoustic privacy is also important to consider, as it will affect the patient's overall comfort if they are able to hear from another room and, thus, know that other people could be hearing them as well. Studies from the emergency department have shown that patient satisfaction is directly tied to their feelings of privacy. In addition, patients have been shown to be less forthcoming and honest when they feel they could be overheard.[6,7] Important factors include a thick wood door, sound galleys, and insulation of the walls to ensure that there is a sound barrier. Should noise from outside the examination room be an issue that cannot be mitigated by physical alterations, consider a white noise device in the affected room(s).

5.5 Potential Pitfalls

As the field of dermatology changes and new technology emerges, the clinic structure will need to be consistently updated and refined. It is important for the physician and the entire supporting team to continue to be flexible to these new implementations and avoid resistance to change.

Ways to Ensure Success

- Be willing to implement a standardized room layout.
- Listen to support staff's ideas/concerns.
- Constantly modify procedure and look for ways to improve.
- Be willing to try new things out; even if they do not work, you can always just return to your original ways.
- Look for ways to improve the system, don't just "get used to" a system.

5.6 Conclusion

Every inch of the dermatology clinic room layout should be focused on physician efficiency. Efficiency increases your ability to provide high-quality care to your patients while avoiding unnecessary hinderances and obstacles. The more efficient you are, the better-quality care you will provide and the higher patient satisfaction you will see. Start with a standardized practice across all your rooms, but also be flexible and adaptive, as your practice evolves to use "speedbumps" to help you figure out a better process and flow. Make sure that you adapt these practices across the entire clinic to increase your efficiency, which leads to increased productivity.

References

[1] Silvis JK. Having It All: New Trends in Clinic Design. Available at: https://www.healthcaredesignmagazine.com/trends/architecture/having-it-all-new-trends-clinic-design/#slide-2. Published 2016. Accessed December 15, 2018

[2] Pati D, Harvey TE, Reyers E, et al. A multidimensional framework for assessing patient room configurations. HERD 2009;2(2):88–111

[3] Paper MW. Rethink the Outpatient Clinical Space: Efficient Exam Room Design. Available at: https://cdn.midmark.com/docs/default-source/documents/white-paper—rethink-the-outpatient-clinical-space—efficient-exam-room-design.pdf?sfvrsn=1703a23e_0. Published 2011. Accessed December 13, 2018

[4] Warren M, Beck S, Rayburn J. The State of Obesity. Available at: https://www.tfah.org/

stateofobesity2018. Published 2018. Accessed December 13, 2018

[5] Freihoefer K, Nyberg G, Vickery C. Clinic exam room design: present and future. HERD 2013;6(3):138–156

[6] Lin YK, Lin CJ. Factors predicting patients' perception of privacy and satisfaction for

emergency care. Emerg Med J 2011;28(7): 604–608

[7] Olsen JC, Sabin BR. Emergency department patient perceptions of privacy and confidentiality. J Emerg Med 2003;25(3):329–333

6 Office Flow

Kavita Mariwalla MD, FAAD

Abstract

The flow of patients in your office is dictated by three processes: check-in, the exam visit itself, and check-out. Understanding each step of check-in can help you streamline how much time patients spend in the waiting room or filling out paperwork. It is essential that check-in occurs as quickly as possible so that patients can spend the majority of their time in your office interacting with you as their provider. Since check-in and check-out are where the transactional portion of your business occurs, it is important to ensure this is done discretely but also effectively so that copayments, balances, and deductibles are collected. Taken together, the elements of office flow can impact the quality of a patient visit by making your office appear coordinated and professional.

Keywords: check-in, copayment, deductible, receptionist, established patient, new patient, check-out

Top 10 Things You Need to Know

1. Understand the intricate processes involved in check-in and check-out, as these are two areas where office flow efficiency can be maximized.
2. A single receptionist at a single desk in the middle of a waiting room can be beautiful and aesthetically pleasing, but is not efficient as he or she is bound by the Health Insurance Portability and Accountability Act (HIPAA) legislation with regard to the tasks they can carry out that may be overheard in the waiting area.
3. Ensure the person checking in patients is not burdened by answering phone calls or other questions and can focus on the patient in front of them, so as to process their information and start the office visit as quickly as possible.
4. Try to direct all patients into filling out paperwork online at all times.
5. Separate surgical procedure visits in time, and preferably space, from general medical dermatology. Similarly do so with cosmetic patients.
6. Position check-out and check-in spaces in separate areas.
7. Choose the type of assistant you want in the room with you.
8. Evaluate how you practice in terms of time you spend in the room for different types of visits to maximize your schedule.
9. A separate nursing schedule which can run alongside you is an efficient way to manage tasks such as suture removals and patch test placement.
10. Craft your templates with great care as "new patients only" over the course of an hour will not flow as efficiently as a mixture of established and new patients. Attempting to spread out skin checks and new patients will ultimately lead to better flow dynamics.

6.1 Introduction

Whether you are building your office space from the ground up or inheriting someone else's design, it is important to think about your flow of patients throughout the day. Although the concept of bringing someone from the waiting room to the examination room seems straightforward, there actually exist multiple processes along the way that can gum up the works. The result can be the difference between the patient having a good experience in your office versus a bad one—little of which has to do with the quality of care you delivered in the room. And while it is true that physicians in a small private practice may have more say over the flow of patients, do not let the confines of an academic institution or a large group practice dissuade you from influencing office flow. The best way to think of this process is to break it down into the following three components: check-in, rooming, and check-out.

6.2 Check-in

Although the title seems obvious, "checking in" to a doctor's office is far from easy. If you have more than one physician schedule running at a time, it may be worth considering having either a separate check-in desk for each provider or several check-in staff working as a team. The check-in process directly influences how many patients are present in the waiting area which can impact their perception of how chaotic the practice is. If the check-in process backs up, the schedule tends to fall apart. For this reason, check-in is where the first decisions from a practice flow standpoint should be made. This is what I recommend considering:

6.2.1 Receptionist

The first observation a patient makes when he or she walks into the office is the waiting area and that includes how many receptionists are behind the welcome desk. (Note the use of the word "welcome" and not "check-in.")

Behind the Glass or Not?

The ideal image of a dermatology practice is a beautiful desk behind which sits a receptionist who welcomes the patient. While this setting conveys luxury, it is not always practical due to space limitations. Keep in mind that HIPAA privacy laws are immediately in effect as soon as a patient enters the office. Therefore, if the people present in the waiting room can overhear a private conversation, there can be an issue. So, if you have one person in an open desk arrangement, bear in mind that this receptionist will need to understand HIPAA carefully and may not be able to perform the same number of functions as someone who sits behind a glass window that can slide shut.

6.2.2 Sign-in Sheet

Many physicians use sign-in sheets for their patients. The HIPAA Privacy Rule explicity permits the incidental disclosures that may result from this practice, so long as the information disclosed is appropriately limited. For example, patients may hear the name of another patient being called but should not see on a sign-in sheet the reason for the patient's visit. Depending on the type of practice you have, the recognition of a patient's name may not ensure their privacy adequately. In my office I use patient sign-in label forms. When a patient signs in, the sticker of the signature line is pulled off and kept by the receptionist so no patient is missed and other patients cannot see the names of others in the waiting room.

6.2.3 New Patients

New patients to a practice often have paperwork to fill out. In the age of electronic medical records, it is best to provide patients access to their portal at the time of scheduling out forms, so that they can fill this out ahead of out forms. Remember that one of the measures of the merit-based incentive payment system (MIPS) is to have these portals open within four days of new patients making appointments. Keeping in mind that patients may still not utilize their portal to fill out history and pertinent medical information prior to the visit, patient kiosks in the waiting room can decrease the time needed to manually enter information. These kiosks should be compatible with your electronic medical record to transfer information seamlessly. We use our patient kiosks for patients to fill out all Allergies, Medications, Past Medical and Surgical History and to sign practice forms such as Financial Guarantee of Payment. The final option (and I truly mean the last) is to hand patients actual paperwork on a clipboard with a pen. While as a practice owner you understand that patients can take anywhere from 5 to 30 minutes to fill out paperwork and then that paperwork must be hand transcribed into your EMR, this is rarely taken into account when the patient themselves thinks about wait time. As a result, in our office, we have implemented a laminated sheet that acts as the cover sheet for all paperwork given out on a clipboard. It simply states "Welcome to Mariwalla Dermatology. We would like you to fill out the following paperwork, so that we can understand your medical history better in order to help you with your skin. From the time this paperwork is completed and handed back to the receptionist the wait time should be no more than 25 minutes, as we have to also enter this information into the computer. Thank you for your understanding."

Although having physical paperwork is important for those who do not feel comfortable on the computer, every effort should be made to steer away from it because it is incredibly inefficient for your staff and also your schedule. A new patient scheduled at 3:00 pm who shows up at 3:05 pm and then has to do all of their intake paperwork manually may not actually be ready to come back to the examination room until 3:45 or 4:00 pm The patient thinks they have waited an hour to see you and, in fact, they have. But from your perspective, they took an hour just to check in, thus upending your schedule. In the end, the patient's perception is the only one that matters and, in their mind, they have already been in your office for an hour.

The other option you have (depending on number of patients) is to dedicate a resource to calling patients who have not done the paperwork online. If for some reason, patients are not willing to log on to their portal, having an area of your website where patients can download forms and fill them out at home is also quite helpful.

6.2.4 Established Patients

For established patients, the check-in process should be streamlined. They should be able to sign in and go through the rest of check-in quickly. It is important to remind your staff that patients who have not been seen in three years are technically new patients to the practice and may need to update their records.

6.2.5 Insurance Verification

Once you have the patient name and can start his or her chart, several other housekeeping items need to be taken care of. The most important task is to ask for insurance cards to verify that all of the information is current and correct. In today's landscape, even Medicare has started issuing new ID numbers, and it is important for downstream processes to have all of this up-to-date. While many patients will simply state "nothing has changed," it is important that your staff ask for the insurance cards, as many patients do not realize the changes that have taken place in their own plans.

6.2.6 Demographic Information

There are certain demographic questions that are part of the patient's chart which are helpful if collected up front. This includes email addresses, secondary phone numbers, and referring physician name. Asking patients who else they can share their information with is important (often a wife will call up re: a husband who has not given permission to share results, for example, and it is important to know this) as is permission to put the patient on any marketing or newsletter email lists from your office. It is up to you whether you want each patient to answer this as part of the check-in process or you plan to do it in the room.

6.2.7 Copay Collection

Some offices collect copayments up front and others after the patient has been attended to by the physician. There are advantages and disadvantages to both. If you collect a copayment up front, you ensure that the patient doesn't walk out of the office at check-out without paying it. If you do it afterwards, you can verify that the patient will actually owe a copay for the visit (for example, some visits that involve procedures like wart treatment with liquid nitrogen may not require a copay) and be spared refunding credits on accounts after they have gone out to insurance. If patients must stop to pay a copay, they also then are more likely to make a follow-up appointment instead of simply stating "I'll call."

6.2.8 Balance Collection and Deductibles

Once uncommon, high-deductible plans are now the norm in most practice settings. Unfortunately, this is also often a surprise for the patient. This is where transparency is key. Verification of benefits should be conducted prior to the patient entering the office and if not possible due to change of insurance, your check-in person should know how to do this on the fly through your medical software. Before being taken back into the exam room is also an opportune time to collect balances owed and store credit cards on file or collect a deposit for the visit if the deductible is high and has not been met.

Billing Office

Asking for money is not only part of an awkward conversation but also a sensitive one. One successful model for tackling this are offices in which a separate billing office is present. Each patient, after registering that they have arrived at the office, goes to the billing office. Over there, a knowledgeable staff member can collect any balance and explain to the patient your office policy regarding deductibles. This person can also print bills for patients who, more often than not, claim to never have received a statement. Because the conversation is out of earshot of the waiting area, it also maintains privacy and respect for the patient and the practice from judgments made by "listeners-on." There are other ways to handle this function but in all successful models the billing discussion is carried out in privacy and discreetly.

Tip

What do you do if a patient refuses to pay a balance? This can be tricky, especially for practices in the beginning. In our office, if a patient claims to have never received a statement, we gently remind them that their insurance company also sends them a statement of what they owe called an Explanation of Benefits ("EOB"). Of note is the fact that most insurers allow online access to these statements as well. In our experience, if a patient owes a debt over 90 days old, they are highly unlikely to make this payment (collection agencies will tell you the same) when they return home. We ask for a partial payment and ask them to leave a credit card on file which we will charge in 60 days if payment is not received. If the balance is greater than $100, debt is more than 90 days old, and patient is unwilling to pay their balance, we have a policy where we reschedule the patient. I didn't do this in my early years in practice, but I was burned by a ballooning accounts receivable at the end of 2 years.

6.3 Rooming

Congratulations! You have a patient on your screen who is ready to be attended to. This is where you, personally, have the most accountability. There are a number of questions to ask yourself in terms of office flow, which depends on the efficiency and skill set of your support staff as well as the type of patients you cater to.

6.3.1 Staff

There are a few models on how to move patients through the process efficiently as discussed below:
- **The "loader":** In this model, a medical assistant simply calls patients from the waiting room, escorts them into the room, and takes a brief chief complaint. He/she is adequately trained to know if the patient needs a gown and is also aware of how to direct the patient to be positioned prior to you entering the room (e.g., taking the shoe off if the issue is on the feet).

This loader can room multiple patients across several providers. The downside of this is that the loader must present the patient to you or your scribe/medical assistant/nurse, which is a process that can take time if you are waiting for them to get out of another room. At the same time however, it can also be cost-effective, since you can potentially have one loader and two scribes/medical assistant/nurse across two providers (3 staff total) instead of 4 staff.
- **The "scribe":** In this model, your scribe enters the room ahead of you or with you and either take the patient's HPI (including confirmation of allergies, medications, and social history), or you do so together. As you examine the patient and diagnose them. This person is entering everything you say into the EMR. The upside is that your note is completed by the time you walk out of the room. The downside is that this person requires a considerable amount of training and all notes must be carefully reviewed. If you have a scribe, it is important to build in a function where the only person who can finalize a note or sign off on scripts is you.

Tip

Hiring an aspiring medical school applicant or physician assistant program applicant is a good way to find that "super scribe" who is truly able to help you work more efficiently. The downside is that you put a lot of time and effort into training and these staff members often leave after one or two years. The advantage is that for the time they are with you, you have a reliable and talented student with whom you can not only develop a mentoring relationship but also practice efficiently with. And, depending on the student, he or she could potentially be someone who you can recruit back to the practice.

6.3.2 Types of Patients

When it comes to attending to patients in the room, there is a certain degree of unpredictability. You may have a skin check that is done quickly or an established rosacea follow-up who suddenly wants to talk about hair loss or a new patient who presents with bullous pemphigoid. Although this cannot be anticipated fully, it can be planned for in terms of office flow. If you think about the types of patients you attend to, it can help you "assign" rooms and space and also understand how long it will take for the patient to leave the room and free it up again once you have left it.

Depending on the type of practice you have, patients may not be attended to by the physician per se. In other words, there are several types of visits which, in our office, we categorize as "nursing visits" or quick visits. Ask yourself if you have an area that can be dedicated to this, where the nurse can run a schedule themselves and call you in for a brief discussion. These are best described as visits that can be delegated. For example, suture removal visits, placement of patch tests, and photodynamic therapy. These sessions are carried out in a small examination room in our office and we have a dedicated space equipped with all supplies for these visits specifically.

New Patients versus Established Patients

Clearly, there are some visits that require less time than others (e.g., wart management or actinic keratosis follow-up). Creating a scheduling template is important. It prevents blocks of new patients from being checked in at the same time which interrupts patient flow by starting charts for all the new people. Similarly, it is important to reserve slots for established patients who need regular follow-up but for whom the visit is relatively quick. Scheduling six total body skin examinations in a row may not only lead to burnout but also ties up the rooms, because these visits take much longer than regular follow-up.

Cosmetic Patients

There is a lot that goes into a cosmetic patient before physicians enter the room and after they leave the room. Typically, this requires more rooms and also a change to office flow from medical dermatology. For cosmetic patients, the check-in process is much more streamlined and less information is required. Where flow differs is in rooming. Do you want a cosmetic coordinator or nurse to go in before you to find out what the patient is interested in? Do you want to conduct the consultation first and then have a coordinator or nurse come in to discuss pricing, detailed procedure, and scheduling? Do you want each person to first

undergo a skin analysis that reviews what they are using in terms of products and then discuss the cosmeceuticals you have in the office? All of these add time to a visit that is not reflected in a schedule and may have to be modified on the fly. Do you have time built in to treat the patient with a neuromodulator or a filler if the patient decides they want to do it that day? Successful models tend to have a combination of touch points for the cosmetic patient. There is no "one right way" to do this and different physicians have different approaches. Some physicians conduct a consultation and then the patient goes to a separate room with a desk/chair consultation setup, where they can look at before and after photos with a cosmetic coordinator and schedule. A cosmetic questionnaire might be handed to each patient while in the waiting area and this can be reviewed by a skilled nurse or cosmetic assistant or by the physician, and once the cosmetic coordinator completes their portion of the visit, the patient is brought to another area where products can be tested and reviewed. By having these touchpoints, the patient avails of the opportunity to ask questions and attend a comprehensive session, while the examination room is open as is your time to attend to other patients. In an ideal setting, you have multiple assistants and all of this can be carried out in one room.

With cosmetic patients, there also exists a sensitivity regarding privacy. Whereas a Mohs patient may not mind being in a waiting room of similarly bandaged patients between stages, a cosmetic patient usually wants to have numbing applied and wait in privacy. Therefore, room turnover is much slower. Successful rooms schedule procedures that require numbing or long procedure time in a specific way, so as to best minimize patient wait time. In our office, we have a dedicated area just for cosmetics and procedures as the needs in those rooms differ from our medical dermatology practice. Our staff for cosmetic procedures is also different than the medical dermatology staff and are trained on all procedures and specifics that go into aftercare instructions, recommendations, and follow-up. Others, however, have cross trained nursing staff who are able to work in all facets of the practice.

Surgical/Mohs Patients

Surgical patients are usually apprehensive when they walk into the waiting area. They may have an understanding of their diagnosis or they may need refreshing on exactly why they are being attended to. It helps with office flow if you have someone assigned to call patients the week of their surgical visit to review basic medical history. For example, things like the presence of artificial valves or joints, use of blood thinners, and of course postoperative instructions regarding travel, heavy lifting, and exercise. You never want to be in a situation where you have a booked Mohs patient who tells you, as you are about to numb them, that they are leaving for their winter home the following day for a period of 3 months. If you are a Mohs micrographic surgeon, you may decide to leave patients in the rooms between stages (one patient, one room) or you may decide to have them wait in a common waiting area. In my experience, patients do not mind waiting in an area with similarly afflicted patients, as they often strike up a conversation with each other. We provide beverages and light snacks and often hear laughter and chatting from our waiting area between stages. We do not cross mix general dermatology and cosmetic patients in this waiting area during our Mohs times. Of course, if a patient is elderly or requires assistance, we provide them with the option of staying in the procedure room with their family.

Tip

If you decide to have Mohs patients wait in a common waiting area with their family members, suggest that they only bring one other family member at the preoperative call. Sometimes, people will come with numerous family members who are concerned that their parent or grandparent is undergoing a major surgical procedure. Similarly, if there is an elderly patient who is unable to have someone with them during their wait, keep the patient in a room where they can be monitored or within sight, so that your staff can make sure they are doing well.

6.4 Check-out

You have successfully navigated the check-in process and attended to the patient. Now all they have to do is leave, right? Check-out is a time that is often overlooked. You want to make sure

that your patients book follow-up appointments and have a process in place for completing any transactions.

6.4.1 Booking a Follow-up Appointment

It is always amazing to me how much information one can forget between leaving an examination room and going to the check-out area. For this reason, it is important that you control the flow of information. If you ask a patient at check-out, "When does the doctor want to see you again?" most of the time (50%) they will get it wrong even if it is the last thing you said as you walked out of the room. In an ideal world, your medical staff is able to book that appointment in the room with the patient and they can literally just walk out of the office. Alternatives to this include a headset system where follow-up information can be transmitted to the check-out desk from the medical assistant to the receptionist.

6.4.2 Separating Check-out

Depending on the number of patients you attend to per day, you may be able to have the same person perform check-in and check-out procedures. I do not recommend this however. The amount of information that must be collected from patients at each step has grown tremendously with time and one person cannot be expected to do both jobs all day without burnout. For this reason, check-out is a helpful station to have before the patient exits back into the waiting room. It should be easily visible and accessible to patients. If there is a backup of patients that results in the formation of a queue, ensure that, wherever it is located, this line does not extend in front of patient rooms where doors are opening and closing.

6.4.3 Collecting Copays

It is a contractual obligation between the physician and an insurer to collect copayments. Doing so at check-out is commonplace in many practices, although you must make sure your staff has a way of going about doing this before a patient simply walks out of the door. In my experience, collecting a copay up front is beneficial for the practice as prior balances can be collected at that time as well. If patients have a deductible and you collect at the time of visit, you may have no choice but to collect at check-out after the visit has been coded.

6.4.4 Cosmeceutical Transactions

If a patient is purchasing products, remember that this can be time consuming because invariably there are questions that arise at the time of purchase. One option is to have a runner get the products for the patient and collect payment in the room, or separately, and then leaves him or her for pick up at the check-out window where the patient can book a follow-up appointment. Alternatively, have more than one staff at check-out, so while one patent is checking out another can purchase products and check-out with another staff member.

6.4.5 Make Check-out a Mandatory Stopping Point

Not all patients realize they must check out. If your office flow in place prioritizes clearing the examination room for the next patient to come in, then completing everything while in the examination room may not be efficient. Similarly, it is often easier to train two people well on the nuances of your templates and booking procedures than it is to train your entire medical assistant staff on how to do this.

6.5 Conclusion

Office flow does not have to equate to herding cattle around in a circle. But how you accomplish these three aspects of a patient visit can certainly not only change the mood of the waiting room but also ensure that the majority of the patient's visit time is spent with you. Checking in and checking out are the required time elements that, for the purposes of practicing dermatology, seem mundane but for the purposes of the business of dermatology are essential, as they are the points at which transactions occur. My last tip is that while computers and electronic medical records can help, ensure that does not mean your office comes to a grinding halt if they go down (as often happens). Have paper copies of everything your EMR requires and a few premade packets that can be distributed on the fly while others are photocopied until your technology situation comes back online.

Ultimately, if you can predict the type of room needs your various patients have, honing in on how your office flows will allow you to maximize your time in the office and lead to a better work environment for everyone.

7 Creating a Practice Ambience

Annie Chiu MD

Abstract

In an ever-growing time of patient choice and aggressive digital marketing, running a successful practice extends far beyond physician expertise. The "look and feel" of your practice are tools that can help promote the comfort and well-being of patients and offer a "first impression." Patients not only want an organized, clean environment but also are looking for it to be personable to the individual practice. Making active choices in setting your practice ambience can create an atmosphere that is inviting and warm. When starting a practice, consider how to harmonize your practice demographics with elements of design that will appeal to patients across the office space. The goal is a well-thought-out reception and welcome area design, incorporation of digital tools, layout, storage, color, and branding that help convey what your practice represents while promoting a feeling of expertise, professionalism, and wellness. Ultimately, the goal is to have an efficient, organized office that still appears welcoming and conveys your specific practice personality to the patient.

Keywords: ambience, design, branding

Top 10 Things You Need to Know

1. Practice demographics.
2. Reception desk design.
3. Furniture choice.
4. Layout.
5. Lighting.
6. Colors and branding.
7. Internet access and technology.
8. Welcoming elements for the waiting area.
9. Creating an atmosphere with music and décor.
10. Entire patient wellness experience.

7.1 Introduction

Patients form an immediate impression of your medical practice as soon as they step through the door to your waiting area and reception. In fact, physician rating sites show most patient reviews will include commentary on clinic ambience as much as a physician's clinical skills. As dermatology is a visual medical field, and cosmetic procedures are often part of a practice, it is important to be cognizant of what you want to convey as a first impression through the setting of your practice.

Comfortable environments in dermatology practices that feel more like a home than a medical facility are becoming the new standard. This means that beauty and comfort are viewed as just as important to a patient's well-being as the physician interaction. Outdated magazines, worn out furniture, and a messy reception area immediately lead to a negative impact on patients'

perceptions of quality of care at a practice. Whether fair or not, patients often judge practices by standards they understand—your décor, the friendliness of your staff, and timeliness—instead of factors such as a physician's medical decision-making.

Hospitals and clinics often hire design firms that employ strategies of evidence-based health care design. In the book Evidence-based Health Care Design, the authors suggest patients' perception of your office ambience directly impacts not just their opinion of the office, but of their own health. Choices you make, ranging from what color schemes you choose to decorate to the layout of your furniture, or the type of lighting used in the waiting area, can impact your patients' and staffs' sense of well-being and mood.

Ultimately, thoughtfully considered practice ambience is a part of patient communication and an end-to-end experience for your patients. Direct and subliminal cues in your practice are communicated to patients: Is your practice up-to-date? Is your practice organized? Is this a calming or chaotic environment? Is this practice more focused on cosmetics or general dermatology?

7.2 Creating a Welcome Area

Most dermatology offices are set up opening into a waiting room with reception. Consider this the very first impression your patients will have of your practice. It should convey a welcoming and comfortable atmosphere and *not* an area to "wait" for your appointment.

7.2.1 Specifics to Consider

Reception Desk

Do weigh the benefits of an open reception versus one that has a distinct check-out area with a physical barrier.
Do design with plenty of storage to keep files and papers out of sight as much as possible.
Don't allow staff to keep food or drinks at the front desk.
Don't allow clutter or a crowded appearance at the reception desk.

Be deliberate in how you want your reception area to be arranged. Do you want an open atmosphere, which can make the practice feel more friendly and approachable, or do you want separate check-in and check-out areas with a physical barrier in between to offer patients more privacy in their transactions? Keep in mind a more open reception would require careful training of staff with respect to the Health Insurance Portability and Accountability Act (HIPAA) and how they communicate to patients. Think through a plan when more than one person is checking in and out to ensure privacy—do you have chairs they can sit in, or a clear delineation of where the next person can wait? Upon check-out, develop a system where specific patient care is not discussed beyond making follow-ups or completion of a financial fee collection. Ambient music or white noise is crucial to keep monetary transactions private in an open reception area.

As important as your décor is how you train the staff. Having a receptionist greet each patient that walks through the door with a smile and a welcome can set the tone for your practice as paying attention to patients as individuals and not a number. Be careful when using a sign-in system for your patients, as this, at times, creates staff that does not make eye contact with patients as they step into your practice, since former are more focused on who is next on the sign-in sheet.

It is crucial that the reception area is not cluttered, as this conveys a sense that the practice is disorganized. Clean, streamlined appearance of the reception desk with as few papers as possible conveys the feeling that the practice is organized, and the physician runs on time. Make sure all the computers and phones at the reception desk are of the same model and make. Consider the appearance of your technology as this can convey to the patient whether you are a dermatologist that is up-to-date. Do not allow front desk staff to have drinks and mugs strewn around these areas. Give your staff binders or notebooks for messages and notes to avoid post-its or scribbles on loose scrap paper.

Welcoming Waiting Room

Do consider your practice population when choosing furniture type and layout.
Do offer items like beverages, Wi-Fi, and easily accessible outlets for patient electronics to help ease waiting time.
Don't allow outdated magazines or an overflow of promotional brochures.
Don't supply drinks or food that are easily spilled or have strong smells.

Choosing the layout and the type of furniture in the waiting room should be a conscious decision and should be planned with the type of dermatology practice in mind. Consider how many practitioners will be working at the same time and how many patients are likely to be waiting at a given time. Do you have the type of practice where the patients are often accompanied by family members? Ensure there is adequate seating to accommodate. Everything about good practices in waiting rooms is for it *not* to feel like a wait. If patients feel like there is not adequate seating, you are already sending the message that there is a prolonged wait in store and the doctor is running behind.

Think about the layout of your seating. To convey more privacy and save space, some practices choose to have chairs in a line, some with their backs to each other. This type of atmosphere works well if you have a more family-oriented practice, as it allows for small groupings of chairs. If your practice is more geared toward cosmetic dermatology, be aware you are trading off a welcoming, warm feeling when you have this linear row of seating arrangements; in other words, it can feel very medical. If possible, arrange chairs like a living room with plenty of seating around the periphery, as this gives the atmosphere of a comfortable luxurious environment. Grouping the seating in clusters versus side by side chairs allows for more privacy.

Think about demographics of your practice when choosing furniture. If you have a high volume of pediatric patients, avoid any glass surfaces like a glass-topped coffee table but do add an area with lowered seating and writing/play surfaces. If your dermatology practice has a higher number of elderly patients with skin cancer, consider higher chairs with armrests, as they are easier to get in and out of. Modern low seating can be hard for elderly patients if this is your practice demographic. Woven furniture collect dust and are more difficult to clean. Look for waiting room seats that are nonwoven, nonvinyl, and easy to clean.

Your waiting room demonstrates to patients how you will treat them and how they should treat your office. Patients expect cleanliness and are likely to respect that more when they see it modeled—instruct staff to pick up dirty cups and other things patients leave behind. Avoid conspicuous trash cans as they look messy—consider not having a trash can in the waiting area, so your front desk staff can help dispose of any trash behind the reception area. Displaying of pharmaceutical brochures and products should be kept to a minimum in the waiting room because not only do they look cluttered but they can also derail the patient visit with unnecessary questions. Keep these types of promotional materials in the patient room where the provider can direct the patients' attention to the right items. Although magazines are commonly found in doctors' waiting rooms, they can look untidy. Nothing conveys an outdated office faster than a two-month-old magazine. Consider more high-tech alternatives like electronic readers as they look sleeker and are always timely.

Welcoming items such as a beverage stations, Wi-Fi, and lots of electrical outlets for laptops, phones, and other electronic devices are often greatly appreciated by all patients. Be mindful of the beverages you offer—will your office smell perpetually like coffee? Is it better to offer bottled drinks to decrease spillage or odor? When you lay out bottled water and healthy snacks, you can send a message of wellness to your patients.

Video Monitors in the Reception Area

When designing a practice space, make sure you have the option of installing a video monitor. However, whether you choose to put one in is highly dependent on what you are trying to achieve and who your patients are. Video monitors can be used for educational or marketing purposes for your practice. Definitely do not just tune into it like a TV show. Look at your clientele. Certainly, video monitors can reduce the boredom of waiting, but it can also add to noise and stimulation if you are trying to convey a relaxing, anxiety-reducing mood. Again, consider more mobile personalized devices such as ipads as an alternative to keep distractions at bay.

Practice Atmosphere

Do consider consistent branding and strategic, tasteful placement of your practice logo.

Do design your office to have natural light if possible.

Don't ignore the demographics of your practice when choosing design elements.

Don't assume patients only care about the physician interaction and that ambience is unimportant.

Patients expect an increasingly sophisticated experience when visiting a doctor's office. In the past, the physician–patient interaction was all that counted, but nowadays dermatology practices are under higher expectations to provide an entire patient experience, as it conveys patient-centered care. This is particularly important if you are considering growing the cosmetic aspects of your dermatology practice. The cosmetic patient considers their treatments to be a luxury and part of the service-oriented industry; accordingly, they expect a comfortable, higher end feel to the practice compared to their family medicine physician's office.

Consistent practice branding and choosing colors that match the branding can help bring cohesivity to the patient experience. Display your branding and logo in tasteful ways, such as with door signage, displays behind the reception, and logos on items like booklets and ice packs. Ideally, a consistent branding experience should extend from the décor of your office to your collateral as well as your website. When all these items are thoughtfully presented, patients will know that you care and are attentive to details.

Evidence-based health care designers place a lot of importance on natural light. Daylight not improves not only the mood of your patients but also your staff. When possible, having natural light in clinic office interiors provides a more calming, open atmosphere for the patient as it can elevate mood and reinforce circadian rhythms. Not every office is designed where this is possible either in the patient room or in the welcome area. In that case, choose LED lighting temperatures that best mimic natural light, and explore atmosphere immersive visual platforms that can bring views, water, and nature into your office.

Imagery you choose to decorate your office should be consistent with the feeling you want to convey to your patients. Colors or artwork can reflect regional sensibilities or the ambience of what you want to establish. Is it a Zen-like atmosphere? Or a more bustling, efficient, and friendly vibe? Music or water features can be consistent with the ambience you want to present, which aid in dampening ambient noise and allowing private patient conversations. Again, be intentional in choosing elements and finishes that contribute to your practice atmosphere. Ask yourself what is the most important feeling you want to convey to a patient when they walk through the doors of your practice. It should reflect the personality and specialty of your dermatology practice as much as the patient demographic you are cultivating.

Patient-Centered Experience

When you thoughtfully curate specific design elements into your dermatology practice, you will naturally be extending patient care not just limited to the examination room, but for the entire time the patient is in your office. With competition from medical spas and increasingly sophisticated patient expectations, creating an end-to-end patient experience, which combines the ambience of your practice along with expert care, can help give your practice a truly patient-centered holistic feel that sets your practice apart. Studies show patients' satisfaction with their care is influenced by a medical office's physical environment. There is no one design element or visit metric that conclusively defines a patients' office experience. Ultimately, it's a combination of the ambience you set for your practice along with the social factors of staff attentiveness and provider expertise that influence patient satisfaction. When considering your practice ambience, the most important thing is to put yourself in the patients' shoes and ask yourself what you would want to surround the practice space with. Be authentic to that vision and you will find out that not only have you created an ambience that promotes patient-centered experience but also your and your staff's well-being.

Suggested Readings

Becker F, Sweeney B, Parsons K. Ambulatory facility design and patients' perceptions of healthcare quality. HERD 2008;1(4):35–54

Cama R. Evidence Based Healthcare Design. John Wiley and Sons; 2009

Kondasni RK, Panda RK. Customer perceived service quality, satisfaction and loyalty in Indian private healthcare. Int J Health Care Qual Assur 2015;28(5):452–467

Narang R, Polsa P, Soneye A, Fuxiang W. Impact of hospital atmosphere on perceived health care outcome. Int J Health Care Qual Assur 2015;28(2):129–140

8 Photography and Space Requirements for Everyday and Clinical Trials

Neal Bhatia MD

Abstract

There is no greater visual medical specialty than dermatology; therefore, there are no more important elements essential to patient care than photography and understanding the requirements of physical space and components indispensable for photography in everyday practice and clinical trials. However, unlike the photos taken of babies, or the amateur shots taken during the family vacation, or even the daily selfie, photography in the dermatology practice requires a fundamental understanding of how to best represent the subject for use. The correct technique, setup, and application of photography are essential for the following reasons: before and after photos for assessing clinical response, clinicopathological correlation after biopsy or surgery, and proof of eligibility and clinical response in research, all of which only serve to scratch the surface. Attention to detail cannot be minimized when it comes to photography. For example, the correct room setup, lighting, privacy settings, equipment, cameras, and software are only part of the equation. The consent process, protection of identity to comply with Health Insurance Portability and Accountability Act (HIPAA) guidelines, and storage of the photos once taken are all pivotal components. This chapter will review the essential tools for successful applications of photography in the dermatology clinic, whether the images are used for medical, surgical, aesthetic, or research-based dermatology.

Keywords: image, pixel, exposure, compression, resolution, consent

Top 10 Things You Need to Know

1. For photography in dermatology, the correct room setup, lighting, privacy settings, equipment, cameras, and software are essential components for success.
2. Keeping in mind that capturing the image is necessary for the medical record, the entire office staff in addition to the clinicians need to be properly trained on the basics of clinical photography.
3. A comprehensive consent process should be in place for taking and storing a patient's medical photograph.
4. Privacy issues begin once the physician patient relationship starts and need to be emphasized once photography becomes part of documentation.
5. Since there is usually one chance to take a photograph at the patient's visit, or post operative condition, the importance of appropriate brightness, contrast, and the exposure settings have to be prepared.
6. Assign a designated room in the clinic that is free of windows, away from the daily clinic traffic, and without excessive lighting for taking clinical photographs.
7. A neutral background such as a black, blue, neutral grey soft fabric should be placed on a wall away from potential distractors.
8. Position patients in the Standard Anatomical Position to ensure that there is consistency in the way photos are evaluated.
9. Smartphones, DSLR cameras, and Complexion Analysis Systems are all being used in today's dermatology clinic as cameras.
10. Photo files should be converted to either a TIFF or a JPEG image which are easiest for storage and for transmission.

8.1 Introduction

The role of photography in the dermatology office setting cannot be taken lightly. There are pivotal steps in the entire process from start to finish that require attention to detail. No matter what the office lays emphasis on, whether the focus is on practice or clinical research, the process from patient consent to image storage has to be handled with precision. More importantly, the entire office staff, including the clinicians, need to be properly trained on not only the basics of operating a camera, but also capturing the image necessary for the translation of the patient experience into the medical record.[1]

The medical photograph not only requires permission to use but also precision to capture, store, and secure in order to maintain privacy and longevity. Clinicians must be trained on correct photography techniques as well as the art of storage of photos in the digital age. Unlike casual photos, the desired image should fill the field of the photograph and be free of distractions. One should consider the size of the lesion being photographed, position of the patient, background that is compatible with the color of skin, and its pathology. In addition, the importance of appropriate brightness, contrast, and the exposure settings of the camera cannot be underestimated, when there is usually only one chance to take a photograph during the patient's visit or postoperatively.[2]

8.2 The Consent Process

Just as a clinic or research site needs to develop a general consent for treatment, and how a HIPAA-compliant patient authorization of protected health information (PHI) must be completed, a similar consent form should be provided to a patient that includes his or her consent to take medical photographs. Although documentation of verbal consent for photography can be used, in most cases the consent process should be comprehensive in order to include any imaging procedure: still photography, videotaping, filming, or other means of recording and reproducing images that involve the patient.[3,4] This documentation should not only account for the HIPAA privacy rule but also the often overlooked HIPAA security rule, which includes security protection for any electronic patient protected health information including digital transmission of photographs.[4]

Any permission granted by the patient, guardian of a minor, or legal representative agreeing to allow the production of photographic images should be well documented, and a copy of the signed consent form should also be photographed at the time of the image capture to be considered complete.[3,4]

The destination and purpose of the photograph should be thoroughly disclosed to the patient. These are included for assessing treatment, publication, presentation, and health care operations purposes where the images might be utilized. Special considerations such as release of photos under subpoena, under criminal investigation, and transfer of care, must also be anticipated. In addition, there may be cultural norms among patients that may lead to hesitation on his or her part to being clicked by a stranger, despite the relationship established with the physician, and also the trepidation that the patient is still not at ease about where the photo is going and what it is being used for. These issues transcend simple consent and should be addressed with every patient as a matter of respect to any concern prior to taking any photos.[2]

In the era of smartphones, where patients and potential research subjects send photos to clinical staff by text, email, or patient portal, the privacy issues that begin once the physician–patient relationship starts need to be optimized for patient protection. These photos are usually of poor quality or poorly capture the necessary image for it to be of further use, but their existence should be accounted for and protected as part of the medical record.

8.3 The Office Setup

A photo studio should be an inspiration to the dermatology office when it comes to setting up the best environment for taking clinical photos. A designated room in the clinic that is free of windows, away from the daily clinic traffic, and without excessive lighting, should be chosen as the patient photography suite. Although it might be easier to take a quick photo of the patient while seated in an examination chair, the lighting and distractions of clothing create only a few of the potential pitfalls that might distract from the desired image. In addition, a room dedicated to photography should not appear intimidating or unwelcome, as the presence of a professional photography equipment might create unnecessary anxiety for the patient.[2]

In similar fashion to the studio, the clinical photography room must utilize various lighting options. There is often a question of when to incorporate flash (which is most of the time, as flash will allow reproducible color temperature balance), what type of flash, and how to avoid overexposure. Various lighting strategies are used for making sure the best photo is taken under any circumstance. For example, axial lighting is used most

55

frequently to provide illumination to most images. By aligning the flash unit adjacent to the barrel of the camera lens, shadows that might interfere can be minimized. Consequently, from the development of light reflections, there is improved definition of texture, color, and highlights of the image. Texture lighting creates a three-dimensional effect by increasing shadow sizes, which are useful in accentuating subtle elevations or depressions of an image. This can be accomplished by holding the flash unit 30 to 45 centimeters from the camera barrel, as adjustment of distance from the subject can alter shadows. Finally, flat lighting, often accomplished with a ring light, is used to demonstrate colors. By placing a flash unit on either side of the barrel of the lens, shadows can be eliminated, resulting in better color display.[5]

In addition to optimal lighting, use of a neutral background, typically with a soft fabric which is either black, blue, neutral grey, or of a similar color, should be available in accordance with how the patient is positioned for images, no matter which body part is being photographed.[4] Usually this background is placed on a wall away from other equipment or potential distractors, so that the patient is free to stand or sit for the image. The background should be far enough away from the subject, so that it is out of focus and offers color without texture which can be distracting. The background should be used to highlight the contrast of colors often seen in clinical images: red, brown, black, and white colors that represent cutaneous pathology, as well as normal skin, need to be accentuated by contrast from the background to best appear on the image. The key is replication: if there are sequential photos to be taken, whether for a before and after capture of a procedure, postbiopsy assessment, or the next visit in the clinical trial protocol, it is critical to have a standardized method for patient configuration in the photo, so that there is no misinterpretation or scrutiny of clinical results (▶ Box 8.1).

Box 8.1
Consistency
• Lighting
• Background
• Positioning
• Framing
• Elimination of distractions within the image
Courtesy: Ashish Bhatia, MD

8.4 Positioning the Patient and Framing the Photograph

To prevent any variations in capturing a sequence of images, positioning the patient in the standard anatomical position is the best way to ensure that there is no inconsistency in the way photos are processed. As a result, consistencies in rotation, distance to the patient from the camera, and adjustment for the image to be photographed can be made with relative ease.[6]

Successful positioning will involve optimizing exposure in order to maximize the image being placed in the camera field. In harmony with the neutral background, the patient should change either into a gown or disposable shorts to minimize the distractions from colors and patterns of clothing, especially if the photos are for a sequence, as the clothing worn will invariably not be consistent. The patient should not be tilted, rotated, or bent (except when the scalp is the desired image), which is something that can be minimized by centering the patient against the neutral background. Long hair should be tied to the rear, and all jewelry and excessive makeup should be removed.[4] If the photo requires an oblique or lateral view, the entire body should rotate not just the head, and the tip of the nose should be used as the most lateral focal point for any facial images to be photographed.[2,6]

The distance from the camera should also be uniform for each photograph to maintain consistency not only for the same patient but, especially for a research trial, all of the patients.[3,4] Photographs used for mole mapping or other clinical conditions might include a full head-to-toe photo, regional body area photos, and then specific lesion photos. Consequently, the lighting, distances, and background all require consistency. Many experienced photographers suggest that the focal point should be to first look at the pupils, using the mantra "eyes reflect the soul but pupils reflect the flash." In addition, the point flash enhances shadows while ring flashes wash them out (Personal Communication. Daniel M. Siegel).

For photos of individual lesions, a simple ruler free of any text should be approximated to the long axis to demonstrate the scale of the photo as well as provide a context for any clinical progression.[6] Adhesive sticker rulers have space for patient identification on them; rulers with color charts are also available. Images should be obtained with and without the said rulers in the field. A natural human tendency is to hold a ruler close enough but not in contact with the patient, so as not to contaminate the ruler; this results in either the ruler or patient going out of focus and forces the photographer to function in "selfie" mode with one hand, resulting in an often blurred image with or without flash.

Framing the image involves positioning to maximize the image in the photograph, but the orientation depends on alignment with either one edge (edge-oriented framing) such as forehead lines or eyebrows that allow a free edge to be variable in size or distance. This could be useful in comparing different patient outcomes for aesthetic procedures or research. By contrast, orient the center of the image, such as the tip of the nose, as a consistency marker for the purposes of comparison with other patient images. For face-on or side-view images, aligning the tip of the nose with the lower pole of the ear lobule enhances reproducibility.

8.5 The Camera: Compression, Focus, and Resolution

Historically, the dermatologist's camera of choice has been the simple point-and-shoot camera for the simple reasons of cost and ease of use.[4] The main disadvantage is that most settings are automatic, but for the novice photographer, the critical need to adjust settings may not be essential. By contrast, the digital single-lens reflex (DSLR) camera offers significant versatility and higher quality of images, which may be important in clinical research, presentations, or publications. The potential to use different lenses, flashes, and settings can offer the trained photographer higher standards of photography of images, but the costs involved and opportunities for use by the entire office staff may be limiting. The use of a DSLR camera with manual focus to a preset mark on the lens barrel will allow excellent reproducibility over time.

The newest techniques include systems referred to as "complexion analysis systems." Primarily used for research purpose, these systems are optimally used to generate photographs using various light sources, including ultraviolet and cross-polarized lighting. These systems are also used to analyze the photographs to quantify the character and integrity of cutaneous manifestations such as lentigines, comedones, and other similar defects.[8] The advantages of this approach compared to the usual photography methods include standardization of images in sequence, details and variable exposures, and accuracy of diagnostic probability from the details.[8]

The modern smartphone continues to evolve both software and hardware with limitless potential. Aside from the ease of use, familiarity of use by the entire office staff, and ease of transmission and storage of photos, there are many applications in use for combining dermatoscopes, UV filters, and other components that can simplify integration for clinical uses.[8,9,10]

8.6 Storage and Transmission

The responsibility of protection of stored or saved PHI is critical to the clinic's integrity. The photographs taken can easily be placed on any desktop, but it is the preservation of those photos, the identities they represent, and their potential use, that warrant attention. Images are captured initially as RAW files which are not standardized like TIFF, JPG, or BMP images. Most inexpensive cameras do not provide the option of capturing in RAW while all DSLRs do. In most cases, camera default settings capture images in the JPG format, with the larger image size settings (large and high resolution are common terms) offering more detail. The images should ideally be stored or converted to either a TIFF or a JPEG image, as these are usually the easiest to send via emails, portals, and texts. A TIFF image is usually the most ideal and the largest file, and can be edited without loss of information if saved as a TIFF after editing or cropping. However, every time JPEG images are either saved, edited, or compressed, they lose some quality of information. In addition, without a system for filing and cataloguing the files, difficulties will arise for the clinic personnel to utilize the images as the need arises. Consequently, files of images should be saved appropriately, as storage sizes may also become an issue.[4]

8.7 Conclusion

Clinical photography may seem intimidating or difficult at first, especially when the practice setting is not equipped or the staff is not familiar with simple procedures. However, with a basic review of the attention to detail of the images, avoidance of distractions in the photo, and correct protection of the patient's privacy, every dermatologist can incorporate taking photos in clinical practice. Even the phone in a pocket can now serve as a camera for the dermatology clinic. Finally, with proper storage and application of the photos, whether they are used for research, before-and-after clinical photos for clinical progress, identification of the biopsy site, or even for simple patient identification, every dermatologist can make photography a routine part of practice.

Acknowledgments

Besides immensely valuing their contributions and friendship, the author wishes to acknowledge the work carried out in this field by Dr. Ashish Bhatia, Dr. Adnan Nasir, and Dr. Daniel Siegel.

References

[1] Stack LB, Storrow AB, Morris MA, Patton DR. Handbook of Medical Photography, 1st ed. Philadelphia: Hanley & Belfus; 2001

[2] Bhattacharya S. Clinical photography and our responsibilities. Indian J Plast Surg 2014;47(3): 277–280

[3] AHIMA. Sample consent for clinical photography, videotaping, audiotaping, and other multimedia imaging of patients. J AHIMA 2010

[4] Blechman A, Mikailov A. Photography. In: Nasir A, ed. Clinical Dermatology Trials 101. Cham: Springer; 2015:195–212

[5] Principles of Medical Photography. Available at: http://www.lbstack.com/photography/Principles%20of%20Medical%20Photography%20-%20 Handout.doc. Accessed October 31, 2019

[6] de Meijer PP, Karlsson J, LaPrade RF, Verhaar JA, Wijdicks CA. A guideline to medical photography: a perspective on digital photography in an orthopaedic setting. Knee Surg Sports Traumatol Arthrosc 2012;20(12):2606–2611

[7] Goldsberry A, Hanke CW, Hanke KE. VISIA system: a possible tool in the cosmetic practice. J Drugs Dermatol 2014;13(11):1312–1314

[8] Wang X, Shu X, Li Z, et al. Comparison of two kinds of skin imaging analysis software: VISIA from Canfield and IPP from Media Cybernetics. Skin Res Technol 2018;24(3):379–385

[9] VISIA Complexion Analysis System: Frequently Asked Questions. Canfield Imaging Systems, Fairfield, NJ. www.canfield.com

9 Corporate Structure: Limited Liability and Taxation

James D. Kelso JD, LLM (Health)

Abstract

This chapter provides background on corporations and provides information on different types of business entities or business organizations. It will address what considerations are important when physicians are deciding what business structure to utilize when opening a practice.

Keywords: corporate structure, business entities, proprietorship, dermatologist

Top 10 Things You Need to Know

1. There are several types of business entities.
2. Each business entity will have different liability protections.
3. Limited liability is important to protect a physician's personal wealth.
4. Each business entity will have different tax implications.
5. When selecting a business entity, you will need to discuss the ramifications of federal, state, and local taxes.
6. Liability and taxation issues differ from state to state.
7. Corporations may be prohibited from operating a medical practice in your state due to the prohibition on the corporate practice of medicine.
8. It will be important to understand if your state requires physicians to use a certain business entity that is limited to professional medical services.
9. If a physician selects the wrong entity, the business might violate the prohibition on the corporate practice of medicine.
10. If you are not absolutely sure, consult an expert on corporate structure. It's easier to do things right the first time than to correct errors once they're made.

9.1 What Does Corporate Structure Mean?

Businesses are run through business entities or business organizations. The terms "corporate structure" and "business entity" are interchangeable. Due to the fact that some people get confused between "corporate structure" and a corporation, business entity will be used. (For clarity, a corporation is just one type of business entity.) There are several different types of business entities that can be used to operate or run a business. Many states regulate what type of business entity can be utilized for certain types of business activities. As an example, Professional Limited Liability Companies (PLLC) and Professional Associations (PA) are the only business entities that can be used to run a small physician owned medical practice in Texas.

An important aspect to consider while establishing a business is that the business is considered a "person" under the law and has rights just like people. You may have heard about the *Citizen United*[1] case. This case lead to one of the most influential United States Supreme Court decisions. This case was significant because the Supreme Court ruled that a business could contribute to federal election campaigns just like an individual person because businesses also have the right to exercise their freedom of speech. To further the point, a business possesses its own assets and liabilities separate and independent from the business owners. A business can operate or transact business when the owners are not present and when the owners are not involved in day-to-day activities.

To operate and function, a business must have assets greater than its liabilities. Business assets might be real property like income (generated from the practice of medicine by its employee physicians), computers, chairs, and lasers. It can also have assets that are less tangible like intellectual property rights or other intrinsic value based on recognition of the business as a leader in the field, which is sometimes referred to as goodwill. If a business is sold, its assets are evaluated and the sales price is determined based on the business' assets less the business's liabilities.

The business can also accumulate liabilities and be forced by a court to pay them. These liabilities could include billing fraud, sexual harassment claims, uncollected bills from patients who did not pay the medical practice, malpractice claims, taxes (federal or state) or loans, or lines of credit that must be repaid to a bank or other lender. As stated above, these liabilities offset the sales price and directly impact the value of a business.

Business entities can either be simple business structures or very complicated business structures. The different types of business entities are: a Sole Proprietorship, Partnership (either a General Partnership or Limited Liability Partnership [LLP]), Hybrid Entity (Limited Liability Company, Professional Limited Liability Company, Professional Association, or Professional Corporation), or a Corporation.

The difference between different types of business entities revolves around two issues, that is, limited liability and taxation. A business entity may retain more or less liability with corporations having the most limited liability. To begin with, if an individual is transacting business without a business entity, that individual retains all liabilities. However, if the individual is an owner of a corporation, the individual's liability is limited to the individual's investment and the corporation retains all liability. If an individual has criminal liability, the individual goes to jail. If the individual has civil (or financial) liability, the individual must pay the liability unless the individual elects bankruptcy. If the corporation has criminal liability, it is subject to criminal fines and penalties. The passive owners will not be criminally liable. If the corporation has civil liability, the corporation is liable and individual passive owners are not liable. If the owners are active individual owners and not just passive individual owners, the individual's actions can be separately analyzed, and the active individual owners may be liable both criminally and civilly. The gage on whether the business has a lot of limited liability or a little limited liability is based generally on the tax status of the type of business entity selected.

Limited liability (or limited personal liability) is the legal protection limiting each shareholder to the par value of the fully paid up company shares a shareholder owns to cover the financial liability of the company's debts and obligations.[2] So, if a corporation makes a dermatology drug that *causes* cancer instead of *treating* cancer, the individual

shareholder of the company who owns $100,000 worth shares of stock (this would be the par value of fully paid up stock) cannot be held individually liable for the drug that caused cancer. If the company has assets of $50 million and those assets are liquidated to pay its debts, but the company has lawsuit liability of $500 million, there is $450 million in liabilities still outstanding. The individual shareholder's shares of the stock will be worthless and the individual shareholder would have lost his or her investment. However, the shareholder cannot be sued and found personally liable for the actions of the business. This means the shareholder cannot be sued and forced to pay for the remaining $450 million in liabilities.

In order to be granted limited liability, a corporation will be exposed to double taxation. Double taxation is the taxation principle referring to income taxes paid twice on the same source of earned income.[3] Corporations pay income tax on the corporate profits annually. They file income taxes returns yearly just like individuals. The shareholders of the corporation will pay taxes again on the same earned income when the shareholders receive dividend payments. Dividend payments are payments made to the shareholders of a corporation when there is a large surplus of cash from profits and the managers and/or members of the corporation vote to pay a dividend payment to the shareholders.

Some business entities do not provide their owners with limited liability. Generally, these business entities have single taxation. An example of a simple business entity that has no limited liability and is subject to single taxation is the Sole Proprietorship. In the example above of the drug that caused cancer, if the business was a Sole Proprietorship, the individual owner would have to pay the balance of the $450 million in liabilities because this business entity does not grant limited liability. This is why there are not many physician practices operating as a Sole Proprietorship. Likewise, General Partnerships have single taxation and do not benefit from limited liability either. In general, it is worth paying a little extra to an attorney to elect the correct business entity because limited liability is very important. Limited liability is similar to an insurance policy, because if business harms a person, the owners are protected and cannot be sued personally for the actions of the business.

9.2 Selecting a Corporate Structure

When establishing a business entity, it is important to consider of limited liability and taxation. Taxation is a very important aspect of the selection of the business entity, because it can directly impact whether a business entity will be viable. Some businesses operate on very thin profit margins and double taxation can destroy the profits.

In ▶ Fig. 9.1, there are two types of business entities in the middle. These are Partnerships and Hybrid Entities. A General Partnership has single taxation and no limited liability for its owners. If one partner is a physician and that partner causes an injury through malpractice, all of the other partners may be required to pay the injured patient. In a General Partnership, partners are liable for the errors and omissions of the other partners. Since physicians are paid based on the amount they collect, this can significantly hurt the other partners because all the partner profits can be taken to offset the liability and, if that is not sufficient, the injured party can go after each partner individually for the balance. As a result, there are not very many General Partnerships that are used to operate a medical practice.

To address this the partnership laws were expanded to allow for Limited Liability Partnerships (LLPs), which protect the partners from some but not all liabilities, while still preserving single taxation. In general, LLPs provide limited liability for the errors and omissions of the other partners. So, the example of partners having to pay for another's malpractice does not occur in this type of business entity. This business entity is utilized by medical practices. There is also a business entity known as a Limited Liability Limited Partnership (LLLP) that provides an even narrower scope of limited liability, but these have never been a good fit for medical practices.

From the other direction, the corporation laws were amended to allow for hybrid entities that benefit from limited liability and have single taxation. The most common hybrid entity is known as an LLC, which stands for "Limited Liability Company." While LLCs and the other hybrid entities have limited liability, the owners must elect single taxation status through an internal revenue service election known as the Subchapter S election or "S Corp election." (Please note: Business entities must be filed and established through the state where the entity conducts business.) The S Corp election is a federal income tax election. There is no "S Corp" as a stand-alone business entity to be filed at the federal or state level. Many physicians ask to set up an S Corp and there is no such entity because it is a federal income tax election. The S Corp election is named after the chapter in the IRS code that has several significant requirements that must be met in order to allow a business entity to have single taxation.[a] In some instances, as an LLC grows, it may no longer qualify for the S Corp election and the business entity can lose the S Corp election.

The other hybrid entities exist to allow professionals to create business entities that are limited to the professional services of the owners. These entities enjoy single taxation through the S Corp election and limited liability. These entities require all the owners to hold the same or similar licenses. The hybrid entities are as follows: professional limited liability companies (PLLC), professional corporations (PC), professional associations (PA), and service corporations (SC). (As there are 50 states that regulate business entities within their respective states, there may be some other options that are not listed.) Since state law regulates these entities, the requirements differ from state to state but, in general, these entities are reserved for physicians, attorneys, engineers, architects, and other licensed professionals.

If a physician is opening a practice, the business entity that provides the most benefits are entities that provide for limited liability and single taxation. The vast majority of business entities selected for a new medical practice would include PLLC, PA, PC, or SC. Since state income taxes will also impact the business entity selection, it will be of paramount importance to work with an accountant in the physician's state to address the impact of state taxes. State taxes can impact the final selection of a business entity. Lastly, some physicians will select to operate as Sole Proprietorships when the medical practice does not operate a clinic and does not have any employees, except the individual physician-owner. This is because there are few liabilities, single taxation provides a higher benefit, and different states can impose increased yearly costs

---

[a] 26 U.S. Code § 1361. S corporation.

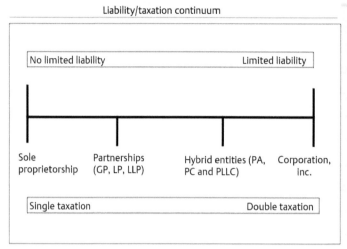

Liability/taxation continuum

No limited liability — Limited liability

Sole proprietorship | Partnerships (GP, LP, LLP) | Hybrid entities (PA, PC and PLLC) | Corporation, inc.

Single taxation — Double taxation

Fig. 9.1 Limited liability versus double taxation.

for operating a business entity. Before operating as a Sole Proprietorship, it would be extremely prudent to research this option and fully appreciate all the potential ramifications.

9.3 Corporations and Medicine: The Prohibition of Corporate Practice of Medicine

For many years, corporations were prohibited from owning and operating a medical practice in most states. Under this prohibition, only business entities owned by licensed physicians could operate a medical practice. The rationale for this public policy decision was to insulate physicians from corporate managers/owners, who may be more focused on cash productivity and profits than patient care. This prohibition was to prevent a corporate manager from asserting undue influence over a physician's treatment choice. The reasoning was physicians who own their own business would be more likely to use their professional judgment and less likely to pick a profit-based solution that did not help the patient. There were processes in place to regulate physicians who did not exercise sound professional judgment. These physicians were regulated through the state medical licensing laws via adverse licensing actions by boards of medicine and also regulated through malpractice lawsuits. This idea of deferring to physicians is noble and more viable when reimbursements are adequate. However, when reimbursements are low, this noble, self-regulating idea may be less supportable.

The prohibition against the corporate practice of medicine began to slowly erode in the 1990s when hospital systems began to push regulators to allow hospital systems to purchase medical practices in order to protect their primary care referral networks. State laws began to change to allow hospital systems to directly employ physicians. As an example, in Texas, a law was passed that granted hospitals the ability to own medical practices. This law was the 501(a) Non-Profit Health Care Organization[b] and soon after many states enacted similar laws. As hospital profits soared, by the mid-2000s, entities supported by private equity[c] began to become interested in medical practices with high-cash flow and low-management requirements. Hospital-based physician practices were targeted and were purchased by the private equity-based entities. The private equity-based entities really do not and often cannot comply with many of the laws that prohibit the corporate practice of medicine, but they have proliferated anyway with the use of "friendly" PAs or PLLCs. These are PAs or PLLCs that are controlled by licensed physician owners who are "friendly" to the private equity entity. If there is an exception like the Texas state law mentioned above, it is difficult for private equity

[b] In recent years, the name "501(a)" has changed to match a re-codification of state law.
[c] Private equity is a general term that is used to describe the funding source of investments, where the funds come from private investment sources as opposed to more public funding sources like publically traded companies (or other regulated securities like mutual funds) that must report ownership or other funding sources.

entities to meet all of the permissible legal exceptions. Further, the Affordable Care Act supported the erosion of the prohibition against the corporate practice of medicine to make Accountable Care Organizations (ACOs) possible. For complex and political reasons, state boards of medicine are not enforcing provisions that already exist to prevent the corporate practice of medicine and are not stopping the further erosion of the prohibition.

As a side note, hospitals are owned by corporations, but the hospitals owned by the corporations must go through rigorous state law applications to obtain the hospital license before the hospital can operate. They are also regulated by numerous federal and state agencies and, many, if not all, follow the Joint Commission standards and requirements. The intense regulatory oversight is designed to protect the patient. The private equity owned or controlled medical practices do not always have the same level of oversight. In the old days, the physician owner lost their license and the business died if the medical practice was operated contrary to public policy. Today, this regulatory scheme does not fit to protect the patient from corporate managers controlling medical practices like those that are seen in a corporate owned hospital. With the rise of procedural based services in outpatient setting, patient safety may be more at risk. However, this risk is unknown.

9.4 Conclusion

For a physician opening a practice it will be important to consider which business entity will provide the most limited liability and be subject to the least amount of taxation. Since these issues are regulated by individual states, the determination of the best business entity will be based on whether the state prohibits the corporate practice of medicine, whether the state limits medical practices to operate certain types of business entities, and the impact of federal, state, and local taxation.

References

[1] Citizens United v. Federal Election Commission, 558 U.S. 310 (2010)
[2] The Law Dictionary. Available at: https://thelaw-dictionary.org/limited-liability/. Accessed October 10, 2019
[3] Investopedia. Available at: https://www.investopedia.com/terms/d/double_t. Accessed October 10, 2019

10 Academic versus Private Practice

Nazanin Saedi MD, Kenneth A. Arndt MD

Abstract

At the end of a multi-year, multi-decade education and training marathon, and having finished the travails of residency or fellowship, it is time to consider how to carry out the rest of your career. Would it be best to stay in or pursue a position in an academic dermatology setting, or consider starting or entering a private practice? There are so many options within each choice, and positive and negative considerations about a potential life in either arena. Both authors have spent parts of their careers in both settings and can comment on the benefits and disadvantages of these career choices.

Keywords: academic medicine, private practice, research, private equity

Top 10 Things You Need to Know

1. Take time to figure out your life goals and career goals.
2. For academics, find out your academic obligations in detail.
3. How many administrative responsibilities will you have to take on in an academic position and how will that impact your teaching and clinical practice?
4. In academics, is the scope of your practice limited by others who are subspecialized?
5. Evaluate the main office versus satellite office options carefully.
6. Conduct research on a practice diligently prior to joining (local reputation, patients, and other colleagues).
7. If starting a solo practice, think carefully about the responsibilities that come with that level of autonomy.
8. Evaluate the available opportunities for becoming partner.
9. Explore options in relation to volunteer faculty positions if you are in a private practice but possess academic interests.
10. There are many different opportunities within dermatology and if one does not work out, there is always the chance to try a different option.

10.1 Academic

We have all become accustomed to the academic setting and sometimes it is the familiarity that makes it appealing. As a member of a hospital and/or medical school dermatology department, there are constant educational, administrative responsibilities, which come with the position. These can include weekly or frequent clinical conferences, Grand Rounds presentations, access to and consultation on inpatient dermatologic patients, easy access to consultation with other medical specialties, interaction with dermatopathologists, access and possible involvement in ongoing research studies, and access and interaction with clinical and research faculty in your department and medical school. The support received from others in your department and within the institution can be comforting, especially early in your career. If your principal interest is that of laboratory research, then a career in academic institution is a great option for career advancement. Alternatively, if your interest is in clinical care and teaching, perhaps with some clinical research, these can take place in an institutional practice setting.

The settings within an academic department can vary as well, as there are hospital-based departments, group practices, and also satellite offices. The different settings can impact your practice. Some university departments house dermatology offices that are part the hospitals. When this is the case, they have to follow rigorous and sometimes restrictive hospital regulations, which are more practical in an operating room setting than an outpatient dermatology practice. The physicians' groups can be located in the hospital campus or university campus, and they can include other departments as well. These groups need to abide by the strict university rules and regulations in place, which will likely impact almost everything that you do. Getting new procedures and devices approved will not only require approval from the department, but also sometimes the institution. The satellite offices are also subject to the university rules, but seem to be more flexible since they are off-site. If your position is primarily in the satellite office, you might not have residents and might be subject to limited teaching opportunities. In addition, if you are not at the main site, you may not be as visible in the department. On the other hand, the satellite offices are often smaller, can be easier to manage, may run more smoothly, and present opportunities for efficient management.

There are some downsides in working in institutional settings that need to be considered. Your ability to make independent clinical or research decisions and bring them to fruition may be frustrating, since having ideas approved is often part of a complex process. As a member of an academic department, you may first report to someone senior within your department who will then report to the departmental chairman. Most new programs and ideas need to go climb a bureaucratic ladder of approval including hospital administrators, physician organization staff and administrations, and at times senior hospital or medical school officers. There is often a lack of autonomy and inability to bring about rapid or any change in many areas. It can also be difficult sometimes to obtain clarity about fiscal matters, since these are taken care of or administered by departmental, hospital, or physician organization groups, which are very large in magnitude and in which dermatology plays a relatively small role. In addition, many academic positions have shifted from fixed salaries to an incentivized compensation model with RVU (relative value unit) targets. Although there lies the potential to gain a higher income, administrators place more pressure on the physicians to attend to more patients, which might detract one from teaching.

In addition to the time required for an active clinical presence, the necessity to attend multiple administrative, hospital, departmental, and medical school meetings may leave little or no time for other activities. Institutional concerns about compliance with federal and managed care requirements, the necessary detailed documentation of records, and the responsibilities of the physician in an academic medical center may dilute the time, enthusiasm, and effort available for teaching, scholarly productivity, and patient care activity. Another consideration is staffing because, in an institutional setting, your staff is often selected through the hospital human resource office. It is not always possible to select the best possible candidate, or let them go if their qualities are not optimal. It can be time consuming and challenging to bring on additional staff members because each position has to be reviewed and approved by the institution.

Although there are many potential drawbacks, life as a practicing dermatologist within an academic medical center can be very stimulating. It is fun and rewarding to have frequent interaction with clinicians within your department and medical school. Clinical and research problems may come up and you may become involved in these studies or projects. With time, it is possible to advance within medical school in the clinician–teacher or clinical research tracks. As you progress, there is also the chance to bag a leadership position within the department and the medical school. There also lies the opportunity to play a mentor to younger trainees and guide their careers. Overall, life in the academic medical center can be very satisfying and rewarding.

10.2 Private Practice: Solo, Dermatology Group, Medical/Surgical Group

As you think about a career in private/group practice, there exist other considerations. Most often, it is appealing to join an established practice, which may consist of several colleagues or be a larger dermatologic group. Dermatologists practice more in the form of a group, whether a dermatology group or multispecialty group, compared to a solo practice in both urban and suburban settings.[1] In rural settings, it is still common to be in a solo practice. It is obviously essential that the type of practice, and personality and quality of the physicians, you will be joining be carefully assessed. Establishing your own independent practice is more fiscally and administratively complex compared to a stable job in a full-time system or joining an active clinical practice.

10.2.1 Solo Practice

After training, you may decide that you wish to establish a solo practice in which you will not only be the solo physician but also own your own practice. You do not necessarily have to be the sole provider and may wish to have physician extenders in your offer, who can enhance the services that are provided. When you are on vacation or cannot make it to work, what will be done about the office? You will be running a business and, therefore, you need to consider the costs of overhead and figure out how to maximize your resources. These responsibilities require quite different skills than those necessary to be an excellent physician. You will possess autonomy, but also have many more tasks to attend to.

In this setting, it is possible to choose your staff and more easily mold a personal, friendly, and smooth working environment in your own image. You can establish expectations for clinical care, administrative oversight, billing efficiency, communication with patients and physicians, and all other practice-related necessities to set the tone for the practice. It is possible to carry out clinical research in a practice environment and many practices do this. In such cases, active interaction with dermatologic or aesthetic industry is necessary. It is possible to build a clinical and clinical research practice of the highest quality.

10.2.2 Dermatology and Multispecialty Group

By joining a dermatology group, you enhance the dermatology services that are offered by the group. You might join a group which provides only general dermatology or one that offers all aspects of dermatology. After hours call, vacations, staff, and overhead will all be distributed among the members in the group. Each group has a different model and compensation plan, so you should research similar practices in the area.

Joining a practice with different subspecialties will offer a great referral source. You might be the only dermatologist, and if so, there could be initial work to start the dermatology aspect of the practice. Often times, other dermatologists are already a party of the group practice. It is essential that you look carefully not only at the structure and function of the multidisciplinary group but also of the dermatologists in the group. The multiple specialties will provide a patient base to start building or course your own patient population. It can also provide collaborative efforts between the disciplines, but there might be problems with procedures that can overlap. These details need to be carefully examined before starting.

10.2.3 Private Equity-Owned Practices

With the rise of private equity-based private practice groups, one should be aware of the benefits but also the limitations. Recently, there has become an increasing interest among private equity groups to purchase dermatology practices across the country.[2] All of the discussion of the possible benefits in terms of independent action, ability to make decisions and act on them, and autonomy are based on the assumption that the practice is independently owned. If a practice or part of a group of practices owned by a private equity or venture capital entity, then almost none of the advantages of a private practice would be present, as the ownership of the practice will always be at least 51% and usually more, and then they could arbitrarily hire/fire all staff, manage productivity, decide what to purchase or not, etc. In such cases, the constraints of the private equity-owned practice become quite similar to the situation of someone in an institutional/hospital setting. Employment in such practices can seem attractive, with higher base salaries; also, late in one's career, it can seem appealing with less responsibility in managing a practice. However, in either scenario, the loss of autonomy needs to be considered.

Ultimately, you have to be comfortable and find the best fit for your personality and career goals. As a resident, one often feels pressure to pursue a career in academics, and often it might also be perceived as a letdown going into private practice; however, this is not the case. You should pursue what fits your personality and not be pressured by external factors. Also, there are so many hybrid opportunities in dermatology that can be created. We are in a growing field with an ever-growing demand. There are many different opportunities within dermatology and if one does not work out in the beginning, there is always the chance to try a different option.

There are options in which you could have a combination of a private practice position and an academic appointment. You can work at a private practice four days a week and then earmark one day for the purpose of administration. At many universities, you can be volunteer faculty for half a day to supervise a resident clinic or a clinic at the VA. This is an excellent opportunity to teach, attain exposure at training programs, and be affiliated to a university. There is the option to engage in this on a weekly or even monthly basis.

References

[1] Ehrlich A, Kostecki J, Olkaba H. Trends in dermatology practices and the implications for the workforce. J Am Acad Dermatol 2017;77| (4):746–752

[2] Konda S, Francis J, Motaparthi K, et al. Future considerations for clinical dermatology in the setting of 21st century American policy reform: corporatization and the rise of private equity in dermatology. J Am Acad Dermatol Published: 2018;pii:S0190–9622(18)32667–7doi:10.1016/j.jaad.2018.09.052

11 Managing the Telecom and IT of Your Business: The Central Nervous System of a Medical Practice

Daniel I. Wasserman MD, David A. Rubin BBA, MPA

Abstract

A practice's telecommunication demands require careful thought toward preparing a business to run efficiently and smoothly in the digital age. It is imperative that preparation starts at a business's inception. The rate-limiting step for anyone's medical practice is establishing a physical address. Not only do the standard administrative obligations require a commercial address, but the electronic operations of the business will require it as well. IT consultants can help design, implement, and manage the technology solutions. At a business's developmental stage, reserving a corporate domain name, email, telephone, and fax numbers are vital. Build-out phases need workable space that flow for their business needs. Communication takes place between all involved parties including the design and construction individuals as well as those managing IT/telecom demands will be crucial to facilitate and manage. Contracts involving service providers, partners, and vendors will need to be reviewed and established. Hardware and its security will need to be carefully purchased and managed. The active participation of the business owner will ebb and flow, but a deeper understanding of the IT process for one's business start-up is expected. This chapter will provide more than a superficial understanding of the IT infrastructure so that owners and managers can make more educated, efficient, and safe decisions.

Keywords: business associate agreement, telecommunications, Internet, domain, voice over Internet protocol (VoIP)

Top 10 Things You Need to Know

Please note the following about establishing your practice's telecom needs:
1. Consider hiring an IT consultant.
2. Establish a physical commercial address for your business.
3. Reserve a web domain name.
4. Establish a corporate email account.
5. Reserve a vanity phone and fax number.
6. Coordinate all communication between build-out partners and your IT consultant during the initial planning stage.
7. Establish service contracts with vendors.
8. Enforce Business Associate Agreements (BAA).
9. Coordinate software specifications and demands with hardware purchasing.
10. Establish a cyber-security system and plan.

11.1 Introduction

Opening a practice requires careful thought toward preparing your business to run efficiently and smoothly in the digital age. It is easy for a physician to be consumed with thoughts about marketing, waiting room design, equipment, decorations, website design, and social media goals for the overall patient experience. After all, medical practices are, to a large degree, part of the service industry business. The less attractive demands, but far greater in importance, are the software and hardware that provide a critical pulse to the daily flow of a business. It is imperative that the preparation starts early if not at a business's inception. The following is meant to provide a chronological *and* conceptual roadmap for the design of a practice's telecommunications requirements: While there is an order to properly establish this component to your business, many of these steps can be carried out in parallel and not necessarily in sequence.

Table 11.1 Recommended timeline for telecom and IT business operations preparedness

Business inception point:
- Strongly consider engaging the services of an IT/telecom consultant.
- Physical address (at business's inception point).
- Reserve vanity business phone and fax numbers.
- Reserve a web domain name.
- Establish corporate email accounts.

At start of buildout:
- Introduce the telecom/IT consultant to the construction team.
- Determine the following:
  - Low voltage cabling.
  - Access points.
  - Hardware locations.
  - A/V needs.
  - Security and alarm requirements.

Throughout the process:
- Establish service contracts (90–120 days prior to operation).
  - Internet.
  - Phone.
  - Merchant processing.
  - Cable.
  - IT.
- Establish software contracts (i.e., EMR, practice management systems, etc.) (45 days prior to operation).
- Purchase hardware (30 days prior to operation).

The content in this chapter is meant as a guide to better familiarize oneself with the process required to prepare your business for daily operations with or without an IT consultant. For a summary timeline of the content in this chapter, please see ▶ Table 11.1.

11.2 Hire an IT Consultant

It is highly recommended that a business owner work with an IT consultant who will help design, implement, and manage the technology solutions. These consultants have established relationships with the premier brands in the technology industry, thereby allowing them to streamline the process, so that you can concentrate on your own professional strengths. If one does engage an IT consultant, then the discussion below should provide an excellent background to help you understand the process to prepare your business for its daily operations. There are IT consultants who provide guidance throughout this process and there are agencies equipped with IT consultants,

which handle all daily technology operational service demands, called managed service providers (MSPs). We recommend that a business hire a MSP. The MSP will provide 24 × 7 × 365 IT support for a fixed monthly price based on the number of devices managed. Given that > 95% of all technology issues can be resolved remotely, the location of the MSP is not important. Whether you hire an IT consultant or MSP, please make sure that you have a current Health Insurance Portability and Accountability Act (HIPAA) Business Associate Agreement (BAA) in place to maintain Protected Health Information (PHI) security and overall HIPAA compliance. There are great MSPs located on the East Coast of the United States that service large medical practices with locations all over the country. If a circumstance arises whereby a technician is needed to be dispatched to resolve a local issue, such a service should be included in the fixed monthly fee regardless of the MSP's physical location. Again, it is important to have a relationship with a trusted IT advisor, that they know your network, and are willing to assist at any moment.

11.3 Reserve a Domain Name and Corporate Email Account

Reserving a corporate domain name and email is just as important as the telephone and fax numbers. Those same applications required to launch a business will now ask for email contact information, and email is the basis for all professional communication. As employees are added, it is expected that they have corporate email accounts for their administrative communication with you and your vendors. The easiest way to reserve a domain name is through GoDaddy. You can visit their website at www.godaddy.com and search to see which domain names are available. Domain names ending in ".com" are preferred, but it is recommended that one should also purchase the ".net," ".org," and ".co" versions of the same domain name to prevent others from buying them. You will host the domain names through GoDaddy and it is industry standard to activate your corporate email through Microsoft 365. These two companies work very well together, providing a seamless transition. The business premium license through Microsoft 365 provides an email address, Office applications on up to 5 devices (Outlook, Excel, Word, PowerPoint, OneNote, Access, Teams, SharePoint, and Publisher), file storage via OneDrive, and a full desktop version of your Outlook via webmail. If an employee is going to be emailing PHI, please make sure to upgrade the MS365 license to include Office 365 message encryption (OME). This feature will encrypt the PHI in transit and at rest (see also Chapter 45).

11.4 Establish a Physical Service Address

The rate-limiting step for anyone's medical practice is establishing an address. Without a physical service address, one cannot file for business licenses, insurance credentialing, and the plethora of regulatory requirements for operating any business, let alone a highly regulated medical practice. The same goes for preparing one's business to operate electronically. The physical business address will determine coverage for local telecom, cable, and Internet providers. Prior to signing and executing a lease, it might be a good idea to find out the type of high-speed Internet that is available at the actual location. Failure to do so might end up costing you more money in the long run. If the location in question does not qualify for cost-effective high-speed Internet solutions, then you might have to overspend on bringing a higher cost Internet solution like Fiber into the building. Establishing these contracts can require time and logistics, and therefore, once the address is known, it is important to communicate that information to your trusted IT consultant.

11.5 Reserve Phone and Fax

The moment an address is established, the herculean effort of opening a new business has officially begun. All of this requires communicating with a spectrum of individuals, businesses, and agencies. It is important to establish a professional vanity phone number (i.e., XXX-XXX-SKIN or XXX-XXX-1234) for your professional phone calls and faxes. The process of starting a business commences with an enormous amount of paperwork requiring the listing of business phone and fax numbers. It is not uncommon to come across an unprepared individual who provided a personal cell phone number only to have other businesses contacting them for years to come. HIPAA-compliant electronic faxing is recommended, if not an industry standard. These electronic faxes help reduce paper, ink, and toner used which translates into dollars saved. In addition, it is much easier to have an incoming fax routed to a key employee or designated group of employees (via shared mailbox or email distribution group). The inbound fax arrives as a PDF file, and the recipient can open the PDF and then choose to print, save, or distribute the fax to its destination. With electronic faxing, you can send the fax through a secure web portal or by composing an email. This process can save a lot of time and money.

11.6 The Buildout

Most new businesses are involved with some version of a buildout in order to create a workable space that flows for their business needs. As this process develops, it is critical that an open dialogue is established between the business owner, architect, general contractor, interior designer (if applicable), and IT/telecom consultant. An important question to ask the IT consultant during the interview process is whether they have experience working with and facilitating the design of the technology floor plan. Space planning is often the first step in professionally designing a commercial space. Most architects will know to have a server room designed into the floor plan, but if not, one is necessary. These rooms have specific climate control, size, wiring, and power demands. They are often referred to as a server room or IT closet. Your IT consultant should be competent in assisting with the design of these rooms.

The IT consultant must work with the architect and electrician to design an optimal low-voltage wiring plan. Some IT consultants possess the professional capabilities to subcontract the low-voltage wiring themselves for your buildout. This would be the most optimal arrangement due to their intimate knowledge of your business's needs and their role in its design. Avoiding the need for a third subcontractor will consolidate responsibility and liability to one subcontractor. Network jacks with low-voltage wiring are required for every phone, computer, wireless access point, network printer, fax, credit machine, video camera, etc., thereby making the design and installation of low-voltage wiring a critical step for a properly functioning technological business. In 2019, the industry officially transitioned to CAT6 low-voltage cabling. CAT5E is still acceptable, but CAT6 is the future and should be considered if signing a long-term lease.

A voice and data network on a CAT6 infrastructure will offer lower crosstalk, higher signal-to-noise ratio, and compatibility with a 10-Gigabit Ethernet network which translates to increased network speed and performance across multiple applications, thereby improving productivity.

Once the space plan is complete, employee stations, expected daily responsibilities, and the technological demands for these employees must be communicated with both your IT consultant and the architect. For instance, the front desk staff who handle the check-in and check-out process will have different IT needs than a laboratory technician; in addition, which employees will be tablet-based, desktop-based, or operate from mobile desktop carts. The technological flow and demands of clinical staff are expectedly different than front-office staff and even different than administrative staff. Importantly, one needs to consider and communicate with their consultants the expected growth in 3 to 5 years out and more. The initial buildout is an excellent opportunity to wire the office correctly for a business's expected growth due to the ease of access the subcontractors will have to such things as wall space, ceiling space, wiring, dry wall, and more that will lower costs later and avoid aesthetic and/or operating disruptions to the business when upgraded later.

Audiovisual systems will also need to be communicated to the involved parties. The wiring needed for these systems is subject to the same access requirements as the data access points. Thus, having the foresight to plan any audio and visual preferences for the business is beneficial at this point.

Finally, security systems will need to be designed at this time as well. This relates to video surveillance, key fab access points, and security keypad access points. Most, if not all, of the aforementioned hardware and software systems are often managed and designed with direct communication by a single IT specialist who is in direct communication with the other construction professionals.

11.7 Establish Service Contracts

The IT consultant will begin reaching out to your preferred local telecom, cable, and Internet service providers (ISP). They should recommend two separate and distinct independent ISPs to establish redundancy. It is very important to have a primary and backup Internet solution with a HIPAA-compliant firewall providing network failover. This allows all your mission critical applications to run seamlessly during an ISP outage which does happen quite a bit with non-service level agreement (SLA) Internet products like cable, asymmetric digital subscriber line (ADSL), and nondedicated fiber products. Selecting only one ISP without a backup is highly inadvisable.

Most applications are cloud based such as your electronic medical records (EMR), practice management, email, and telephony. These applications require Internet service to access the cloud. It is equally important to select a reputable, hosted voice over Internet protocol (VoIP) provider for your telecommunications needs. An IT consultant should learn about your current and future business plans with regard to staffing and growth. The industry standard for small business phone systems is VoIP. VoIP is the technology that converts your voice into a digital signal, allowing you to make a call directly from a computer, a VoIP phone, or other data-driven devices. The initial setup and ongoing costs are generally less for operating a VoIP system than a more traditional phone system and obviates the need for a traditional phone line. This can consolidate expenses between Internet and phone systems. The expenses for VoIP phone calls usually have a lower cost than traditional landlines as well. In addition, traditional phone services have a selection of extra features which can add cost. Many times, VoIP will come with a wide selection of extra features that do not add cost. Some of the disadvantages are obvious, such that Internet connection is a must. If you operate a VoIP network and the power goes out, you no longer have an Internet connection, so you no longer have access to your phone system. Quotes from at least three different hosted VoIP providers should then be provided. To optimize management of your hosted VoIP provider, it is best to select a hosted VoIP provider that will include a quality of service (QoS) device known as an EdgeMarc or SD WAN appliance. These devices maintain the quality of every phone communication. Your hosted VoIP provider should automatically failover between Internet service providers during an ISP outage and during a complete power outage failover to a smartphone, iPhone, or tablet-based app so you will never miss a phone call. These hosted VoIP apps are also a great option for medical staff to call patients during off hours, so the office identity is reflected on the outbound caller ID. This is much better than using a cell phone.

These disaster prevention and recovery methods do add an additional cost to the overhead expense of daily operations, but the opportunity cost of having your business's phones, computers, practice management systems, and EMR fail at once can cause a catastrophic disruption to one's daily operations. When considering the cost of an hour or day of disruption, the additional cost of a second provider as backup should alleviate any concerns regarding additional overhead expenses.

Merchant accounts will need to be established. A merchant account is better known as the credit card processing platform. Some businesses use a credit card terminal while others use an iPad- or tablet-based solution with a wedge reader. The most important thing to do is make sure your payment processing solution is Europay-, Mastercard-, or Visa (EMV)-compliant which is the global standard for cards equipped with computer chips and the technology used to authenticate chip-card transactions. It is recommended to work with an independent sales organization (ISO) rather than work directly with your bank. ISOs can quote multiple payment processing providers and can offer more attractive rates while concomitantly offering better customer service. The Payment Card Industry (PCI) data security standard is a set of data protection mandates developed by the major payment card companies and imposed on businesses that store, process, or transmit payment card data. It is required for your business to conduct an annual PCI compliance assessment, questionnaire, and scan. Businesses that are not PCI-compliant can incur hefty fines.

11.8 Business Associate Agreement

You should have all your partners and vendors sign a HIPAA Business Associate Agreement (BAA). Under the HIPAA privacy and security rules, these third parties should only use the provided PHI in a secure and established manner. It is highly recommended that a responsible administrator ensures all vendors and visitors expected to have access to PHI sign the business's BAA. Importantly, the BAA should be reviewed by a health care attorney. When doing business with cloud service providers (CSPs), an administrator should review the respective CSP's BAA. It is inadvisable to assume the CSP's BAA would meet your attorney's standards.

11.9 Hardware

While hardware ultimately needs to be purchased, it is important that throughout the entire start-up process, one needs to establish EMR and practice management service contracts. These systems will have specifications requirements for any hardware utilized to operate their software. These are the two biggest software systems that will be employed by the company, but any additional systems must be considered, such as photography software. Once that has been established, as a continuum of the dialogue previously mentioned between the business owner and the IT consultant, the number and types of hardware will need to be determined. Discussions will center mainly around job description and mobility of staff. For instance, a staff member who is mobile between workstations or offices may benefit from having a laptop computer, while a more stationary position would likely benefit from desktop computer systems. There are considerations that will be made when determining the purchase order such as security (i.e., a desktop is harder to be stolen than a laptop). Laptop computers may be taken home by a staff member and used for insecure purposes such as Internet transactions that may open the business to network invasions. It is very important that you don't rush through the hardware purchasing process. In addition, it is strongly recommended that you do not purchase computers through retail outlets such as Best Buy, Costco, Walmart, Office Depot, or Staples, despite their aggressive marketing tactics. It is very helpful to work with an IT consultant to design the perfect computer for your practice. They will help you determine some critical decisions such as which users can get away with an i5 processor and 8 GB of RAM versus which users need an i7 processor and 16 GB of RAM. You might think that these are little decisions, but when your key employees are slowed down by a sluggish computer, it ends up costing your business money. It is recommended to have your computers shipped to your IT vendor, so they can wipe them clean and then load them with all the important software and programs that you need. Typically, computer manufacturers load a bunch of free software onto new computers known in the IT industry as crapware, bloatware, or shovelware. Just do yourself a favor and stay away from the supercheap bargain computers.

11.10 Cyber Security

Data breaches cost the health care industry almost six billion dollars every year. There is nothing you can do to fully prevent these cyber-security threats, as there are new cyber vulnerabilities discovered daily. Cyber criminals use malware, ransomware, phishing attacks, cloud threats, and misleading websites in an attempt to lure innocent people into their costly traps. The best form of prevention is education. It is very important for a business to establish a security culture with ongoing cybersecurity training and education. Every device that touches your network needs to be protected. This is a critical component that should not be subject to frugal habits by opting for a cheap or free antivirus protection. Make sure you establish a strict password policy and enforce it. It is also a good idea to have your MSP lock each computer from employee downloads and installations.

As I mentioned earlier, it is very important to install a HIPAA-compliant firewall. Industry experts find such devices as SonicWALL and Meraki as the most reliable. Meraki wireless access points are highly recommended, as they include a dedicated security radio that continuously scans and protects against security threats, senses the radiofrequency environment, adapts to interference, and automatically configures radiofrequency settings to maximize performance. "Free" Wi-Fi that comes with the business class Internet from Cable and ADSL providers is not recommended. You do have to purchase the firewall and an annual license to make sure you are consistently upgraded to the latest and greatest firmware. In addition, your IT vendor will be able to always obtain additional support from SonicWALL and Meraki when complex issues arise. It is important to understand that just because the recommended

firewall is purchased, it should not be assumed that network intrusions will not take place. The firewall is one small step in the right direction. All devices on your business network are part of a next generation-unified endpoint protection platform from a company like SentinelOne. These endpoint protection platforms use artificial intelligence to predict malicious behavior, rapidly eliminate threats, and seamlessly adapt defenses. If you think these recommendations are overkill, please reconsider! Your employees will be glued to their smart phones, tablets, and computers. They will be connected to the Internet and eventually be fooled by would-be hackers. Make sure you are properly protected when this happens. You owe it to your patients to protect their private health information.

11.11 Conclusion

The technological backbone of a business is no less critical than plumbing, room size, HVAC, or any of the additional myriad layers of construction specifications required to operate a business. Many of the necessary decisions can be streamlined and made more easily by utilizing an IT consultant. Mistakes will happen, technology will fail, power will go out, and Internet service will go down. Ensuring that you have a well-constructed infrastructure will mitigate stress and operating costs when these circumstances arise. A well-trusted relationship with an IT consultant will help you navigate these times relatively smoothly. If one chooses to develop the technology infrastructure of their business on their own, we hope this chapter provides you with the necessary tools and understanding to make more educated, efficient, and safe decisions.

12 Choosing and Implementing an Electronic Medical Record System

Robin Travers MD

Abstract

Electronic medical record (EMR) systems manifest significant advantages over traditional paper records systems, including rapid receipt and response to new information, tracking data and patient needs over time, and enhancing information sharing among providers and with patients. Unfortunately, the full potential of such systems is rarely realized due to a multiplicity of platforms that impede system communications. In addition, physician and support staff workload may be increased and efficiency may be sacrificed at least temporarily during the implementation process. This chapter outlines the steps that a practice may follow to successfully implement an EMR. These include pre-implementation steps such as articulating the value of the system from the top down, setting a tone of realistic optimism, and creating a multidisciplinary implementation team that incorporates members from all practice and management arenas. This team will review EMR system selection, configure the selected software, and identify the hardware and personnel needs for implementation. Once software and hardware requirements are well-established, timeline development, training plans, and disaster protocols are developed in the next steps. Finally, strategies to potentially enhance physician–patient communications using the EMR are explored.

Keywords: meaningful use, quality improvement, electronic medical records

Top 10 Things You Need to Know

1. Plan, plan, plan, and then plan some more. Much of an electronic medical record (EMR) system's implementation eventual success depends on the preparation you engage in long before you go live.
2. Set a confident tone for your EMR system implementation.
3. Set a realistic tone for your EMR system implementation.
4. Develop an implementation team with EMR champions belonging to all facets of your practice.
5. Use your EMR implementation as a valuable opportunity to critically evaluate workflows in your practice, even those which have been entrenched for years.
6. Perform your own Health Insurance Portability and Accountability Act (HIPAA)-compliant risk assessment, and consider going beyond the "out-of-the-box" HIPAA compliance standards with your EMR system.
7. Develop disaster protocols and file this under "If you bring an umbrella, it won't rain."
8. Go slow and steady with the training. It takes time to figure an EMR system, just as it takes time to learn to drive a car.
9. Plan for ongoing training needs by employing a "weekly huddle."
10. No matter what system you ultimately choose, take the "golden minute" and make the start of each patient visit entirely technology-free.

12.1 Introduction

The path toward computerization of medical records began in the 1960s, with the advent of problem-based medical record-keeping. The creation of the problem oriented medical record (POMR) by Larry Weed, MD, set the stage for the use of electronic methods to maintain medical information within the standardized format of the "SOAP" note, that is, subjective impressions, objective data, assessment, and plan. Dr. Weed was a trailblazer in his effort to develop an electronic version of the POMR. These earliest data processing systems focused specifically on leveraging burgeoning computing technologies and power to develop an organized and systematic approach in order to manage structured clinical data within a hospital setting.

By the early 1970s, the first EMR systems were developed. These systems were cumbersome and expensive, and used mainly by governmental hospitals and institutions such as those within the Veterans Administration. Innovations in personal computing and emergence of the Internet laid the groundwork for faster and easier access to computerized information, paving the way for making health information available online and developing web-based EMRs.

Sometimes the terms EMR and electronic health record (EHR) are used interchangeably, but they are not truly equivalent. An EMR forms the nuts and bolts of an EHR, equivalent to the role the old paper charts played within a larger health care system. EMRs manifest significant advantages over traditional paper record systems. They can allow a dermatologist to track data over time, for example, easily identifying which melanoma patients are overdue for preventative skin cancer screenings or which psoriasis patients on biologic medications need to have their tuberculosis screening. They allow the dermatologic surgeon to track postsurgical infection rates within their clinic, and identify and respond to spikes in a timely manner. They also allow for rapid receipt, integration, and response to dermatopathology reports. However, the information contained within EMRs is not easily conveyed outside of the individual practice. In fact, the patient's record might even have to be printed out in order to be communicated to other specialists and members of the patient's care team.

An EHR, in contrast to an EMR, is a broader system that focuses on the total health of a patient. An EHR goes beyond the standard clinical data collected within a single dermatology practice by offering a more inclusive view of a patient's overall care. EHRs offer the potential for direct distribution of robust health information among individuals who need it immediately: primary care physicians, the pathologists in the laboratory, other specialists, and, perhaps most importantly, the patients themselves. Indeed, this is one of the core measures in the Stage 1 definition of meaningful use (MU) of EHRs, in that patients be provided timely online access to their own health information.

With EHRs, dermatologists can capitalize on reciprocal information sharing among providers. They can e-prescribe, monitor drug interactions, and obtain timely pathology reports from outside laboratories. Although this vision of a seamless EHR system is almost never fully realized. The myriad EMR platforms available actually impede maximal functionality as interoperability concerns loom large. If a dermatology practice within a hospital setting is required to use the generic

hospital-specific EHR system, the dermatologist's specific requirements for effective record keeping may not be met. Dermatologists might easily get lost in the dreaded morass of drop-down lists necessary to arrive at the fairly esoteric diagnoses and plans that comprise day-to-day dermatologic practice. Alternatively, if a practice implements a dermatology-specific EMR, the gateway to the hospital's larger repository of patient information may be obstructed.

I cannot recommend a specific EMR system here, for one size does not fit all. In selecting a best-fit EMR system for your modern dermatology practice, the foremost concern must be the introduction of patient-centric systems and services that allow the delivery of optimal patient care within your specific practice arena. Thoughtful implementation of an EMR system offers the promise of accomplishing all this, while, at the same time, maintaining workflow and caregiver satisfaction. Managing the EMR adoption process should follow a series of incremental steps to ensure success.

12.2 Step One: Set a Tone

Change is difficult. Articulation of the value that an EMR system will bring to a practice is essential from the top down. This is perhaps made easier by the fact that adoption of an EMR system is commonly driven by external regulatory forces: no single person in the practice can be painted as the "bad guy" forcing the issue. A multidisciplinary approach incorporating physician, nursing, management, and administrative staff is crucial. Presenting a united front to communicate the EMR system's benefits for patient care and the practice's goals from the start can establish buy-in and excitement from the organization as a whole. Providers' attitudes have been shown to be a critical driver of EMR implementation success. Influential peers becoming visible early adopters can go a long way in diminishing resistance among other providers. Setting a tone of thoughtful confidence in the EMR implementation process can help overcome fears about the adverse impacts on the doctor–patient relationship or personal ability to master a new technology.

The flip side of setting a tone of optimism is setting a tone of realistic expectations. If an EMR system is purchased with the expectation of immediately making more money without any substantial increase in workload, it sets the stage for a perception of implementation failure. The fact is that EMR systems *do* necessitate extra work for most users during their first year. Financial expectations to break even might be best set for no fewer than 2 to 3 years after EMR implementation. Government incentives in the form of MU may support part of the initial cost outlay of EMR purchase, but maintenance costs and changes in workflow dynamics contribute to lost productivity and revenue. Although the time, effort, and expense involved should not be underestimated, they may also be framed in the same manner as the purchase, implementation, and training required for any new piece of revenue-generating equipment. The expert care undertaken for the acquisition of any new device should be replicated for the implementation of an EMR system, albeit on a larger scale.

12.3 Step Two: Create a Multidisciplinary Implementation Team

A practice's EMR implementation team should incorporate physicians, nurses, medical assistants, management, billing, technical, and front-office administrative staff. This team is delegated with the responsibility of identifying, prioritizing, and articulating the practice's system requirements, and effectively evaluating the various EMR vendors' abilities to meet these needs. The "physician–champion" role is often deemed critical, but, in our practice, champions from within nursing, IT, and administrative staff proved equally valuable to the success of EMR implementation through a consensus-driven process. The implementation team is essential for developing realistic expectations, facilitating compromise, and using their passion with regard to practice and patient-care end goals to rally employees through the process. Candidates for your practice's implementation team should be enthusiastic, broad-minded, receptive to new ideas, respected in their areas of expertise, analytical, unflappable in the face of setbacks, and effortless in relation to technology.

Super users will be essential components of your implementation team. These clinicians should be selected for their aptitude with computer technology and a powerful commitment to the successful launch of your EMR system. They must not only be intimately familiar with your practice's workflow but also capable of critical analysis of this workflow. Workflows denote the processes through which a practice provides care to patients. A patient visiting your office is guided through a series of workflows, from the moment they contact you to schedule an appointment to the time when they visit the check-out desk to schedule their next visit. All paper forms related to these tasks should be critically evaluated.

EMR implementation actually offers a valuable opportunity to reevaluate workflow paradigms that may have become entrenched and unquestioned over years of clinical practice. For each task in the workflow, the team should inquire: is this essential? Are we adding value to patient care? Are the steps being performed in the right order? Are the steps being assigned to the right person? Does this require the skills and training of a physician or can others be entrusted with this task? It is essential that your implementation team avoid the "because we've always done it this way" mindset.

> ### Personal Anecdote: Letters to Referring Physicians
>
> One element of our practice that my partners and I took pride in was our timely delivery of consultation letters to our patients' referring clinicians. These letters were personally dictated, well-crafted, and hand-signed. They often included collegial personal references to these physicians, with whom many of us had forged personal relationships over the course of years. Our new EMR system allows us to construct and send across letters to referring physicians on the fly, based on templates that derive information from the structured clinical data entered at the time of the visit. These letters can be faxed immediately to the referring physicians, placing information directly in their hands at the time of a patient's visit, and obviating the need for transcription services, printing, and postal costs. However, these letters lack the personal touch which many of us were used to while communicating. We had to ask ourselves: what is more important? The timely and inexpensive delivery of information or the personal touch and hand signature of the traditional letters? Most of my colleagues have opted for the electronic version for all of our consultation letters, with only the most complex cases that fit less well within the templated structure left for dictation.

12.4 Step Three: Choose the Software

Well, this is the real crux of the matter, isn't it? Which software platform will you choose for your practice's EMR system? Financial considerations obviously play a prominent role in decision-making. The average initial cost of adoption of an EMR system is estimated to be between $25,000 to $54,000 per clinician, and maintenance costs range from $3,000 to over $20,000 per clinician per year. The variability in these numbers relate to hardware and software choices, implementation models, and service plans. Hidden costs of EMR implementation include loss of productivity and long-term storage of existing medical records. These costs may be offset by incentive payments and eventual improved efficiency, but these may not be fully realized until several years after implementation.

There are some specific software considerations to lay special emphasis on, as they may be of specific relevance to the practice of dermatology. Does the EMR solution offer the ability to use specialized dermatology templates or machine learning algorithms to personalize examinations and documentation according to your own workflow preferences? Dermatology is an image-intensive medical specialty, and the ability to easily access and obtain digital photography within a patient encounter is essential. Skin findings should be easily and precisely documented via an intuitive interface, such as a homunculus diagram, rather than inaccurate and cumbersome drop-down lists. Dermatologists rely heavily on dermatopathology reports to guide their decision-making: if an EMR system is integrated with your chosen laboratory, results will be delivered swiftly and seamlessly to the patient record, allowing rapid development of a treatment plan. EMR solutions should have an integrated practice management system or easily interface with the one you have in place. Autogeneration of bills during the actual patient encounter will allow more accurate coding and rapid reimbursement. Some practices report discovering that they had been chronically undercoding patient visits and realizing financial gains simply by more appropriate capture of the visit and services rendered.

Take steps to fully inform yourself about the EMR vendors under consideration. Join vendor listservs and watch vendor-hosted webinars. Insist on demonstrations in office and then conduct live site visits to observe the clinical workflows in action. Members from all facets of the implementation team should be prepared to attend these live site visits for the fullest appraisal of all facets of the EMR system. Assess the financial health of the vendor to ensure its longevity and obtain legal representation when reviewing any contracts.

Very importantly, your EMR implementation committee should determine the ease of facilitating reporting requirements for the merit-based incentive system (MIPS) as well as advanced alternative payment models (APM) payment tracks under the Medicare reforms laid out in the Medicare Access and CHIP Reauthorization Act of 2015 (MACRA). The centers for medicare and medicaid services (CMS) will pay dermatologists on a curve under MIPS. Practices that score above average can earn bonus payments, while those who fail to report will likely incur a penalty. An EMR system can capture your MIPS data in real time, allowing the practice to benchmark your performance and identify areas for improvement.

12.5 Step Four: Configure Your Software

Congratulations, you are the proud owner of an EMR platform! Now comes the heavy lifting for your information technology vendor or staff to configure the system to meet your own practice's requirements. You may perform a Health Insurance Portability and Accountability Act (HIPAA) risk assessment, and go above and beyond the security protocols, of the out-of-the-box that your EMR system provides. Discuss customization options and costs with your vendor, such as creating practice-specific templates, to support documentation which your providers feel most confident with. You've spent years developing workflow patterns that work for your office, its clinicians and their personalities, can these be incorporated into your new system? Alternatively, be prepared to relinquish some of these patterns in the name of greater efficiencies that might be realized by the new system.

12.6 Step Five: Identify Hardware and Personnel Needs

What hardware might best support the clinical processes under the new EMR system? A printer in each room may seem a significant financial outlay, but if it diminishes the need for multiple trips in and out of each examination room in search of printed materials, it will be well worth it. How best to minimize the distractions and disruptions to enable the delivery of safe, effective patient care? "Distracted doctoring" refers to clinicians who are more focused on capturing information on their devices than on the actual delivery of patient care. Choice and placement of appropriate hardware can help create a "triangle of trust" with the patient, clinician, and device at points of a triangle, so that eye contact with the patient is maintained while also allowing interaction with the device. Laptop computers may be placed on a cart that can be wheeled into a position anywhere in the examination room to facilitate doctor–patient communication. EMR systems that offer an option for iPad-based data entry are easily portable and unobtrusive.

To scribe or not to scribe? That is the question. In our practice, we use a melded model, where our medical assistants and nursing staff assume some data entry responsibilities related to the patient encounter, while the physicians assume others. Rooming procedures were expanded for our clinical staff, where they now enter a chief complaint and history of present illness for each patient, review and record past medical history including skin cancer interval history, examine medication lists and drug allergies, and verify preferred pharmacies. During the patient visit, clinical staff play a more active role during procedures, pulling up and reviewing the appropriate consent forms in the EMR, and documenting the lot number and expiration dates of any injectables being used during the visit.

Scribes prove to be an imperfect solution. Full-time live scribes in the examination room (unlike the melded model in our practice) are often underpaid and undertrained, and the turnover rates are often quite high. Having medical documentation occur in real time reduces error rates in general, but the error rates in scribe-recorded data remains high. Clinicians using live scribes must be prepared to carefully review and edit any scribe-generated notes, and the resultant loss of productivity must also be taken into account during decision-making. Virtual scribes offer a relatively new option: IKS Health in Mumbai currently employs 400 physicians on staff, transcribing thousands of patient visits a day in clinics across the US. Using the Scribble service, physicians can record an entire patient visit and then transmit the recording online to India, where the scribe listens to the encrypted visit and frames a first draft of the office note, which is tailored to the style and specialty of the provider. This note is then subsequently reviewed by a second physician and an insurance coding expert.

12.7 Step Six: Transfer Data

The EMR implementation team must determine the optimal approach for migrating data from the former recordkeeping system to the new one. Paper records may be scanned and made accessible in digital form. Some information can and should be migrated freshly into a new EMR system. In our practice, the patient's primary care physician, preferred pharmacy, medication list, allergy list, past medical, family, and social and cancer interval history are entered the day prior to a patient's visit. Thus, clinicians possess a fully functional electronic chart the very first time they see a patient after "going live." As time passes, and return visits have increasingly become the norm, this task has become less onerous. We have maintained our old EMR in read-only mode to allow continued access to older detailed records.

12.8 Step Seven: Decide on the Launch Approach

Once software and hardware requirements are well-established, your EMR implementation team should create a detailed timeline. The "go-live" date should be set and communicated widely both within and outside your practice. Patients should be made aware of the implementation of a new system, and every effort made to reassure them of the safety of their health information and the maintenance of their solid relationship with their clinicians. The "go-live" date will dictate the entire roadmap of implementation.

Some practices transition all users over to the fully-functioning EMR on the same day. While this "big bang" approach confers the advantage of minimizing the time spent managing a paper record and the new electronic system simultaneously, it can also be highly disruptive and anxiety provoking. Even small, unexpected bugs in the system can be magnified. Alternatively, other practices introduce their EHR incrementally, turning on certain functions in a step-wise approach. In our practice, we adopted the "little bang" approach. We went live for all users on the same date for almost all EMR functions. Only a select few functionalities were turned off. For example, we turned off the automated prescription refill request because ease of use depended on the initial prescription having been generated within the EMR. Now, a year after our "go-live" date, this function has been turned back on, and it has worked consistently well for all of our providers.

12.9 Step Eight: Develop Disaster Protocols

Even the best of systems may fail at times. What will your practice do in the event of a natural disaster, or even something much more mundane such as a power failure? Physicians and staff should have clear instructions about workflows when the EMR becomes unexpectedly unavailable. Downtime procedures and supplies should be available electronically and on paper. Protocols should be developed in advance for documenting patient visits and transmitting prescription information to pharmacies in the event of an EMR malfunction.

12.10 Step Nine: Initiate Your Training Plan

Training your staff and providers is the essential component for EMR implementation safety and success. Go slowly but steadily with the teaching of the basic skills prior to the "go-live" date. Do not underestimate the length of time it will take physicians and staff to get up to speed with the EMR system. I like the process of learning how to use an EMR to the process of learning how to drive. You don't just hop in the car and turn the key and expect to be driving on the highway right off the bat. After studying the driver's manual, a novice driver will take a test and obtain their learner's permit. They then learn how to drive a car by sitting at the wheel of a car with a proficient driver by their side, guiding them as they drive. First, they may drive slowly in an empty parking lot with few challenges, then on quiet suburban streets, and finally into more urban

or highway traffic. Basic competency can easily take 6 months to achieve while driving, and it is no less for learning the intricacies of a new EMR system. Even after passing the road test, a fully licensed driver becomes even more proficient only by spending hours on the road and encountering new situations.

Find out what training assistance you can expect from your EMR vendor and use them. It is difficult for new EMR users to absorb much information abstractly without having a chance to "drive the car." Consider written and online materials and videos to be like the driver's manual: essential for laying the groundwork to becoming a safe driver, but not enough to actually teach someone how to drive. Your EMR vendor may offer a mock system or "sandbox" to play in and simulate patient encounters. This will allow users to develop and hone templates and protocols for the most common types of encounters well before launch.

Super users will form the backbone of the "at-the-elbow" support required by staff and clinicians as they learn more about your chosen EMR system. These can be considered the accompanying drivers for those with a learner's permit. While playing in the "sandbox," and during the first few weeks of implementation, these pretrained super users should work alongside new users, serving as roaming support to bridge the gap between the resources that are needed and those that are provided by the EMR vendor. There is no better way to learn than to learn by doing. Super users will require dedicated time during which they could fill their usual roles of attending to patients or performing clinical support work, so even if they are comfortable with the new system, their schedules should be lightened to allow them time to serve as resources for their colleagues.

Just as a newly licensed driver will develop a sense of mastery as they log more hours behind the wheel, so will the new EMR user. After several months, users will develop shortcuts or find new functionalities that they can share with colleagues. Over time, there will also be EMR updates which will require additional ongoing training. Practices should encourage users who are constantly interacting with the system to actively engage in improving the EMR system and their interactions with it.

In our practice, we convened open weekly lunch meetings during which all interested EMR users were invited to discuss EMR-related quality and safety concerns, as well as workflow optimization. Super users were present to facilitate, but other physicians and clinicians often discovered tips and workarounds which they shared and disseminated in this informal environment. We called this our weekly huddle. Whereas the traditional IT approach to a software problem is to put in a ticket and wait for a response, our weekly huddle often revealed that another user in our practice had already worked out an innovative answer, offering swift and often creative workflow solutions to inevitable glitches we encountered.

12.11 Step Ten: Enhance EMR-Related Communication Skills

It is possible that the EMR system could reduce the amount of time necessary to complete a dermatological examination by allowing a more complete review of prior visits and laboratory data, and thus increase the face-to-face time during a patient encounter. However, many dermatologists express concerns regarding depersonalization of the office visit during the course of data entry into the many systems. In the event of a poor clinical outcome, might this depersonalization and interruption of the interaction between doctor and patient be enough to spur a patient to consider legal action? The best practice of dermatology requires patient-centered communication that enhances the quality of care while at the same time allowing dermatologists to fulfill professional competencies and reduce medical errors. Might the use of an EMR systems interrupt these best practices?

The fact is that there are mechanisms by which an EMR system might be incorporated into the daily practice of dermatology in such a way, so as to enhance the doctor–patient interaction. Physicians can be taught to integrate patient-centered communication strategies while using the EMR, just as they were taught to use patient-centered communication strategies with old-fashioned paper charting. One of the most important strategies is to incorporate the "golden minute" into your patient interactions. The first minute spent with a patient is critical to establishing rapport, so make the start of your visit completely technology-free. Greet your patient, offer them your full attention, and actively listen to their concerns. Once an agenda has been established for your visit, examination and data recording can begin. Note that this differs very little from the patient-centered practice of medicine with paper charting. Introduction of an EMR system offers us the opportunity to reevaluate and improve our patient interactions in the examination room.

The previously alluded to physical arrangement of the examination rooms in order to create a "triangle of trust" between physician, patient, and device is essential. Your examination room setup should be optimized to allow you to look at both the patient and the screen without shifting your body. Interestingly, with old-fashioned paper charting, many patients reported barriers to interaction with their physicians who were taking notes at a desk during the encounter. EMR implementation actually offers advantages for physical positioning which may not have been available with paper charting! In the EMR-compatible examination room, your patient should also be able to view the screen and be engaged in decision-making in this manner. Pulling up a photograph of a nevus taken a year ago and comparing it to the current appearance offers opportunities for patient engagement that did not exist with paper charting.

12.12 Conclusion

Like it or not, EMR systems represent the future of the modern practice of dermatology. Thorough planning and careful selection of a system can afford a dermatology practice not only the opportunity to incorporate an EMR successfully, but also use the implementation process as an opportunity for reflecting on and improving current practices and workflows! When properly implemented, an EMR needn't depersonalize the doctor–patient relationship, and can be incorporated into a powerful model of shared decision-making.

Suggested Readings

Arndt BG, Beasley JW, Watkinson MD, et al. Tethered to the EHR: primary care physician workload assessment using EHR event log data and time-motion observations. Ann Fam Med 2017;15(5):419–426

EMR. The progress to 100% electronic medical records. University of Scranton's Online Resource Center. Available at: https://elearning.scranton.edu/resource/health-human-services/emr_the-progress-to-100-percent-electronic-medical-records. Accessed November 19, 2018

Farina L. Tips and lessons learned for a successful clinical EHR implementation. Health Management Technology. Available at: https://www.healthmgttech.com/tips-and-lessons-learned-for-a-successful-clinical-ehr-implementation. Published June 28, 2018. Accessed November 16, 2018

Gawande A. Why doctors hate their computers. The New Yorker. Available at: https://www.newyorker.com/magazine/2018/11/12/why-doctors-hate-their-computers. Published November 12, 2018. Accessed November 16, 2018

Kaufmann MD, Desai S. Special requirements for electronic health records in dermatology. Semin Cutan Med Surg 2012;31(3):160–162

Kreimer S. Team-based approach puts dent in physicians' EHR "pajama time." American Association for Physician Leadership. Available at: https://www.physicianleaders.org/news/team-based-approach-puts-dent-in-physicians-ehr-pajama-time. Published October 3, 2017. Accessed November 16, 2018

Lee W. Distracted digital doctors: the need to rehumanize medicine. Gold Foundation. Available at: https://www.gold-foundation.org/distracted-digital-doctors-the-need-to-rehumanize-medicine/. Published July 24, 2014. Accessed November 16, 2018

Lee WW, Alkureishi MA, Ukabiala O, et al. Patient perceptions of electronic medical record use by faculty and resident physicians: a mixed methods study. J Gen Intern Med 2016;31(11):1315–1322

Wald HS, George P, Reis SP, Taylor JS. Electronic health record training in undergraduate medical education: bridging theory to practice with curricula for empowering patient- and relationship-centered care in the computerized setting. Acad Med 2014; 89(3):380–386

Wheeland RG. Separating EMR implementation hype from fact. Dermatology Times. Available at: http://www.dermatologytimes.com/modern-medicine-now/separating-emr-implementation-hype-fact. Published July 1, 2012. Accessed November 16, 2018

13 Private Equity and Venture Capital-Backed Practice Models

Editor's Note

The field of Dermatology has been undergoing a dramatic change in its financial structure over the last few years, driven principally by the infusion of private equity-backed capital into the space. With the acquisition and consolidation of practices, there has been a significant shift in practice type and model from solo practitioner-and physicians-owned small group practices to equity-backed, consolidated, large conglomerated practices. Whether this is good or bad for dermatology as a specialty and for individual practitioners depends on your perspective. This is a hotly debated and emotional topic for many. Without a doubt, this is the transformative issue facing the specialty of dermatology.

Given some of the polarity in opinions on this topic, we felt it only fair. Our attempt is to provide you, our readers, two sides of the argument to be sure to give both perspectives. Our attempt in this particular topic is to provide you with enough information to help guide you regarding which is the best fit for you. We are aware that some of the opinions provided in this chapter may be controversial and will likely ignite debate, but without discussion, good decisions are never made. Ultimately, our goal is to empower you, our reader, with information to ask more questions and come up with the best decision for you.

Jeffrey S. Dover MD, FRCPC
Kavita Mariwalla MD, FAAD

Abstract

There are many ways to make money practicing dermatology. The employment choices you make can have a huge effect on your autonomy, happiness, and sanity—not just your bank account. Private equity-backed dermatology groups have experienced a boom during the last decade. This chapter will discuss the pros and cons of private equity (PE) in dermatology, including valuable testimonials from those who possess firsthand experience with PE-backed groups. The ins and outs of selling an existing practice and what happens if you are acquired by PE are also discussed. The corporatization of dermatology has proven to be one of the most divisive issues in our field. While some view it as a savior, others warn of the effects greed and profiteering have already had on dermatopathology. This chapter presents a balanced discussion of both sides of this controversial issue.

Keywords: corporatization, dermatology, private equity, venture capital, testimonials, consolidation, monetization

13.1 Part A: The Corporatization of Dermatology

Joseph K. Francis MD

Top 10 Things You Need to Know

1. Private Equity (PE) groups believe that they can apply business principles to the way you practice in order to maximize profits. Think about what that means.
2. PE groups insert themselves between the generations by buying the practices of older physicians and hiring younger dermatologists to staff the offices. Take a look at the job postings in any dermatology journal or magazine.
3. Noncompete and assignment clauses are two ways in which you can get trapped into signing a PE contract if your practice is sold.
4. PE and large dermatology groups depend on exemptions to the Stark law in order to legally self-refer. This not only provides the basis for much of their profits but also drives overutilization.
5. The corporate practice of medicine (CPOM) is illegal in California and to varying degrees in other states. A true example of this would be a PE firm that wanted to increase utilization of Mohs surgery, so they hired a nonphysician to determine which biopsy reports to schedule for Mohs.
6. The biggest difference between a profession (us) and an occupation (i.e., nurse) is the level of autonomy. To accomplish their goals, PE firms strip you of this autonomy and place decisions in the hands of administrators.
7. The real value of your medical practice lies in your patients and your relationships with them. The essence of a noncompete clause is to capture this value from you.
8. Physician-run hospital systems like Mayo and The Cleveland Clinic are consistently rated the top hospitals in the country and have the highest patient satisfaction.
9. Spokespeople are relatable. PE groups have been known to recruit influential dermatologists and even overpay residents from prominent programs in order to spur recruitment. The push for disclosure of these conflicts of interests among dermatology leadership is gaining steam.
10. All PE-backed dermatology groups say they focus on quality and are different from other bad actors. In actuality, they all have a primary fiduciary responsibility to their investors. The needs of you and your patients are secondary concerns.

13.1.1 The Elephant in the Room

I would like to start out by introducing myself. My name is Joseph Francis and I am adjunct faculty at the University of Florida College of Medicine. Prior to medical school, I worked as a management consultant for PricewaterhouseCoopers for a period of 3 years where I was primarily a computer programmer.

Working as a consultant was probably the best and worst experience of my life. I was able to save some extra money which allowed a person with no means to live comfortably throughout all the years of my medical training. I was also able to travel around the country and work with a diverse group of people at several fortune 500 companies. The constant travel wore me down and I began to appreciate the value in work-life balance and routines. I also became disenchanted with corporate America and its focus on monetary gain over basic human values like honesty and responsibility. Most people I worked with really hated their jobs but were trapped by debt and obligations. My successful escape from the seeming glamor of airline statuses and reimbursed meals is something I thought about often during those tough nights on call as an intern and motivates me to this day.

After the first Medicare physician payment data release in 2014, I got a call from my mentor Dr. Richard Bennett. He has been keeping detailed records on patients and Mohs case logs since the 1970s and postulated that this data could be mined for research. He explained to me a formula he would use with his case logs to determine the average number of stages per case. The first stages of Mohs are only billed once, which can be used in place of the number of cases (denominator). If you add the first stage to the number of subsequent stages, you get the total number of stages (numerator). Dividing the two numbers during the period of a year will give you the average number of stages per Mohs case in that year.

On day one of my fellowship, I realized that it was my job to do the billing for the entire day from the paper charts by hand. I absolutely hated it at first and during the first few weeks I got frequent reprimands for making errors. Later, I came to realize just how important a skill this would be when doing my own billing and analyzing Medicare data.

My first attempt to open the Medicare dataset resulted in my computer running out of memory and crashing. I was ready to give up once I realized that SAS software costs $2k, and I didn't know if I had a computer powerful enough to handle it; however, I was confident that I knew how to do it. I eventually discovered the free software program "R" and began writing programs to analyze almost all dermatology procedures.

The data release was part of the Affordable Care Act and was done in the spirit of increasing transparency. The AMA was blocking the release of the data for several decades due to concerns over inaccuracy and possible misinterpretation (We have actually found some mistakes in the data and developed ways to detect them). *The Wall Street Journal* won a Pulitzer Prize for creating a searchable online database using this data, which they have continued to update as new data is released every year. Since 2015, Medicare has improved the accuracy of the releases and reports an error rate of "0.01% or less."

Back in 2014, we discovered several Mohs surgeons, including a few fellowship directors, who were billing 3 to 4 standard deviations above the mean in number of stages. I had seen some of the toughest cases in LA during my fellowship (my opinion), and our average number of stages was within one standard deviation of the mean, as were surgeons at almost all academic referral centers. It was obvious that something was awry with the practice patterns of these physicians and they had been caught red-handed by data. We shared our findings with the ACMS leadership, and I think that the application of "Improving Wisely" methodology to Mohs has been a very proactive way of dealing with the problem. Medicare seems unwilling to do anything besides cut reimbursement in response to abuses. Investigating each individual physician is an onerous and expensive task. Physician outliers can usually run circles around Medicare RAC and ZPIC auditors and then go right back to their old ways. I hope that in the future Medicare will make more use of data analysis conducted by subject matter experts.

In addition to Mohs, I started looking into dermatology procedures such as biopsies and cryotherapy and realized that many of the highest outliers in the country practiced down the street from me! I went out of my way to meet most of them, trying to discreetly sit next to them at dinners and meetings. I learned the term "productivity-based practice" which some of you may already know is a practice model based on doing as many procedures as you can on someone before they can run out the door. This form of practice was something pretty much all of them had in common. "This is the way I've always done it" was another common refrain. Not to imply that all the outliers were older, but if I were to characterize them, I would say that they didn't seem to act like any of the physicians I'd ever met. They were highly intelligent people with sociopathic tendencies. They all had a strong disdain for evidence-based medicine, standards of care, and very firm beliefs in their own way of doing things such as $3500/lesion radiation treatments for all skin cancers. These men and women practiced medicine with the same ethical standards as the shrewd businesspeople I knew at PricewaterhouseCoopers.

Some of the residents at the hospital next door to my office figured out that I was one of the dermatologists they could call for consults who would actually show up. I saw victims of cherry-picking and overtreatment and could almost guess what procedures where done on them based on who their dermatologist was. Patients who had multiple benign lesions biopsied and skin cancers adequately treated were left with bad psoriasis, photosensitivity, and chronic wounds. I felt like I was doing the right thing by seeing these forgotten and abandoned patients who were never going to go back through the ringer.

In 2017, I read the *New York Times* article on Dermatology by Hafner and Palmer that detailed the abusive practices of some dermatologists, including inadequate supervision of midlevel practitioners, and patients being pushed toward aggressive treatments I sort of knew Sailesh Konda at the time and he told me that he was also inspired to do something after reading the *New York Times* article. I told him about what I knew of the Medicare data and he explained the PE connection to me. He told me that he signed up for a date to give grand rounds on the topic at the University of Florida and invited me to join him. We agreed that the talk should be geared more toward explaining these concepts to residents.

Afterward, I stood in the hallway with Stanton Wesson, the since retired program director at the University of Florida, who told me "Joe, the data you presented was very interesting but I want you to imagine Medicare as an enormous dead whale at the top of the ocean. While it slowly sinks, more and more sharks and other fish circle around it, ripping off pieces of fatty flesh to eat. By the time it gets to the bottom of the ocean, there is nothing left but an empty carcass. That's how the health care system works in our country." I imagined ways to keep the whale afloat during my four-hour drive back home.

A couple of weeks later I met up with Sailesh and gave him an article I had just read by Arnold Relman, former editor of the NEJM, warning about the corporatization of medicine that was happening in the 1980s. He shared with me that he had spoken to Jane Grant-Kels about our talk and she was interested in hearing more about it. Later, we would form a group together with Kiran Motaparthi, who had left a PE-backed dermatopathology group and taken a position at the University of Florida. The purpose of the group would be to research the effects of PE on derm, with each one of us bringing our own perspectives and experience. Sailesh and I got to work using Relman's concepts as our guide.

I began to really dive into the available Medicare data and noticed that some of the biopsy outliers I had identified years ago were now retiring and selling their practices to PE-backed derm groups. Well that isn't entirely true. One of the ones I stalked ended up getting caught and is now serving time in prison for Medicare fraud. At first, it was only 3 of the top 25 biopsy outliers in the country who had sold to PE, as of February 2019, it's now 6! Have PE firms figured out that you can make millions on unnecessary procedures with very little oversight? Many of the PE companies have adopted and expanded upon the abuses highlighted by my analysis. Corporate interests were forcing their way through the door and applying their lower ethical standards to dermatology, restructuring it to mirror the outlier practices that attracted them in the first place. A new school of sharks had found the whale. I thought that everything I worked so hard to get away from was back. The difference was that this time I understood the game much better than they did.

13.1.2 A Short and Simple Chronology of PE in Dermatology

PE derm groups evolve through these steps:

1. Physician consolidator—a physician decides to use his or her personal wealth or team up with an investment bank to start purchasing practices of retiring physicians. Usually this occurs as a regional phenomenon. These physicians

are usually excellent salespeople and the three I can think of off the top of my head have been wildly successful. A physician can be much more convincing and is much more relatable when acquiring practices. At this point, the physician can also say his or her entity is not affiliated to PE, even though it is obviously his or her intention to flip the organization to PE in the future. Physician consolidators take risks and are rewarded greatly. Using borrowed money, or their own personal wealth, they pay a retiring physician 2 to 3× EBITDA (EBITDA is a way to measure profitability) for their practice. Why is it worth that much? Why are there now multiple groups lining up to bid on them? Often times, the practice of a retiring physician is in slow decline with loyal, highly payed long-term employees who don't use newer technologies as part of an office workflow. The key is that the physician consolidator understands that once he or she pays 2 to 3× EBITDA for a practice, it instantly becomes worth 8 to 12× EBITDA when he or she flips it as part of his or her larger organization. The consolidator may know that you are an outlier and your high EBITDA is based on the fact you average a ridiculous 6 biopsies per patients every year. He or she will pay the inflated cost for your practice and when he or she flips it, it becomes the equivalent of flipping six practices on paper to the next buyer who can't tell the difference. One consolidator who ran out of practices to buy in my area opened a new one in the parking lot of my second favorite Chinese restaurant. It was staffed by a newly graduated family practitioner and physician assistants (PAs) with several years of dermatology experience. Growing with reckless abandon without care for inefficiencies or quality is okay because everything becomes a multiple of 8 to 12. Once the calf is sufficiently fattened, it is shopped around to many different banks who attempt to decipher what is real. Sometimes the consolidator bows out but most of the time they stay on as a valuable spokesperson for the new entity. The consolidator may retain equity in the new corporation and so may some of the doctors who sold. This is equity that they can hang on to forever. Eventually, we may all be working for their children and relatives. Sometimes the consolidator is not a physician but a PE firm manager who wants to enter the dermatology "space." Since they don't know anything about dermatology, they will try and pair up with what is known as a "platform practice." The owners of the platform practice will recruit other doctors to sell to the PE firm in return for a larger share of the equity in the new organization. They won't do as well as the physician consolidator who did it all alone but will have the same pressures to grow the organization and accomplish the first flip or their shares in the new entity will have no value. If you need help understanding their motivations, go to Google and type in "multilevel marketing herbalife amway." It's a very similar concept with a few subtle differences.

2. After the first flip, the organization will need to grow in order to flip again. As the organization matures, it will have to do a better job at economies of scale in order to remain solvent. Some of these organizations are sold as a value proposition with potential to increase profits with the right management.

3. After the second flip, larger organizations may start to close offices that were opened just to boost EBITDA on prior flips. They may also become more concerned with compliance. Usually this is the point where the focus is more on profits and everyone has become an employee. The more flips, the less autonomy. A wise mentor of mine once told me that PE firms are like McDonalds. I didn't understand what he was talking about until I started looking into the mature PE-backed practices: standardization, branding, uniforms, conformity, franchising, mandatory smiling, commercialization, consistency, but not very healthy for consumers. The doctors become replaceable drones: accountable to the nonphysician administrator and most of the patient management decisions are made for them—their licenses "maximized" to comply with CLIA laboratory and extender supervision laws. Part of the ruse is a concerted effort to obscure the credentials of the providers. You can't tell who's who but it doesn't matter because everyone is the same. There is an endless supply of extenders lining up to don a long white coat with a brand new dermatoscope in the front pocket and work alongside you as your perceived equal, or even replace you. There are many trends that show the effects of this in the Medicare dataset.

What is the endpoint of this cycle? What cuts off the oxygen fueling this wildfire of consolidation and stops the flipping in its tracks? Large cuts in reimbursement to dermatology CPT codes stops the music and pulls the chair out from under the consolidators. This is what happened to dermatopathology. Also, maybe enough younger generation dermatologists are unwilling to wear the uniform and work the drive-through window.

13.1.3 A Bad Value Proposition for Older Dermatologists?

Dr. Rao is approaching retirement and is approached by a PE firm offering to purchase his practice for 2× his EBITDA. As part of the terms in the deal, Dr. Rao must stay on for another 5 years while they transition the practice to a younger associate and work at 38% of collections. He must also supervise two PAs who have recently graduated and are eager to learn. After 5 years, Dr. Rao has missed out on approximately 100% of collections and has assumed the liability of supervising extenders. As a salaried physician, he was no longer eligible for the tax breaks allowed to small businesses. His long-time office manager was terminated by the PE group that caused a disturbance with staff which was felt by patients and Dr. Rao. He also lost the flexibility of charging patients a need-based rate for his services, as all billing was taken over by new management. The PE firm was unable to find a physician to take over for Dr. Rao and he ends up leaving his practice in the hands of the two PAs who will be remotely supervised by another doctor in a neighboring state. If you factor in opportunity cost, how much does Dr. Rao really get for his practice? Do you think he feels true to the patients who supported him over the many years he has been in practice?

13.1.4 List of Dos and Don'ts

- Don't lock yourself into a contract with a non-compete and assignment clause.
- Don't believe that anyone else is looking out for your best interest.

- Do work with people who share your values.
- Do get a clear idea of the retirement plans of the older doctors in your group.
- Do spend the money on a lawyer when dealing with a large organization to make sure you don't end up in a bad situation.

13.1.5 List of Challenges

Larger firms in certain areas may have negotiated complete exclusivity with specific insurance companies which stifles competition. This is especially challenging in certain communities where Kaiser-Permanente and some large employers or academic centers control large swaths of the market.

Personal and student debt after many long years of training may leave you no choice but to accept the best offer available.

Research has shown that physician extenders practicing independently do significantly more biopsies than dermatologists. PE derm models that over-leverage extenders for revenue growth will not pass scrutiny in the age of data and value-based care.

Consolidation cheerleaders have ulterior motives, mainly their own bottom line. It is designed to move through dermatology like a virus where each infected person tries to infect others. Knowledge is the antidote.

To-Do Checklist

- ☐ Look at publicly available data on the practice such as paid malpractice cases, billing patterns, and employee litigation.
- ☐ If applicable, speak with the person who had the job before!
- ☐ Online review sites such as Glassdoor, Yelp, Google, and Healthgrades can sometimes provide real insights, although be aware that many of the positive reviews and ratings can be faked.
- ☐ Social media sites for dermatologists are a good way to find jobs and communicate with colleagues.

13.2 Part B: Testimonials from Dermatologists Regarding PE-Backed Practices

Sailesh Konda MD, FAAD, FACMS

My name is Sailesh Konda and I am an Assistant Clinical Professor of Dermatology at the University of Florida (UF) Health System, where I serve as Medical Director and Director of Mohs Surgery and Surgical Dermatology. During my time at UF, I developed a special interest in the evolving role of PE within dermatology. I have researched, published, and lectured extensively on PE-backed dermatology groups. In addition, I have served as an advisor to the American Academy of Dermatology Emerging Practice Models Committee.

The lecture circuit has taken me to over 25 local, regional, and national settings to (1) discuss PE pearls and pitfalls with residents and practicing dermatologists in different stages of their careers and (2) debate physician consolidators from some of the largest PE-backed groups. Dermatologists from all over the country have shared with me their experiences with PE-backed groups. Many of them are afraid to share their experiences publicly, as they are restricted by nondisparagement agreements. I have selected some of their testimonials to share with you and provide these dermatologists with a voice. These testimonials contain information which would prove to be valuable for all residents and practicing dermatologists.

13.2.1 Testimonial One

Coming out of residency, I evaluated multiple practice models but was not aware of the implications of joining a PE-backed practice. Ultimately, I signed with a smaller group, at which time I was promised complete autonomy in building my practice and plenty of financial support to remodel and update two highly outdated practice settings in order to suit my tastes and clinical interests. I was never informed of the possibility that they may sell or add midlevels, and I certainly didn't think to ask. I simply didn't know those were options.

One month prior to graduating residency, a colleague mentioned to me that my soon-to-be practice had hired a PA for one of my clinic settings. I was taken aback that they would hire someone new so soon before I was to join them, and this

had never been mentioned to me as a possibility. I was reassured by the group that she "wouldn't be there for very long," yet when I started working three months later, the PA was still there, practicing without an onsite supervisor several days a week and complaining to management that I was attempting to "steal her patients" by insisting my schedule be filled preferentially. Our professional relationship was never repaired as the PA continued to refuse to speak to me for the next 2 years. She never once asked my input on a patient and never once referred a patient to me.

A mere 10 days into my employment, I received a phone call from the CEO and was informed the group would likely be sold to a PE-backed practice. I was told it "developed quickly" and they had "no prior plans to sell when they hired me" but wanted to "put me in the best situation." The next day I had a contract in my inbox from the PE-backed practice, with an overwhelming number of stipulations that went far beyond the scope of my original contract. My attorney and I were dismayed to see that the PE-backed practice was attempting to lock me into a longer contract with a larger restrictive covenant and, most notably, refused to provide any clarity whatsoever on their bonus structure. During this negotiation period, I was once again reassured by the senior executives that the costs that were required to bring both practice locations into the 21st century would not hit my overhead. Overall, I spent twice as much money on attorney's fees negotiating this contract than I did with my first.

Once the sale was announced, all spending on my clinics was frozen. I could not even get an order for sutures approved for nearly 2 months, so I had to defer surgeries during the sales period. Following the sale, I noticed that I was being charged overhead (which counted against my collections for the sake of determining any production bonus) for desperately necessary updates to the clinics (painting, basic repairs, replacement of broken furniture, and even clinic signage for the new ownership). When I complained, only the signage was ultimately reversed. The transition period was chaotic and undersupported for both physicians and staff. The "team" in charge of the transition made one site visit over the 6-month transition period and was generally unresponsive to concerns—they were too busy locking in their next acquisitions. A substantial number of my emails were simply ignored. In a 2-year period, I went through four regional clinic managers (none of whom were ever stationed onsite). When on multiple occasions I complained about lack of structure and incompetency, I was admonished by the president of the company that my tone was "too harsh."

Overall, my experience with PE-backed practices was a professional misadventure filled with empty promises, inadequate supervision, and a "pay no attention to the man behind the curtain" culture. My working hours were filled with a sense that I truly lacked autonomy to make decisions that impacted clinic culture and workflow. The implicit message from the PE-backed practice was that I was not a colleague, but a tool to further their mission. Two years couldn't pass fast enough.

13.2.2 Testimonial Two

After working in private practice for 4 years at a successful dermatology practice, the owner was approached by a PE firm for buyout. As per the owner, this would be a positive opportunity for not only him but for me. As I walked into the initial meeting, I had open ears and an open mind. I knew I always wanted to be an owner, but maybe this would be a good opportunity for me and help the practice to grow. My mindset quickly changed when I realized this deal was completely one-sided.

Here was their proposal:
- The owner would receive a sizable payout; I would receive nothing. This was quite confusing as I was the primary producer working full-time, 5 days a week, while the other practitioner worked on average 3 to 4 half days a week.
- The owner and I would discuss what compensation I would receive but they were clear that it would likely be continuation of my current percentage of profits.
- I would continue to run my patient care as I saw fit (as I was already very successful), however they expected incremental increases in profitability annually over the next 5 years.
- A 5-year commitment—no negotiability.
- Approval would be necessary for any equipment purchases or practice expansion.
- Vacation days would be limited.

I went into the meeting with open ears and an open mind and left the meeting with a clear understanding of my future. I was going to walk away and start my own practice and empire. A 5-year commitment, with limitation on vacation days, an expected profit margin (more pressure!), and no financial incentive, while the owner, who

was much older, would be able to walk away with a big payout and continue working minimal hours while I worked day in and day out. This was one-sided and it was clear they would be in full control.

So, here I am today, a new practice owner and happier than ever!

13.2.3 Testimonial Three

I was in my first or second year of practice when approached by a PE or VC group. They were based out of state but didn't go too in depth into management or the business side. In my case, I did not meet a physician, but their corporate representatives which I was OK with either way since it was preliminary and initiated by them. They continually, via email or phone, praised my business acumen, courage, influence, decisions, research, etc., in deciding to start my practice and locate it where I did. I had not yet shared any significant information that I remember (possibly my office manager gave some basic information but I don't recall). After a few exchanges, they requested to meet for dinner. I made it clear from the outset that I wanted information but wasn't actively looking to sell and they were OK with that (supposedly). They again reviewed how I was an amazing practice and all of the positives of my situation. They said that I was a priority for their company to help improve their overall stance, reputation, etc. They had brought a contract to sign at dinner. I do not remember being at that point in discussions, so I am either recalling incorrectly or they had hoped that I would feel obligated to sign to avoid wasting their time and taking me to dinner for no reason. I told them that I'd been thinking it over and was very impressed with their plans and that they seemed to be focusing on my practice potential. Then I said as good as it was that I just didn't think that the time was right, since I was still in growth mode, but that I would certainly keep in touch and call them with updates and if I decided to take another step closer to joining. They were visibly bothered and then pressed a little more, but still a polite push. After more talk, they asked me not to count them out and to sleep on it and make sure that I was making a wise decision. I told them that I would do that since I owed myself, the business, and them, a very critical review and the best decision possible. Again, I really don't remember ever even having a specific offer or exact details of a contract. It's speculation but possibly they were hoping to catch me as a new solo physician with minimal/no business smarts (and no financial savings to hire an appropriate attorney for review) who was easily influenced and would sign a generic, vague contract. After reconsidering all of the pros and cons and discussion points, I called and said I still thought that I should wait for now. They asked if I was really making the decision to pass on their offer and I affirmed. In seconds, their smiles and compliments disappeared. They told me that I just made the decision that would shut my practice doors. They said that they would buy all of the local practices and overpower with numbers and other methods to choke me out of business. They said I could never survive without their referrals (from presumed other practices) and that with decisions like I made, my practice probably wouldn't survive anyway. I believe they still left their card (I'm sure to give me the "scary" side to consider instead of the "rosy outlook"). I did not hear from them or contact them afterward. Within the year, their company had sold to another PE/VC company and no other practices in my area had been acquired. Obviously, I'm still plugging along super busy and still growing.

13.2.4 Testimonial Four

I worked for a PE company for a few days per month for approximately a year as a Mohs surgeon while building my own practice. I was recruited to do cases on a straight collections basis. I will describe some of the pros and cons of my experience:
Pros:
- The income was extremely useful, particularly in helping build my own practice.
- The company was able to provide an adequate number of cases for each of the days I worked there.
- The company was somewhat responsive to my needs for instruments, sutures, and other items needed to do my job.
Cons:
- There was extremely high turnover of the staff. The company did not pay its employees well and could not retain the better ones. Some clinics were understaffed or had inadequately trained staff, making it very hard for me to do my job properly.
- The company did not desire any feedback from me in running a clinic. The C-level management did not seem to really care about details on the ground.

- The company was not forthcoming in providing requested financial and charge information. While I am not concerned that there was any withholding of payments in the end, I would have liked to have more information on my production.
- I heard mixed reviews of the company's billing practices and handling of patients directly from the patients. I was not proud of the way the company handled some of these things.

Overall, the experience worked well for me and my situation for the year that I was there, but I would not want to have continued employment there afterward. The focus on profits and cutting costs undermined the reason I became a doctor in the first place, which was to take care of patients and those around me.

13.2.5 Testimonial Five

My experience with PE began when the physician-owned practice I originally joined was acquired by a PE group. This transition was swift and little was revealed about the changes to come.

Slowly and abruptly, the changes manifested. Some examples of such changes are:
- Discontinued 401K contribution match and loyalty bonuses.
- Elimination of support staff with subsequent increase of patient burden on physicians (i.e., wound care nurse suddenly removed from role, resulting in all suture removals and wound checks to be attended to by physicians).
- An expectation from staff and providers to build new office locations (2–3 new office locations annually) regardless of productivity loss.
- An increase in the number of unsupervised physician extenders (i.e., PAs) with corresponding decrease in the percentage amount of compensation to supervise PAs.
- New employment contracts had greater restrictive covenants and a decrease in fringe benefits.

The recurrent theme in these scenarios is that change, be it small or large, can have large consequences. Without transparency and a protocol to facilitate the transition, the consequences of these changes increased tremendously in magnitude. I felt devalued, taken advantage of, helpless, and trapped. Each day I wondered what was next. It was made clear to me that I was replaceable, so if I wasn't happy, there were plenty of other candidates who would take my position.

I spent 1.5 years in the practice after the PE acquisition. While my volume did increase, I could not tolerate being treated as a puppet. The last straw for me was when I was presented with an ultimatum to either build a new practice that was outside of my contracted requirements and was negatively impactful toward productivity or I would be terminated without cause. I chose to be terminated. While at first, I was scared that I would be without work for an extended period of time, I was happy to see the support of fellow board-certified dermatologists. There have been several opportunities to do locums and join physician-owned groups. I don't feel trapped or afraid anymore. Instead, I am excited to explore opportunities that have a mutually vested interest and offer profit sharing, instead of the PE model that focuses on the bottom line, often at the expense of its employees.

13.3 Part C: Selling a Practice: The Viewpoint from Someone Who Sold

Edward (Ted) Lain MD, MBA

The current wave of private equity (PE)-backed consolidation in dermatology shows few signs of slowing and can prove to be a life-changing opportunity for a physician. The purpose of this chapter lies not in a discussion of the effect of consolidation on our specialty, but rather to provide a roadmap and highlight decision inflection points to a practice-owner considering a sale. I include learnings from selling my own practice, being a founding partner in a consolidation, and advising many of my peers as they ponder whether joining a consolidation is the correct next move in their career. As a practice owner, I have felt the burden of being one, experienced the hardships of dealing with human resource issues, attempted a solo navigation through the sea of CMS-mandated compliance regulations, lost sleep due to the spiraling costs of providing benefits to my loyal employees, and managed relationships with vendors as I tried to negotiate costs to more sustainable levels in the climate of annual declines in insurance reimbursement.

Yet while administering a practice is becoming increasingly difficult, and expensive, I have learned that the reason many dermatologists sell is much more nuanced. Some are interested in receiving the value of their practice in cash (monetization of the practice), so they can take capital that was once tied up and utilize it for other investments or to reduce liabilities. Others believe the investment in their practice remains the most lucrative in their portfolio, but would like to join and invest in a consolidation in order to diversify their investment across geography, subspecialties, and ancillary services. Still others, especially younger practice owners, are concerned about the future of private practice in the United States, and see that the best opportunity to successfully navigate any changes will be as part of a larger group with the resources and regional clout to ensure survivability. Finally, but certainly not comprehensively, some owners nearing retirement wish to ensure their patients have continuity of care and join a consolidation in order to avoid closure of their practice when they stop working.

There are those in our specialty who aim to vilify the corporatization of dermatology. There are many threats to the survivability of a private practice physician, including the growing independence of midlevels, increasingly narrow prescribing and practice boundaries imposed by insurance companies, greater penetration of government regulation and oversight into the physician–patient relationship and visit. Many see corporatization as hammering one more nail into the coffin of the independently practicing physician. In addition, they fear that a corporate team, and board of directors, with financial oversight and accountability, reduce the patient to a widget and the provider to a factory worker.

Again, while the purpose of this chapter is not to act as a rebuttal or justification, I think that responding to these fears helps inform a practice owner's decision of whether to join. The fact is that dermatologists, and physicians as a group, have never truly had a unified voice or vision that allowed them to push back against the competing and conflicting interests of various stakeholders in medicine. Consolidation helps with that. Consider, for example, the small practice's inability to negotiate contracts with an insurance company. With scale and density, a consolidation brings more power to the table and allows for at least a dialog to occur, if not true negotiation. In addition, the scale of larger practices, with corporate leadership and support, forces cosmetic vendors to reconsider their pricing structure and support, making them more a partner in the success of a practice rather than just a supplier. When a practice with numerous locations dictates terms to an aesthetic company, the balance of power shifts in favor of the customer (the consolidation), which leads to greater innovation and competition.

Perhaps the greatest homegrown challenges to the survival of our specialty are the increased independence and practice scope of the midlevel provider. I say "homegrown" because midlevels are not inherently competitive or threatening to physicians. It is my belief that their prevalence and increasingly elevated stature in our specialty is our responsibility, or lack thereof to be exact. Many "supervising" dermatologists fail to properly supervise or provide a limited scope of practice to their midlevels, yet they speak of and regard their midlevels as highly as a board-certified dermatologist. Shouldn't we expect that midlevels, buffeted by our high regard, push for their own independence and equal footing?

Numerous reasons exist for the prevalence of the midlevel in our specialty. The profitability of a midlevel cannot be disputed; their lower compensation but oftentimes similar revenue generation to a physician leads to a greater margin for the practice owner. The prevalence and ease to hire also play a role. Hiring a new physician requires copious time, resources, and a hefty guaranteed income, as they build their practice over the first 1 to 2 years. Midlevels, on the other hand, are much easier to find and hire, especially in areas of the country that are less desirable for physicians. Finally, most states impose few restrictions on the scope of practice for a midlevel, allowing them full license to practice much like a physician.

13.3.1 The Sale

The first step in selling a practice is deciding on the right partner, or at least the concept of the right partner. Consolidations come in many flavors, and deciding which philosophy matches your own narrows the field of candidates and will save you much time and effort. I consider consolidations to be grouped as follows:

1. Toe-dippers: Many practice owners feel uncomfortable selling their entire practice, but realize the benefit of the administrative support and back office functionality of a consolidation. One business model of consolidation takes advantage of this by offering partial ownership; the practice owner sells only a fraction, usually a minority stake, to the consolidator, and in return is able to benefit from some, if not all, of the consolidator's management process and procedures. After the sale, the consolidator receives a percentage of the annual revenue, concomitant to the fraction of ownership. The benefits to the practice owner are obvious, such as access to the billing, marketing, human resources, and other resources. The benefit to the consolidator lies in the limited risk of a minority stake, and the ability to have access to, and learn about, the practice's performance over time. If, for example, the financial performance of the practice wanes after the partial

sale, the consolidator has limited its exposure and would not acquire additional ownership of the practice. Conversely, if the consolidator's resources and leadership add value to the practice, such that the financial performance improves, there would be greater probability on both sides for a full sale in the future. Therefore, a partial sale may benefit the consolidator more than the owner in terms of limiting downside risk and exposure to the performance of the practice over time. Despite this, many owners feel more comfortable "dipping their toe in the water" of consolidation in this fashion. I would hesitate to advise an owner to agree to this structure, primarily because of the imbalance of power in the relationship.

2. Grab baggers: This relates to the degree of operational integration a consolidator decides to accomplish with its practices. Full integration involves assimilating all practices on the same software (both practice management and electronic medical record [EMR]), centralizing billing, having a call center, distributing the corporate HR manual to all locations, etc. Essentially, all practices act as one, allowing the corporate management company to achieve all possible economies of scale. Partial operational integration is anything less than this, and I consider partially integrated consolidators as having a "grab bag" of practices. Theoretically, one would assume that all consolidation would involve full integration, since profitability derives from both growth and the avoidance of duplicative functions at the practice level. However, full integration requires an investment on behalf of the corporate team which many not pay off for years. The cost to build a call center, develop a billing team with revenue cycle management (i.e., minimizing accounts receivable), install layers of management, and build a cohesive marketing strategy along with human resource management of all the employees is tremendous. Indeed, while this integration needs to be accomplished while the consolidation is relatively small in order to support future growth, it absolutely squashes profitability until the corporate team achieves substantial growth in revenue.

Hence, partial integration allows for a corporate team to show profitability earlier, but may limit the profitability potential overall. As a practice owner, the partial integration could be appealing since your legacy processes, procedures, and even practice name and logo may go untouched after selling. However, I would urge you to consider the reason for selling; if the reason is to monetize and act as an employee, then partial ownership makes sense. On the other hand, if the reason is to both monetize and invest in the consolidation, then the question is why would you invest in a company whose strategy literally limits profitability in the long term?

3. Going whole hog—the term I use for a fully integrated consolidation—usually attracts practice owners interested in investing in the parent company and playing an active role in its success. It requires patience on behalf of the private equity investors, keen oversight on behalf of the board of directors to ensure the corporate leadership exhibits careful investment in key people, technology and equipment, and willingness on behalf of the practices to undergo the changes necessary to achieve this goal. The short-term pain endured by all parties hopefully pays off in smoother practice operations (which translates to better patient care), quick installation of best practices, and, ultimately, higher profitability.

After deciding on which consolidator(s) you would like to work with, the next step in selling is getting to a Letter of Intent (LOI).

13.3.2 LOI

The process that culminates in an LOI involves a varying degree of diligence by the consolidator. Some dive deeply into the financial data, usually asking for trailing twelve-month (TTM) financials as well as year-end financial statements for the previous 2 to 3 years. Assessing profitability of the practice allows the consolidator to determine the EBIT-DA (earnings before interest, taxes, depreciation, and amortization), a multiple of which comprises the valuation of the practice and what will be stated in the LOI.

Most practice owners pay themselves a salary and take net earnings/income as a distribution or further regular income. Consolidators, however,

pay providers based on a percentage of collections, meaning providers receive a percentage of the top line (revenue) of the income statement, and cease to benefit from the net earnings (bottom line of the income statement), which now belongs to the consolidator. This incentivizes both parties correctly; the provider to maximize revenue based on their capacity, and the consolidator to both assist the provider in maximizing revenue (through marketing, clinic support systems, etc.) and control costs in order to maximize its own profits.

Since a provider will be transitioned to this new compensation model after joining the consolidator, the analysts will take the financial data and "normalize" it, meaning that they will simulate a provider's income as if they were already on the new compensation model. In addition, analysts will look for "add backs," or expenses that could be considered either one-time extraordinary (e.g., laser purchase), or duplicative to the efforts of the consolidator, such as billing and marketing personnel labor costs, unless these workers are absolutely essential to the running of the practice. This process usually requires quite a bit of communication between the analysts and practice owner to both ensure correct understanding of expenses and, ultimately, deliver an LOI with a valid EBIT-DA value.

13.3.3 Papering the Deal

Upon receiving the LOI, the practice owner now has a choice to make: either agree with the valuation and sign or walk away. Signing does not bind the owner to a sale of the practice; rather, he or she enters into a "silent" period during which he or she agrees to:

1. Not share the LOI with any other Consolidator.
2. Not enter into any negotiation or process with another consolidator.
3. Proceed with good faith into the next step of diligence.

This next phase of diligence requires a hefty investment on the part of the consolidator, thus the requirements mentioned above. Third-party consultants and analysts are usually hired to not only perform documentation and billing audits of a sampling of charts but also prepare compliance audit of human resources, OSHA, and HIPAA processes and procedures within the practice. Some will hire companies to contact referring physicians in order to better understand the practice's (and providers') reputations in the area. Finally, an accounting firm may be retained to further analyze the financial performance of the practice and ensure that the EBIT-DA included in the LOI is absolutely correct.

Once all this has been completed, which requires months, and the consolidator and practice owner are comfortable with results and valuation, the two sides would agree to "paper the deal." Both sides retain attorneys to negotiate employment agreements and sale documents which are voluminous. The percentage of the proceeds of the sale that the practice owner wishes to invest back into the consolidator is determined at this stage as well. Consolidators require a minimum percentage investment from practice owners and may allow other providers to invest as well. Indeed, consolidators encourage investment, because not only does it show confidence in the viability of the new company but also minimizes the risk of losing providers postsale. Finally, investing in the consolidation requires providers to act as employees and owners, meaning they have the best interest of the corporation alongside their own.

13.3.4 Life after the Sale

Practice employees experience a high level of anxiety during and after a sale of their practice, but communication is the key to pacifying these concerns and allowing the practice to continue to perform successfully. Changes are not made on the first day after a sale, but are incorporated slowly and thoughtfully. Perhaps the most stressful is the transition to the consolidator's EMR and practice management (PM) system. The bridging of data, learning new software, and changing standard operating procedures, as required by the new systems, engenders stress and requires flexibility. I have learned that the process tests the leadership abilities of the office manager (OM)— those who have these abilities flourish and the office will transition smoothly, culminating with an even stronger OM leader and partner with the corporate team.

The first changes likely to be made involve human resources. Implementation of the consolidator's HR manual, with its policies and procedures, along with transitioning to new (and usually more generous) health insurance and retirement plans, requires employee information

sessions and trainings. These are usually welcomed by smaller practices that have never had the wherewithal to develop a full complement of policies and procedures, not to mention a full benefits portfolio.

After HR changes, come operational modifications. While every operator differs in terms of the degree of operational integration, expect at least software changes and possibly phone system changes. Most will also centralize marketing and billing after the software changes. In parallel, depending on the assets of the consolidator, efforts will quickly begin to internally capture the practice's Mohs referrals and dermatopathology. While the initial HR changes primarily benefit the employees, these operational changes truly benefit the patient. For example, internalized Mohs and dermatopathology allows for greater communication and transparency between providers, which enhances patient safety and care. A larger group also allows providers to develop referral specialty clinics based on their interests, such as contact dermatitis, hair disorders, pigmented lesions, or autoimmune diseases, another way that patients benefit.

The importance of marketing cannot be understated. After acquiring a practice, in order to justify the multiple paid, and achieve a return on the investment, the consolidator must increase revenue in the practice. While this is important for the management team, it is equally so for the providers, especially for those practices with open schedules or the desire to build a cosmetic practice. In fact, some consider that the primary purpose of the operator is to market the practices, ensuring that everyone is busy and maximizing their own incomes. I think most experienced practice owners agree with the importance, and difficulty, of marketing. Handing that function over to a consolidator relieves much pressure from the (former) practice owner's shoulders.

13.3.5 What's Next

As with any equity investment, the desire and expectation is that the value of your stock grows or stays stable with an annual dividend. The same holds true with an investment in a consolidation. As an owner and employee, the former practice owner has the dual incentive to maximize his/her own income while maximizing the value of the investment. This incentivizes many to get involved in business development, leading them to approach their friends and colleagues about joining their consolidation.

After (hopefully) 3 to 5 years of growth, the private equity investors will need to realize a return. The corporate team will start looking for strategic partners either in terms of a larger private equity investor or a larger consolidator. Many providers convey a lot of trepidation about this step, since they will likely become a part of a much larger organization and have to deal with possible changes in the corporate team and structure.

My response to this is the same as my response to every concern about administrative changes in a consolidation: providers are the absolute most important members of the organization. Without them, the revenue vanishes and operation ceases. The corporate team of any consolidation recognizes this. Your value is never higher than as a busy provider in a well-run consolidation!

Section II

Human Resources

II

14 Essential Components of an Employee Manual

Cynthia Forbush BA, SPHR

Abstract

An employee handbook serves multiple purposes: from setting expectations for new employees to showcasing company culture and values, meeting legal requirements, and providing a way to keep all of this important information in one place. Providing a consistent message to your team, a well-written handbook becomes a go-to resource for all employees on a wide range of topics including practical details like company policies, benefits, pay practices, and legal notices. Take the opportunity to create an employee handbook and it will be time well spent.

Keywords: handbook template, legal notices, company culture, acknowledgment of receipt

Top 10 Things You Need to Know

1. Yes, you need a handbook. The handbook is your forum for outlining your business' rules, policies, and expectations for employees, as well as letting the employees know what they can expect from you.
2. Use clear and simple language so there is no confusion about your message.
3. Federal notifications: Many federal laws require employee notification, which must be in writing for legal purposes, and the manual is the perfect place to go about doing this.
4. State notifications: Some states have additional laws that must be disseminated among employees.
5. Employee policies: Remember that these are adults who want to do a good job and you hired them for a reason. Make sure your policies are positive and not punitive. Instead of defining "tardy," state that employees are expected to show up on time. Give leaders flexibility in terms of dealing with specific situations that arise.
6. Benefits: Get your employees excited about what you offer.
7. Legal review is a must! An employment attorney should review and approve the handbook prior to publishing.
8. Accessibility: The handbook must be accessible to all employees in a format that is easy to use.
9. Keep it current: Review and update the handbook once a year or when a new law is passed that requires employee notification, whichever comes first.
10. Acknowledgment of receipt: Ask employees to sign a form saying they've read the handbook and agree to the terms upon hire, and each time the handbook is updated.

14.1 Introduction

You are busy running your business and it's paying off. Your client base is growing, you have reliable staff that is happy at work, and you are even thinking of adding another provider or two. You've done all of this without getting bogged down by paperwork and you're grateful for that. So why should you spend time putting together an employee handbook? After all, your employees are happy without it.

Even though there are no legal requirements to have an employee handbook in place, all businesses should employ one as a tool for both employers and employees. The truth is that it's never too early to start writing down your policies and values. As your business grows, it'll help you stay consistent and organized, and everyone will be on the same page. Whether you decide to spend more time focusing on your company's culture, policies, or both, getting it all down in writing is always a good idea. Instead of viewing it as a chore, the best way to view the entire handbook process is as an *opportunity*. This is your opportunity to get your message across to every employee in the practice.

An employee handbook has important legal purposes, which include avoiding liability and satisfying legal requirements set by federal and state laws. A well-written handbook provides legal protection for both your company and your employees, and can protect you against employee claims. By communicating relevant information about federal and state laws in writing, you show that your business understands and complies with these regulations. For example, if an employee is let go, having an at-will policy clearly documented in the handbook can help show your company was legally in the right. Communicating workplace policies and expectations clearly will help to avoid conflicts, and if they do arise, resolve them as efficiently as possible.

Writing an employee handbook is quite an undertaking. It is more than just a guide to your company policies and procedures—it's also an introduction to your history, values, and culture. Your handbook sets the tone for your management style, outlines workplace expectations, and provides essential information about working for your practice. In this chapter, we walk you through what an employee handbook looks like, offer tips on how to write one, and give you an idea of what to include.

Do Employees Actually Read the Handbook? According to a 2014 survey[a]:

- Almost half of workers between the ages of 18 and 29 or "millenials" didn't read their handbook.
- 11% didn't open it at all.
- 36% didn't know where to find it.
- 86% believe benefits play a significant role in choosing to stay with an employer.
- 56% don't fully understand their benefit options listed in the manual.

Personal Anecdote

Writing or editing an employee manual is not the most exciting task, but it is an important one. The worst type of manual is long and wordy, with lots of legal language and is not well organized. The best ones are interesting, entertaining, informative, easy to understand, and well organized. I've written both kinds.

In my early days as an HR professional, I was tasked with writing the first official employee manual for a 200-person company. I jumped right in and gathered everything I could possibly think of. I thought that legal wording was the best choice because it was "official," and I thought it important to include every detail of every policy, benefit, etc. When the very long, detailed handbook was complete, I had it bound and handed out copies—paper was still the publishing method of choice at the time. Eventually I collected an acknowledgment from every employee and filed them away for safekeeping.

Not long after the manual distribution, I realized that most employees didn't read the manual, nor did they use it for a reference when they had questions. I was still receiving the same volume of questions on the same topics which I had so meticulously described in the new manual. I didn't mind answering employees' questions—in fact I enjoyed it—but this company operated 24/7, so it meant that employees who really needed an answer couldn't always get it in a timely manner. And those who wanted to figure things out on their own were faced with deciphering a challenging resource. This manual also did not reflect our culture, which was quite casual and friendly. Technically, this manual got the job done, but that's about all it did.

Skipping ahead to the most recent employee manual I compiled, which was assisted by lessons learned over the years as well as advances in technology, it is lightyears beyond my original attempt. I learned to be discerning about when to use legal terminology—only when specifically required by law—and use simple, straightforward, easy-to-understand wording whenever possible. The manual, now an electronic version, includes hyperlinks from the Table of Contents to each topic listed, making it easy for employees to find their answers. This company is also casual, and possesses a clear mission and values, so I took that into account when writing.

In addition to the required policies, employees will find a message encouraging employee interaction with peers, leaders, and physicians both within and outside an employee's team, and informing them of the availability of both leaders and human resources personnel for clarification on anything without hesitation; all of this along with friendly tips. It is still a work in progress. My goal is to make the leap from a standard employee manual to a form of culture book. As our culture falls somewhere between casual and professional, it will be carefully crafted, including real-life anecdotes from our team laced with some humor. I'm looking forward to the day I get to distribute that culture book and receive feedback from employees who read it from cover to cover voluntarily.

---

[a] Date from GuideSpark, 2014

Based on the data above, creating a manual that employees will actually read can prove to be a challenge. In answer to this challenge, and to make the most of this time-consuming undertaking, an increasing number of companies are going beyond the standard approach to handbook writing and turning the old fashioned handbook into a clear articulation of the company's vision and culture, with some style thrown in for good measure. If this is done correctly, it will help your new employees feel like part of the team and may even become a recruiting tool. Whether you want to improve your existing handbook or need to develop one from scratch; whether you want to have a handbook that just covers the basic requirements or one that contains a more personal touch, you can use this outline to simplify the process.

In this chapter, we'll follow a step-by-step process to create a handbook from scratch. We'll talk about the different aspects of assembling a handbook, including the basics such as legal requirements, company policies, and expectations for employees, as well as focusing on how to get the most out of it by showcasing one's unique company culture. When it is complete, you will have a handbook that creates an accurate impression of your company and communicates expectations as clearly as possible.

this is your opportunity to send a message to everyone in your practice, so take advantage of it. What can you include that is unique to your organization? How can you show off your branding and company culture? Do you have core values or a greater purpose that you want to communicate? These messages should be spread across the manual not only highlighting your company culture but also helping your new employees feel like part of the team.

> **Tip[b]**
>
> Even the little details, such as tips for the onboarding process or a letter from the president of the company, make your handbook so much more personal. Every company has a section dedicated to required legal policies. Not every company has a section about in-house traditions or volunteer causes. Some handbooks stick to text while others include images and illustrations to get their ideas across. Even if your brand is more reserved, you can still get the message across. You just have to be you. Every employee will receive your handbook, so if you create something that's a great resource and successfully conveys your employer brand, you have a better shot at fostering a great culture.

14.2 Step One: Why Are You Doing This?

The first step in this process is to decide why you're creating this handbook. Take a moment to consider the following:
- Is it just to cover your practice legally or do you want to get more out of it?
- Should it serve as a guide to your new employees as they acclimatize to your culture?
- Should it be a visual example of your branding? Possibly even serve as a recruiting tool?

Keep your answers to these questions in mind as we go through the process; they will serve as a guide to creating the employee manual that works for you.

14.3 Step Two: Who Are You?

The next step, before putting any words to paper, is to think about who you are. Regardless of the reasons as to why you are creating this handbook,

14.4 Step Three: Gather Your Policies

Now that you've put in some thought about what your handbook will look like, it's time to gather your unique company policies which will go in it. Spend time in scanning the work environment for common practices that are currently in place. If there are no policies in place, they should be developed. Once you have updated the policies and formalized the common practices, have legal counsel review them. These policies, as well as those mandated by federal and state governments, will take up a large portion of the employee manual. Employment laws can be complicated and vary in accordance with business type and location. As an employer, it's critical that you understand your obligations, and the proper legal counsel will assist you with this.

---

[b] Company policies should focus on what employees SHOULD do, and not what they can't do.

14.5 Step Four: Choosing a Template

There is no need to create an employee handbook template from scratch when there are so many websites that provide well-organized templates free of charge. Rocketlawyer, NFIB legal foundation, and Society for Human Resource Management (SHRM) are companies that offer this resource. These templates typically include an outline of suggested items for inclusion in the employee handbook and options for a basic template (free) or a customized version (for a fee). Choose one that works for you and edit based on your business needs.

14.6 Step Five: Creating a Welcome Message

Once you have chosen your template, the next step involves creating a welcome message. Every employee in your practice will view this message, so take this opportunity to make the right impression. For new employees, this is an introduction to the company, and employees are more likely to become productive, faster when they feel welcomed and accepted. Use this forum to your advantage by formally welcoming new employees to your team, creating a sense of community, and building a foundation for a positive employee relationship. For current employees, this message should be a confirmation of what they already know.

Here is a generic example of a Welcome Message:

Welcome to _____ !

On behalf of your colleagues, I welcome you to _ (company name) _ and wish you every success here.

We believe that each employee contributes directly to _ (company name)'s_ growth and success, and we hope you will take pride in being a member of our team. _(Company name) _ takes special interest in the well-being of everyone in its community. The policies, benefits, and services available to eligible employees, as well as the expectations of our employees, described in this manual reflect that concern. Please familiarize yourself with the contents of the employee handbook as soon as possible for it will answer many questions about employment with _ (company name) _. Feel free to discuss any questions you have regarding this manual, or any policy, with your supervisor or the human resources department.

We hope that your experience here will be challenging, meaningful, and rewarding. Again, welcome!

Sincerely,
President and CEO

14.7 Step Six: Table of Contents

While an employee handbook cannot possibly include everything, it does need to contain a wide range of information. A good rule of thumb is that to be effective, the handbook should include a high-level overview of everything a new employee should know in simple and clear language, and laid out in a format that makes sense, with a Table of Contents that makes the information easy to find.

By clearly setting out company policies, employee handbooks can help promote a positive, productive, and safe work environment, thereby avoiding improper and unlawful conduct. As a result, the handbook can help to protect the company from sexual harassment, wrongful termination, and discrimination lawsuits, and can help you should you ever need to defend a lawsuit.

As we move through the meat of the handbook, keep in mind that everything you write should reinforce one or more of the following:
- Smoother assimilation for new hires.
- Legal protection for your company and employees.
- Demonstrated compliance with state laws.
- A sense of community.

The challenge will involve including all required policies and procedures without losing the personal touch. Think *Welcome, Communicate, Inform*…You can do this!

14.8 Step Seven: Handbook Topic Selection

What follows is a list of suggested topics for the Table of Contents, which are broken down by like subjects. Those marked with an asterisk (*) are required. The rest are optional and it is up to you to pick and choose which to apply to your practice. This is not a complete list and you should consult an employment attorney when making your selections.
- **Company history, vision, mission, and values:** As mentioned already, this warrants repeating, think of it as telling your new employees *what* you do as well as *how* and *why* you do it.

Include a brief history of the company's origins, founder, current leader, and details that are important to the company's legacy.

- **Employment information and required notices**: This list will vary depending on the size and location of your practice. Important factors to consider are legal mandates for federal and state laws that affect employees, such as the Family and Medical Leave Act (FMLA)*, Consolidated Omnibus Budget Reconciliation Act (COBRA)*, and the Fair Labor Standards Act (FLSA)*. Depending on your business and where it is located, you may have additional legally required written policies, such as anti-harassment* for California employers and the Pregnant Workers' Protection Act* for those in Massachusetts. The notices listed here generally need to be in writing for legal reasons and should therefore be placed in the handbook, so everything is conveniently located in one place. If an employer fails to communicate these in the employee handbook, there may be confusion and noncompliance with the laws.
- **At-will employment*, equal employment opportunity (EEOC)*, reasonable accommodation (ADA)*:** As a form of legal protection, your handbook should state that everyone who works for you is an at-will employee, which means the relationship can be ended at any time, without notice or reason, by either party. This section should also state that your business is an equal opportunity employee and that you will provide reasonable accommodation for employees that require it.
- **Harassment and discrimination:** Policy*, Reporting Procedure*, and Investigation Process.*
- **Employer-specific employment-related policies:** Employment Eligibility, Open Door, Employment of Relatives, Access to Personnel Records, Standard Operating Hours, and other employee-specific, employment-related policies should be grouped together.
- **Attendance:** Attendance Policy, Employee Classification Definitions—Full-time, Part-time, Exempt, and Nonexempt, and other attendance-related polices such as Emergency closings, Business hours, Overtime, and Telecommuting.
- **Workplace expectations:** This section outlines expectations for employee conduct and workplace behavior in the form of Code of

Conduct and Business Ethics. It may include items like health and safety, dress code, drugs and alcohol, workplace violence, conflicts of interest, business travel, use of company property, weapons at work, workplace visitors, and other relevant topics such as Health Insurance Portability and Accountability Act (HIPAA).*
- **Payroll:** Pay schedule, start and end of payroll workweek, recording time worked, overtime eligibility, and meal and rest periods.
- **Eligibility, benefit descriptions, COBRA (if COBRA applies to your practice, this is a required notification for every new employee), Unemployment compensation, and Workers' compensation.**[c]

This section will be very important for your employees. It is here that you fill them in on the basics of your time off policies, insurance programs, retirement plans, and other benefits, and get them excited about the perks you offer. This section should include a *high-level overview* of all the benefits offered by your practice.

> **Tip**
>
> *Instead of listing benefit details in your employee handbook, create a separate benefits booklet with details such as employee premiums, copays, and other detailed information. This will save yourself from having to update your handbook every year as your benefits change.

- **Performance and expectations:** Explain what is expected of your employees, how your management team measures success, when performance reviews take place, and anything else related to ongoing performance assessment. Regular performance reviews allow you to optimize productivity by ensuring your star employees are motivated to shine, and it also allows you to document poor performance should an employee need to be let go in the future.
- **Acknowledgment clause:** At the end of your handbook, include an acknowledgment of the receipt page that every new hire needs

---

[c] People often don't think of these employee protections as benefits, but as an employer you pay for them, so take the credit!

to sign. By signing their names, the employees acknowledge that they have received and read the handbook, agreed to the employment terms, are aware of and understand the policies, and have availed of the opportunity to ask follow-up questions. Keep this important document in the employee's file.

A sample acknowledgment of receipt is as follows:

ACKNOWLEDGMENT OF RECEIPT OF HANDBOOK

1. I have received and read the _(company name)_ Employee Handbook. I understand that human resources will answer any questions I may have regarding the contents of the handbook.

2. I understand that the policies contained in the handbook are intended for information and guidance only, and may be unilaterally changed or amended by _(company name)_ without notice. I understand that the handbook does not make any promises or guarantees.

3. I further understand that the handbook does not create a contract of employment, but rather my employment with _ (company name) _ is on an at-will basis. As such, I am free to resign and _ (company name) _ may terminate my employment at any time, for any reason or no reason at all, with or without notice. My at-will status may only be modified by a written contract of employment signed by the _ (title, ex. COO) _ stating a specific term of employment. No verbal or written statements by

any other representative of the company shall alter my at-will status.

_____   _____
Employee Name (Print)   Employee Signature/Date

14.9 Step Eight: You're Done!

Almost… After you've written your employee handbook, you need to publish it in a format that every employee can easily access. Most businesses save their employee handbook as a PDF and/or have it available on their company intranet. This is typically the easiest way; just remember to make physical copies available to employees without access to the Internet or as per employee request.

14.10 Step Nine: Updates

It's imperative to create a system to save past versions of your handbook and record the dates of all updates. You may need to refer to these materials in the event of litigation.

Suggested Readings

HR daily advisor. hrdailyadvisor.blr.com
SHRM. www.shrm.org
US Department of Labor. www.dol.gov

15 Vision and Mission Statement

Heather Hamilton MD, Jeffrey S. Dover MD, FRCPC

Abstract

This chapter delves into the vision and mission statements for your practice. We discuss what they are, why you need them, and how to write them. Examples are included. We also discuss how they may change over time.

Keywords: vision statement, mission statement

> ### Top 10 Things You Need to Know
>
> 1. A vision statement says what the practice wants to be like in many years' time.
> 2. A mission statement says what the practice aims to do now and in the near future.
> 3. Vision and mission statements help practices make decisions.
> 4. Having a mission statement in place allows employees to measure how their work moves the practice closer to achieving the practice's mission.
> 5. Vision and mission statements are personal and should reflect the desires, ethics, and values of the practice.
> 6. Your mission statement should reflect your practice's style and what your practice represents.
> 7. A mission statement is not fixed; it can and should be changed as your practice changes.
> 8. Be bold.
> 9. Be personal.
> 10. Just like you would never start a practice without a business plan, a mission statement is essential to every practice.

15.1 Introduction

Nearing the end of the long road of education, you are suddenly in the job market, looking to join a practice or go out on your own. Your roadmap up to this point was fairly straightforward with few variables. You may not have considered all the possibilities for the posttraining world. Alternatively, you may have been out in practice for a while and are considering opening your own practice or moving to a different practice. Perhaps you have pondered a lot about what you envision, particularly if you have been in practice for some time.

The objective of this chapter is to help you formulate a vision and mission statement for your practice. This chapter focuses on private practice; entering into academics, a worthy pursuit, is beyond the scope of this chapter.

15.2 What Are Vision and Mission Statements?

Vision and mission statements are personal and should reflect the desires, ethics, and values of the practice. One might ask, "what is the difference between a vision statement and a mission statement?" Given the lack of business education in medical school, it is no surprise that many of us do not know. Graham Kenny wrote in a 2014 *Harvard Business Review* article: "A **vision statement** says what the organization wishes to be like in some years' time. It's usually drawn up by senior management in an effort to take the thinking beyond day-to-day activity in a clear, memorable way."[1] For instance, Apple's vision statement is, "we believe that we are on the face of the earth to make great products and that's not changing. We are constantly focusing on innovating. We believe in the simple not the complex. We believe that we need to own and control the primary technologies behind the products that we make, and participate only in markets where we can make a significant contribution. We believe in saying no to thousands of projects, so that we can really focus on the few that are truly important and meaningful to us. We believe in deep collaboration and cross-pollination of our groups, which allow us to innovate in a way that others cannot. And frankly, we don't settle for anything less than excellence in every group in the company, and we have the self-honesty to admit when we're wrong and the courage to change. And I think regardless of who is in what job, those values are so embedded in this company that Apple will do extremely well."[2]

Graham Kelley goes on to say, "the **mission [statement]** describes what business the organization is in (and what it isn't) both now and projecting into the future. Its aim is to provide focus for management and staff. A consulting firm might define its mission by the type of work it does, the clients it caters to, and the level of service it provides. For example: "we're in the business of providing high-standard assistance on performance assessment to middle to senior managers in medium-to-large firms in the finance industry."[1] Apple's current mission statement is: "Apple designs Macs, the best personal computers in the world, along with OS X, iLife, iWork, and professional software. Apple leads the digital music revolution with its iPods and iTunes online store. Apple has reinvented the mobile phone with its revolutionary iPhone and App store, and is defining the future of mobile media and computing devices with iPad."[2] Dermatology practices might wish to have both a vision and a mission statement or perhaps only a mission statement.

15.3 Why Do You Need a Vision and/or Mission Statement?

First, vision and mission statements help practices make decisions. For example, if you are considering buying the latest laser and your mission statement is to offer cutting-edge technology, then you should seriously consider buying it. If your mission statement does not include offering cutting-edge technology, then you may not need to purchase it. Second, having a mission statement in place allows employees to measure how their work moves the practice closer to achieving the practice's mission. Every new employee should learn it and let it guide what they do.

15.4 How Do You Write a Vision Statement?

As discussed above, a vision statement is more forward looking, that is, where you see your practice in several years. Your day-to-day mission will be to provide excellent patient care, but where do you envision your practice to be in 5 to 10 years and how might your practice contribute to the advancement of the field of dermatology? If you plan on participating in clinical studies, and research & development initiatives, your vision statement should include that goal. If you plan on incorporating the latest technology and treatments into the practice, then your vision statement should include that goal. The vision statement may discuss how you want to contribute to the science of dermatology, art of patient care, and education of your community and peers.

15.5 Examples of Vision Statements

"The Vision of Art of Skin MD is to shape beauty as the preeminent leader, patient partner, and passionate educator in dermatology and cosmetic surgery."[3]

"Windsor Dermatology will be a model practice which promotes outstanding patient care and advances medical knowledge while enriching the lives of its employees and the surrounding community."[4]

15.6 How Do You Write a Mission Statement?

Before putting a pen to paper, you have to decide what style you want your practice to be and what your practice represents. Keywords and phrases may include kind, warm, family style or new age, edgy, modern, young vibe, efficient, new technology, or cutting edge. More examples include safety-focused, ethical, high-quality, and patient-focused. It probably goes without saying, but examples of words and phrases not to be included are expensive and highly profitable.

Do you specialize in a specific demographic? If so, include this in the mission statement, e.g., women, families, and pediatrics. If not, then you may wish to include that by saying you treat all patients from pediatrics to geriatrics, and everyone in between.

15.7 Examples of Mission Statements

"Our mission is to deliver personalized service along with ethical, skilled, and comprehensive care."[5]

"The Mission of Art of Skin MD is to be a full-spectrum dermatology and cosmetic surgery center, delivering natural, comprehensive and groundbreaking solutions to patients in a safe, caring, and state-of-the-art environment."[3]

"The Johnson Dermatology Clinic strives to deliver efficient, quality, compassionate, comprehensive, patient-centered skin care. We endeavor to provide a team-oriented, productive work environment. We strive to be a responsible corporate citizen and contributing member of the community through education and service."[6]

- To provide the best medical dermatology and cosmetic treatment available not only in NWA but in the country.
- To provide a friendly, caring, and professional office environment.
- To treat each patient as we would want to be treated.
- "To provide exceptional service and conduct ourselves with integrity."[7]

15.8 Should a Mission Statement Change with Time?

A mission statement is not fixed; it can and should be changed as your practice changes. You will probably want to reassess the statement every 5 years or whenever the practice changes significantly. Your core principles/purpose/values, however, should remain the same.

A mission statement should be communicated to employees during the hiring process. You want to make sure prospective employees can commit to carrying out the practice's mission statement. It can also be used as part of employee evaluations to highlight what they are doing well and how they can improve. A mission statement can also be communicated to patients through a variety of ways including the practice's website, social media, electronic and written correspondence, and on the phone through hold messages.

Words to consider in a mission statement	
Include	**Don't include**
Kind	Expensive
Warm	Making a lot of money
Family style	
Modern	
Efficient	
Cutting-edge	
Safety-focused	
High-quality	
Ethical	
Patient-focused	

15.9 Conclusion

Vision and mission statements are what your practice strives to achieve. While not written in stone, they help guide you and your employees in providing optimal care to patients. The statements provide current and prospective patients an idea of what type of care to expect. With that in mind, physicians should put some thought into crafting these statements and we hope this chapter helps with their formulation.

References

[1] Kenny G. Your Company's Purpose Is Not Its Vision, Mission, Or Values. Harvard Business Review. Available at: https://hbr.org/2014/09/your-companys-purpose-is-not-its-vision-mission-or-values. Accessed January 20, 2019

[2] Rowland C. Apple Inc.'s Mission Statement and Vision Statement (An Analysis). Available at: http://panmore.com/apple-mission-statement-vision-statement. Accessed January 20, 2019

[3] Art of Skin MD. Available at: https://artofskinmd.com/about/values/. Accessed January 19, 2019

[4] Windsor Dermatology. Available at: http://www.windsordermatology.com/mission-statement/. Accessed January 19, 2019

[5] SkinCare Physicians. Available at: https://www.skincarephysicians.net. Accessed January 19, 2019

[6] Johnson Dermatology. Available at: https://johnsondermatology.com/about/. Accessed January 19, 2019

[7] Premier Dermatology. Available at: http://www.premierderm.net/about-us/mission-statement/. Accessed January 19, 2019

16 Employees versus Independent Contractors

George J. Hruza MD, MBA; Gabriel J. Martinez-Diaz MD, FAAD; Kyle Kieffer BA; Briana Paiewonsky BS, MS2

Abstract

Working as an independent contractor may not be ideal for every dermatologist. You must reflect on your goals, values, and practice style to determine whether pursuing work as an independent contractor will suit you. If you like the idea of possessing more autonomy and ability to move from various contracts, and being separate from office policies and procedures, this may be a fitting route of employment. However, this position also comes with less job security, an obligation to file your own quarterly taxes, and a responsibility to obtain the benefits you would ordinarily gain through an employee–employer relationship. Consider conversing with your mentors and physician peers to gain insight into their experiences before making your decision. There is opportunity to learn from each type of work you pursue and there is certainly time to alter your course of employment if need be.

Keywords: independent contractor, employee, self-employment tax, internal revenue service, autonomy, 20-factor test, employee–employer relationship, payer, compensation, benefits

Top 10 Things You Need to Know

1. As an independent contractor, you will be responsible for your own benefits traditionally reserved for employees. These include self-employment tax, health, dental, vision, life, disability and malpractice insurance, as well as a retirement plan. As an employee, you will have some or all of these benefits provided by the employer.
2. As an independent contractor, you will not have paid vacation or paid time off (PTO) provided by the employer. Of course, vacation and PTO are moot for an employee if one is paid purely on the basis of productivity.
3. As an employee, one possesses more job security and legal protections which are not necessarily afforded to independent contractors.
4. As an independent contractor, you will typically enjoy more physician autonomy with fewer repercussions if your way of practicing is different from the employer's methods.
5. As an employee, you will have some of your professional expenses, such as malpractice insurance, medical staff dues, professional society dues, and continuing medical education (CME) expenses, paid by your employer. However, any expenses above the employer allowance will not be deductible. As an independent contractor, you can deduct such expenses as business expenses.
6. The Internal Revenue Service (IRS) 20-question statutory employee status versus independent contractor needs to be considered. If an independent contractor is determined to be a statutory employee, the employer may be subject to back taxes, interest, and penalties.
7. Covenants to not compete in jurisdictions where it is legal and upheld by the courts should be as limited as possible in distance and time. A straightforward financial payment instead of an injunction is preferred.
8. An independent contractor is required to pay estimated taxes quarterly, including self-employment tax (both the employee and employer parts of social security and Medicare taxes).
9. Disagreements between independent contractors and practice owners are settled based on breach of contract arguments.
10. In either an independent contractor or employed situation, compensation is usually productivity-based (percentage of net collections). An employed physician may also have a minimum income guarantee for 1 to 2 years.

16.1 Introduction

The dermatology practice landscape is changing with rapid consolidation and various practice models coming to the fore. Fortunately, there is a great demand for the services of those residents who are finishing their residency, allowing them to choose among multiple practice settings. After finishing my (GJMD) residency in July 2014 at the University of Pittsburgh Medical Center, I pursued employment at a private dermatology practice in the metropolitan Atlanta area. I chose to work for a private practice rather than in a hospital environment in an effort to maintain my newfound physician autonomy and make decisions based on my idea of best patient-care practices rather than hospital policy. However, I quickly discovered that, at this particular private practice, I was not given the opportunity to express my honest medical opinion about my patients' care without resistance from the owners and practice management. I was pressured to perform a certain number of biopsies and procedures per patient encounter, whether indicated or not. In addition, I was required to refer patients to the most senior dermatologist for Mohs micrographic surgery, regardless of whether or not I felt it was the best option for the patient. All aspects of my first employment opportunity were controlled by the practice administrator and after one year of experiencing the inability to control and direct my own work, I decided to pursue an opportunity in the metropolitan Chicago area at another private dermatology practice. Unfortunately, I left this practice after 10 months of dissatisfaction due to similar issues. This experience allowed me the opportunity to self-reflect and recognize that the autonomy I valued at the start of my medical career had been compromised. I decided to use my exit from the Chicago practice as an entrance into entrepreneurship as an independent contractor.

Such negative employment situations are not necessarily reflective of other practice settings. In my (GJH) case, I joined the Washington University in St. Louis as an employee and found my 11 years there to be free of interference in my clinical decision-making, allowing me to practice so as to provide optimal care to my patients as a Mohs surgeon. I then built up a very successful private solo practice that I ran for 17 years. Three years ago, I joined a private equity-backed dermatology group where I have been able to continue to take care of my patients without interference from my employer. The decision about whether to become an employed physician, independent contractor, or owner of your own practice is a very personal one and relates to one's risk tolerance and need for autonomy.

16.2 Step One: What Exactly Is an Independent Contractor?

An independent contractor is defined by the IRS, as a situation in which the payor has the right to control or direct only the *result* of the work and not what will be done or how it will be done.[1] In dermatology, it means that the practice management at the practice one works in cannot tell you which lesion you biopsy, how long you freeze an actinic keratoses, or what medication you prescribe to your patients. Of course, very few employers would do that to an employed physician. They hire you because of the training you have as a board-certified dermatologist.

Because of the desire of employers to preferentially designate their workers as independent contractors in order to save on taxes and fringe benefits, the IRS has developed a detailed process to determine if a worker is an independent contractor or a statutory employee, with the main thrust to reclassify independent contractors to employee status. If the IRS reclassifies an independent contractor to a statutory employee, the employer becomes subject to significant back taxes, interest, and penalties. The "nannygate" scandal also derailed some promising politicians' careers due to such reclassification.

The IRS defines an independent contractor based on three categories or rules regarding the relationship of the worker with the payer. The first rule is based on behavioral control the employer exercises over the worker such as training, instruction, and hours worked. Dermatologists come equipped with all the knowledge and training required to perform their job and usually work until the job is done, not based on exact hours, so that they could qualify as independent contractors based on this rule. The second rule investigates the degree to which the company exercises control over the business aspects of the work performed. This could trip up an independent contractor if the employer reimburses certain expenses such as malpractice insurance and provides tools such as lasers or even supplies such as sutures necessary to perform the job. The third rule looks at whether employee type benefits such as retirement plans or health insurance are provided to the worker.

If that were not adequate, the IRS has developed a 20-factor yes/no test with detailed criteria to discern the difference between an employee and independent contractor. To further muddy the waters, it is not clear how many yes answers will lead to the switch from independent contractor to employee. If after looking through all this, one is still not certain if they qualify for independent contractor status, one can file an IRS SS-8 form to be sent to the IRS in order to determine one's employment categorization on an individual basis. As the risk rests primarily with the employer, they should be the ones to send such a form in.

As a practical matter, if you work for more than one practice, in more than one practice setting, or part-time (especially to fill in), you can qualify as an independent contractor. If you work full-time for only one practice, then you are at some risk of being reclassified by the IRS as an employee.

16.3 Step Two: Deciding If Becoming an Independent Contractor Is the Right Step for You

Employment in medicine is shifting as fewer physicians are now owning their own practices. Physician employment by physician-owned practices now only make up 47.1% of all practicing physicians. We also see that independent contractors in medicine are on the rise. According to the 2016 American Medical Association Physician Practice Benchmark Survey, the distribution of independent contractors among physicians is 5.9% compared to 5.0% in 2012.[2]

16.3.1 Things to Consider When Choosing between Employment or Becoming an Independent Contractor

- First and foremost, consider how much autonomy and self-direction you would like to have. Would you like to follow established practice regulations or create your own guidelines? As an employee, I (GJMD) experienced restrictive employer–employee contracts with strict enforcement of practice procedures not aimed at individualized patient care, instead placing a strong emphasis on protecting the integrity of the business.

- If you want the freedom to move from one contract to another, the ability to change employment based on your evolving lifestyle, or have another passion you would like to pursue, becoming an independent contractor may be a favorable option. You will be able customize your schedule to fit your needs and may work for multiple companies at a given time without limitations. After my second private practice job, I recognized that I had not yet found my optimal employment position, and I needed to find the type of practice I wanted to be part of for the long term. As an independent contractor, I was able to explore various avenues until I found what worked best for me.

- Reflect on your interests in specific areas of dermatology you would like to gain more experience in. What cases do you want to attend to? Are there certain procedures you would like to gain more experience in? I was interested in performing Mohs and laser surgeries, but these procedures were not available for me to perform at my first two employment opportunities. By working as an independent contractor, I was able to access other practices and conduct these surgeries, further growing as a physician.

- How quickly can you adapt to change? When working as an independent contractor, you must be able to adapt to the way in which your employer practices medicine. The process will certainly become easier over time, but keep in mind the multiple generations of physicians currently in practice, each with distinct differences in their medical training.

- If you are considering starting your own private practice in the future, you can gain experience as an independent contractor in a multitude of practice settings. You will expose yourself to different practice management styles and can decide which styles work well for you and which do not.

- I (GJH) consider an independent contractor position very helpful as a try-before-you-buy model. However, many of the issues outlined above with specific employment situations can be mitigated through good due diligence on you part. With the shortage of dermatologists, many employers are willing to modify their employment contracts to address some of these concerns. Also, the degree of independence or autonomy as an independent contractor will depend on the contract that you work out with the practices you decide to work at.

- Understand that you will not likely be immersed in the practice operations nor will you be involved in policy decisions. For example, the practice may have very specific scheduling, cancellation, and no-show policies that may clash with your own concept of good patient care. As an independent contractor, you will have little opportunity to effect change. As an employee, your impact will depend on the employer and the culture of the practice. As most dermatologists, under either model, are compensated based on productivity, incentives of the employer and employee or independent contractor are mostly in alignment, making it in the employer's interest to listen to either type of dermatologist with regard to suggestions of improving patient care (better outcomes, happier patients, more return visits, and more referrals) or improving revenue generation.
- Contemplate whether you have the patience to work with employees and office staff members who may not see you as an authoritative figure and may be unwilling to collaborate with you due to your "temporary" status.
- How would you like to be financially compensated? First, consider the opportunities you are exploring and if your compensation, in addition to productivity, will be tied to patient-satisfaction measures as some forward-thinking practice now do. Your job as an independent contractor involves providing medical services and your compensation will likely be strictly productivity-based.
- While independent contractors enjoy more freedom, they also possess fewer workplace protections. You will not be protected by The Fair Labor Standards, Title VII, Family Medical Leave Act, Americans with Disabilities Act, Age Discrimination in Employment Act, and state workers' compensation laws.
- The only worker protections you will have are the ones you negotiate in a legal independent contract agreement. If your employer breaks the agreement, you will have to sue for breach of contact instead of asking for assistance from the Department of Labor. This may be difficult, but at least you will have some legal recourse to try and obtain money owed.[3]
- If your goals include guaranteed income, employment security, and/or relief from duties such as finding your own health insurance and outlining your own retirement plan, employment may be the better option for you.
- As an independent contractor, you will be able to deduct any "ordinary and necessary" business expenses as outlined by the IRS publication 463.[4] These expenses may include malpractice insurance, professional travel expenses, CME, professional licenses, cellular phone costs, a portion of rent for a home office, Internet expenses, professional memberships, medical staff dues and subscriptions. If you work at more than one office location, some automobile expenses may be deductible when traveling between offices (commuting expenses between home and the office are not deductible). Essentially, most expenses that are necessary for conducting your business can be deducted.
- When comparing an independent contractor versus employment contract compensation, adjust for the value of benefits the employment contract includes such as payroll tax, malpractice insurance, and workers' compensation. Employment contracts may also include employer contributions to health disability, life, dental, and vision insurance, retirement plan employer contributions or match, and professional expenses (cell phone, Internet, CME, professional dues, etc.).
- If you like the practice you are working at and are interested in ultimately becoming an owner in the practice, you would usually first move from independent contractor to employed physician. As part of that change in status, you need to discuss and hopefully agree on the potential of becoming an equity owner, including the timeline, cost and percentage ownership.
- Finally, consult other physicians, colleagues, and mentors you trust. Those who know you best may be able to provide unique guidance on your future endeavors based on their prior experiences and personal relationship with you. When doing so, ensure you ask sensitive questions such as their own personal constraints in medical practice or compromises they have made, as these are pertinent considerations during your decision-making process.

- If you plan to work full-time for only one practice, the independent contractor route is not a realistic long-term option due to IRS regulations.

16.4 Step Three: Once You Have Decided on Your Preferred Employment Model, What Are the Next Steps?

You will need to begin searching for a job that meets your needs and desires.

16.4.1 Important Factors to Consider When Conducting Your Job Search

- Who is the business owner? Who is "calling the shots"? In my experience, some practice managers are given too much control over day-to-day operations and can overstep their boundaries with their colleagues. Ensure your values are in line with not only the practice owner, but also the office manager and other integral staff. Focusing on this aspect will likely decrease potential conflict and dissatisfaction at your new job.
- Consider the schedule you will be working and the location of the practice. Does the schedule seem too restrictive? Will you have a say in how your patients will be scheduled? Will you be able to maintain the work-life balance you envisioned in this new setting? Will you be fulfilled outside of work in this particular location?
- Demonstrating the need of a service that is not currently provided will give you an advantage when applying for new contracts or jobs. For example, I (GJMD) was able to secure a longer term independent contractor opportunity because I was able to work on Saturdays, which the owner was not willing to do.

16.4.2 Your Independent Contractor Contract

- You will be responsible for creating your own contract. Regardless of whether the practice or agency you are working with has a shared agreement, you must be sure to highlight your compensation and how it will be paid

(i.e., the frequency of payment and the structure of reimbursement). If possible, eliminate a restrictive covenant and include resolutions if disagreements should occur. Working with an employment lawyer who has experience negotiating physician agreements is crucial when forming a new contract.
- When negotiating your pay, speak to experienced dermatologists who possess real-world experience. You may also consider using market research to conduct your own research.
- If you are using a staffing agency, you will likely make less money and may still be held responsible for additional fees such as credentialing and malpractice insurance. In my experience, you are better off negotiating on your own and accepting a higher reimbursement rate.
- A percent-of-net collections model for compensation is certainly riskier and subjective, but may be a better option for physicians who enjoy compensation dependent on their performance and efforts rather than a set rate. Productivity-based compensation is the norm in independent contractor contracts in private practice settings. In some hospital or other facility settings, a fixed "per clinic" rate is an option.
- There should be no contractual pressure to refer patients to any specific physician for specialty services such as Mohs surgery or dermatopathology due to potential Stark law and anti-kickback law violations.

16.4.3 Other Independent Contractor Responsibilities

- You will be responsible for filing your taxes and will be subject to the self-employment tax. On a quarterly basis, you will be accountable to pay your income tax, Federal Insurance Contributions Act (FICA; self-employment Social Security and Medicare tax) and, in some states, unemployment and workers' compensation taxes.
- You may also be responsible for your own malpractice insurance. If you are working for a locum tenens service, this will likely be part of the agreement. If not, you may obtain your own malpractice insurance directly through an insurance brokerage company.
- You will be responsible for your own health, dental, vision, disability, and life insurance. In addition, you will be responsible for creating your own retirement plan. This can be

beneficial as you will be given the opportunity to customize your own benefits to your individual needs and potentially be able to put significantly more into your retirement plan than you could as an employee.

- It also makes sense to consider setting up a limited liability company (LLC) for additional liability protection. It can be set up without an attorney and, as a single member LLC, there is no difference in tax-reporting requirements. An LLC does not shield you from professional negligence claims, but it can protect you against general business liability claims.

16.4.4 Independent Contractor IRS Forms Checklist

Determine net profit or loss from your business (including any travel or home office deductions). You can fill this out on the Schedule C or Schedule C EZ form. Reconcile your business revenue with Form 1099-Misc that you receive from the practice by the end of January of the following year. It is best to keep an up-to-date ledger of all income and expenses in an electronic spreadsheet such as Excel or simple accounting software such as Quicken. Be sure to store all business expense receipts. Consider a separate checking account for your independent contractor "business."

File quarterly form 1040-ES to determine and pay your estimated income tax and self-employment tax (and companion state forms in states with state income tax).

File Form 1040 to report individual income tax return (annually).

16.4.5 Your Employee Contract

- The future employer will probably hand you a "standard" contract. Due to the shortage of dermatologists, never consider the contract "standard." Make sure to negotiate with the help of a health care attorney changes to the contract that address any concerns you might have.
- The compensation formula should be clearly spelled out. A common scenario is a guaranteed base with a productivity incentive. With due diligence, find out what the going rate is in your community, so that you can make sure that the proposed compensation is reasonable.

- What happens when you leave to the accounts receivable (the money for services you performed that had not been received by the time you left)? Who pays the malpractice insurance tail if you leave the practice, and under what circumstances would you be responsible to pay it?
- Duration of contract? What notice on either party's side is required to terminate the relationship? What represents termination for cause?
- What are the employee benefits? How many hours are you expected to be at the office? Vacation, sick, maternity/paternity leave (if on strict productivity, not really important)?
- Make sure that there is a robust CME and professional expense allowance spelled out in the contract and expenses usually paid for by the employer such as malpractice insurance, license fees and medical staff dues are enumerated in the contract.
- If there is a noncompete agreement in the contract, it needs to be carefully negotiated. It needs to be "reasonable" in the states where noncompete agreements are enforceable. Ideally, a noncompete agreement should have a buyout option rather than an injunction type.

16.4.6 From the Employers' Perspective

I (GJH) ran a private practice for 17 years and my associates and I were always employees.

- The main reason to consider hiring an independent contractor is the flexibility it affords the employer with a lot less responsibility and often a very flexible work situation. The independent contractor comes in only as needed and gets paid only if they generate revenue. They are usually very easy to part with if things are not working out as hoped for. Often the cost to the practice of an independent contractor is less than an employee.
- So, why did I always hire employee associates? True integration into the practice; loyalty to the practice and its patients; and longevity in the practice. I want the employed physician to be interested in the success of the practice as well as their own success. There is also a risk of patient "leakage" to other practices the independent contractor might be associated with. Employees can be encouraged to refer within the practice without violation of Stark and other antikickback laws.

- As I was hiring my associates full-time, an independent contractor relationship would put the practice at risk of IRS sanctions. I underwent an IRS audit of my practice payroll in 2014, and they were very interested in the arrangement I had formed with my associate.
- I found that the cost of the various benefits that employed physicians get as part of their employment contract more than pay for themselves in the goodwill such an arrangement engenders. The employed physician can feel that they are treated at par with the other employees as well as the owner.
- The only setting I could see hiring an independent contractor is as a locum tenens situation when I or one of our other dermatologists are not able to work for a period of time for issues such as temporary disability, maternity or, in my (GJH) case, taking on the duties of American Academy of Dermatology presidency for a year.

16.5 Conclusion

In the final analysis, the structure of the relationship between the practice and the dermatologist, independent contractor versus employee, is less important than the culture and practice style of the practice you chose to work for. Examining, with due diligence, potential practices you wish to work for is most important, so that you do not end up experiencing some of the cautionary tales outlined above.

References

[1] Defined IC. Internal revenue service. Available at: https://www.irs.gov/businesses/small-businesses-self-employed/independent-contractor-defined. Published April 24, 2018. Accessed October 25, 2018

[2] Kane CK. Policy Research Perspectives. Chicago, Illinois: American Medical Association; 2017

[3] Rakoczy C. Your legal rights as a freelancer or contract worker: 5 crucial things to know. interfaith worker justice. Available at: http://www.iwj.org/blog/your-legal-rights-as-a-freelancer-or-contract-worker-5-crucial-things-to-know. Published April 19, 2017. Accessed October 25, 2018

[4] Publication 463. Internal revenue services. Available at: https://www.irs.gov/pub/irs-pdf/p463.pdf. Published January 16, 2018. Accessed October 25, 2018

17 Salaried versus Hourly Wage: Which Is Better and for What Positions?

Murad Alam MD, MSCI, MBA

Abstract

Most US workers are hourly workers, expected to show up to work at prescribed times and for specified durations. A smaller proportion of workers are exempt from minimum wage and overtime requirements. Routine tasks are usually performed by hourly workers. Exempt employees in a dermatology office may be either managerial staff who supervise others, or other cognitive workers responsible for specific job functions.

Keywords: hourly, exempt, minimum wage, overtime

Top 10 Things You Need to Know

1. The hourly rate is specified in dollars and cents.
2. Hourly rates cannot be lower than federal, stage, and possibly local minimum wages.
3. Hours must be accounted for at least in increments of 15 minutes, but more precise accounting is allowed.
4. Travel during work hours, conferences and meetings during work hours, and short breaks are counted as work time.
5. If an hourly employee performs work even when you don't specifically ask them to do, if you are aware of this occurrence and do not explicitly forbid this, it is work time.
6. Overtime is work beyond 40 hours per week (i.e., 168 consecutive hours), and must be paid at a rate of at least 1.5 times the standard wage rate.
7. Workers exempt from minimum wage and overtime requirements are less common than hourly workers, with the former typically in executive, administrative, and professional role.
8. Exempt workers must be paid at least $455 per week, and their salary cannot be reduced based on the quality or quantity of their work, unless they are absent for one or more full days.
9. Hourly employment is more appropriate for workers who perform routine, repetitive tasks during a prescribed interval.
10. Exempt status is better when work hours may vary significantly for a particular employee, as in when that employee is required to perform cognitive work and is responsible for an entire job function, regardless of when this might occur.

17.1 Introduction

So you need employees. But you are uncertain regarding how to proceed keeping in mind the nitty-gritty. How many do you need, what type, for how many days and hours, and how much should you pay them? While how *much* you pay them is an individual negotiation predicated on market forces, where you work, wage rules, and the prospective employees' individual skills and capacities, one question that you can address more generally is whether they should be hourly or salaried workers.

17.2 The Hourly Worker

Let's begin with definitions. An hourly employee is, as the term implies, paid for every hour of work. The hourly rate is specified in dollars and cents, and beyond this there is typically some amount allotted for benefits like health care and retirement. How much you pay is not entirely within your control. The amount is restricted by federal, state, and sometimes local minimum wage requirements. In other words, you can't pick any number you want, and the amount must be greater than or equal to the most restrictive law. For instance, if the national minimum wage is $7.25, the Illinois minimum wage is $8.25, the Cook County, IL, minimum wage is $11, and the Chicago minimum wage is $12, and your practice is in downtown Chicago, which is in Cook County, then you must pay…you guessed it, $12/hour or more.

How hours are counted for hourly employees is carefully prescribed by the government. As per the Fair Labor Standards Act (FLSA), all hourly (aka "nonexempt") employees must not only be paid the minimum wage, but their hours must be accounted for by using standard rules. Hours worked must be measured with some precision, at least, in increments of 15 minutes. Time from 1 to 7 minutes can be rounded down, but time ranging between 8 and 14 minutes is required to be rounded up and accounted for as an additional quarter hour. Travel time during the workday, as in from one hospital or practice site to another, is counted as work time. Time required to get to work before the start of the workday, or time to return home after the end of the workday, is not considered work time. Training sessions, meetings, conferences, and such are generally considered work time for the hourly employee. For such events *not* to be counted they must meet all of several criteria concurrently: they are outside regular work hours, are truly voluntary, do not directly pertain to the employee's job functions, and no useful work is done by the employee during these sessions. For most hourly employees in dermatology, these conditions will rarely exist, as training sessions and meetings are usually designed to convey new skills or improve efficiency. Meal breaks of at least 30 minutes are not considered work time, provided the employee does absolutely no work during the entire period. Shorter breaks like 5- to 10-minute rest breaks for phone staff, or bathroom or refreshment breaks, are generally counted as work time. Importantly, time during which the employee is "suffered or permitted" to work must be counted as work time. In other words, even if you do not ask the employee to do any work, if you have reason to believe that such work is being done and have not expressly forbidden it, you must pay for this. This is designed to avoid abuses in which employers hide behind the assertion that they didn't ask for certain work and so don't need to pay for it, when they know the employee is performing such work, and may have to do so to meet their work requirements.

Hourly employees are entitled to overtime pay. According to federal law, overtime pay is earned when an employee works more than 40 hours in any workweek, meaning a predetermined period of 168 consecutive hours that is fixed but does not need to begin on any particular day. Pay for overtime hours must be at least 1.5 times the regular hourly rate. The number of overtime hours required by the employer is not limited. In addition, overtime is not required for time worked on weekends or days that an employee typically has off, unless overtime is actually incurred on such days. Importantly, hours worked cannot be averaged over 2 or more weeks to avoid overtime. For instance, if an employee works 30 hours a week for 3 consecutive weeks, and then 50 hours a week for the fourth week, she is entitled to 10 hours of overtime even though the 4-week average of hours worked is less than 40.

The federal overtime provisions are contained in the FLSA. Unless exempt, employees covered by the Act must receive overtime pay for hours worked over 40 in a workweek at a rate not less than time and one-half their regular rates of pay. There is no limit in the Act on the number of hours employees aged 16 and older may work in any workweek. The Act does not require overtime pay for work on Saturdays, Sundays, holidays, or regular days of rest, unless overtime is worked on such days.

The Act applies on a workweek basis. An employee's workweek is a fixed and regularly recurring period of 168 hours—seven consecutive 24-hour periods.

17.3 The Salaried Worker

While most US employees are hourly, federal law does recognize a category of employees who are exempt from minimum wage and overtime requirements. These employees include those in executive, administrative, and professional roles. In addition to satisfying these work function requirements, exempt employees must be paid at least $455 per week. Their salary must be paid weekly or less frequently, but cannot be reduced based on the "quality or quantity" of work performed. The full weekly salary must be given for any week in which any work is performed, even if this is far less than 40 hours. Should an employee be absent for one or more *full* days, which are not covered by sickness, disability, or vacation time, then their salary *can* be reduced for that week. However, if the employees are present, and willing to work, they must be paid their entire salary even if there is no work for them to do.

17.4 When Hourly Is Better

Hourly workers are more appropriate for routine, repetitive tasks that require the workers' physical presence. For instance, receptionists, schedulers, and laboratory technicians may be best maintained as hourly staff. The front desk and the scheduling lines need to be covered continuously. Hours can be modified, so that multiple employees are performing these key functions when there is high demand, but at least one is available at all times during work hours. Similarly, a Mohs or dermatopathology laboratory may require workers to gross tissue or prepare slides at particular times, when workers will need to be present and available. None of these jobs entail significant planning or managerial functions, and so the associated workers do not require unstructured time to think or plan or work outside the office.

While hourly workers typically have steady hours, the fact that they are salaried also makes it relatively easy to redeploy when the practice's needs change. For instance, if an early morning or later evening clinic is added, medical assistants' and receptionists' hours may be changed to ensure adequate staffing. In general, it may be best not to be understaffed with hourly employees, since although their hours can be extended through overtime, it is an expensive proposition.

The classification of clinical support staff, like medical assistants and nurses, is more variable. Often, such staff may be hourly, as they too perform defined functions during specific periods. However, more senior clinical staff, such as RNs, may possess managerial roles and need to also perform less defined work that is better accommodated by a salaried position. Moreover, such senior clinical staff may find an hourly classification demeaning and not suitable for their role.

17.5 When Salaried Is Better

Salaried positions are more appropriate for senior staff, managers, and those performing mostly cognitive work. Such positions are also best for those whose work intensity may vary significantly over time. Specifically, nursing managers, front desk managers, laboratory managers, senior administrators, and practice managers may appropriately be salaried. If the practice maintains a biller or an IT support expert, they may also be salaried. While they are not managers in the sense that other staff do not report to them, they are nonetheless each responsible for entire functions, which may, more or less, consume time over the course of a week or month. They are not employed to be present for a particular period of time, but rather to make sure the work gets done.

17.6 Incentives, Emotions, and Unintended Consequences

The performance of hourly employees may be easier to monitor since their physical presence during work hours can be ascertained. In addition, since such workers typically perform repetitive tasks, the rate at which they complete these, and the associated accuracy, can also be assessed. Some phone staff may answer more calls in an hour, and certain medical assistants may be able to turn over more rooms in the same period. For salaried staff, appropriate incentives may be necessary to ensure that the desired level of performance is attained. Compensation for salaried employees may need to be tied to more subtle, productivity benchmarks. As mentioned previously, issues of equity and status may enter decision-making pertaining to staff classification on the basis of hourly or salaried. Some high-performing employees may request one designation or another. Disparities in classification or perceived unfairness in the same can result in resentment from other employees.

One benefit of recruiting hourly employees is that those so classified may be hired for part-time work. When many lower level staff are required, having a large number of part-time hourly workers at different times can allow for practice needs to be met without wastage of excess hours that cannot be usefully allocated.

18 The Practice Administrator

Christine E. Foley BA

Abstract

Many of us remember or, at least, have heard the stories of the newly graduated dermatology resident renting a small office with two examination rooms and a just big enough waiting area. The only other person who worked in the office besides the physician was a "Jack or Jill of all trades." He/she would answer the phones, check in the patients, clean the rooms, tidy up the waiting area, do the billing, and even assist during a biopsy. The individual often was someone related to the physician. The practice was small and personal, and insurance billing comprised of Medicare, Blue Cross Blue Shield, and maybe one HMO. Our current litany of acronyms did not exist nor did the myriad of state and government regulations and compliance requirements. Historically, many physicians practiced as solo practitioners in these small and less complex settings, but over the last 30 years, and especially in the last 10 years, physicians have been increasingly joining larger single or multispecialty groups in order to meet the increasing demands and resources required to run a successful practice. Today, with this trend of building larger practices showing no signs of slowing down, it is essential to have exceptional practice leadership, both administrative and physician, at the helm, managing the complex business of medicine.

Keywords: practice manager, administrator, leadership, strategic planning, practice growth, operations

Top 10 Things You Need to Know

1. Your practice administrator is your partner. He/she may not be your financial or medical partner, but a partner in providing a high-quality patient care and employment environment.
2. You need to know who you are and where you are going before you can have the right people join you. Take the time to develop both a short- and long-term strategic plan.
3. Your practice manager/administrator does not need to be an expert in everything, but he or she does need to know who the experts are and how to quickly find them.
4. A high-emotional quotient (EQ) is essential in management, but search for someone who has both a high EQ and intelligence quotient (IQ).
5. Practice managers and administrators are not the same, so make sure you hire the right one.
6. Commit to continuing education for your practice manager/administrator, as you do for yourself. Invest in their professional development.
7. Physicians need to understand their own leadership potential, and shortcomings, in order to hire the right practice manager/administrator.
8. When hiring, seek an individual who values continuous learning and quality improvement, possesses the right balance of empathy and understanding, and yet can make difficult decisions.
9. Make sure your practice manager/administrator has a comprehensive job description, employment contract, and noncompete.
10. You get what you pay for.

18.1 Things to Consider When Assessing the Need for a Practice Administrator

As a physician evaluates the need for, and level of, practice management expertise when recruiting a practice manager or administrator, it is necessary to not only look at what the current practice setting incorporates, but to also think strategically about what the physician wants the future practice size and scope to be, or may need it to be, in the next five years. Developing a simple yet formal strategic plan will help in determining the direction of the practice and the leadership required to achieve the desired results for both short- and long-term business goals. If the plan for the next 5 to 10 years is to stay small, employ only a few providers, and mostly utilize outside resources or consultants for compliance or more complex issues (accounting, HIPAA, billing, human resources, and marketing); then, the need for a "practice manager" simplifies considerably. In this case, one would consider employing the more traditional "Jack of all trades" individual who may manage the vendor relationships but not possess as much operations or complex business expertise. In this scenario, the owner physician is usually much more involved in the day-to-day administration of the practice. The physician would be the regular decision maker and the practice manager would implement those decisions. The goal of a practice manager in this setting is more of a coordinator who "tee's up" all of the specific practice needs and then requests the physician owner to decide on the path of the practice and required allocation of resources. However, if the goal involves building and expanding the practice over the coming years, then a more strategic investment in an experienced "administrator" is warranted. In general, practice managers are more hands-on in the day-to-day operations of the practice and often perform the duties of staff when they are absent. In larger practices, multiple managers oversee different departments such as finance, billing, clinical, human resources, and administrative efforts, and they all report to the administrator. An administrator occupying an executive-level position is someone who has served some time in various manager roles, has significant knowledge of legal, HR, and strategic planning, and reports to the physician owners and/ or the board of directors.

18.1.1 Physician Involvement and Leadership

In my years of experience, I have seen the following scenario play out multiple times. An entrepreneurial physician starts his or her own practice, quickly becomes successful, and grows at a brisk yet manageable pace. Often the physician owner enjoys the business side of running the practice, and for some years the practice runs efficiently with the physician owner being extremely hands-on and "managing" the practice. The physician is always present in the office, and maintains control over the majority, if not all, of the decisions. At some point, as the practice continues to grow, an official practice manager is employed and supervises a dozen or so support staff, usually performs the job of absent administrative staff (answering phones, checking in patients, ordering supplies, etc.), and is the coordinator of consultant and vendor resources. When it comes to the finances or other oversight, it is not unusual to see a spouse or other close family member or friend involved. This scenario can work wonderfully for years until the owner physician thinks about slowing down, taking more time off, and wanting the practice to be able to run more independently without his or her day-to-day decision-making and close oversight. Now what? Does the current practice manager have the time and, more importantly, the ability to take on a greater role in overseeing the practice at a higher level with a more strategic vision? Is it time to recruit a more experienced administrator? How does a potential management change affect the morale of the existing manager and staff? Will the physician feel like they can ever slow down and sleep soundly at night with the confidence that the administrator can handle the complexities of the practice in the way they would want in their absence? In my opinion, this is the most important factor in deciding how to determine the need for a practice manager or administrator with the right amount of experience. How involved does the physician owner want to be, for how long, and is there accurate self-reflection and understanding of the physician's respective management and leadership skills? Medical management of patients, managing staff, and leading the business are very different. It is fundamentally necessary for a physician owner to understand this difference in order to determine the need for the appropriate-level practice manager or administrator. Most physicians strive to be leaders in their respective fields of medicine, yet leading a business and managing employee performance and complex operational issues require a different set of skills and expectations that medical training did not provide. Intellectually understanding what leadership means versus practicing it on a daily basis are two completely different things. However, it cannot be stressed enough that the physician owner will always be perceived as the practice leader, period (▶ Table 18.1). Physicians are respected and looked up to by staff, as well as expected to set the tone of the workplace. Physicians, whether they are just out of training, or in their 30th year of practice, set the example in their practice. Remember that physicians

Table 18.1 Perception of physician versus administrative leaders

Physician	Administrator
Often sole expert issuing an opinion	Gathers experts with multiple opinions
Solves shorter, episodic problems	Coordinates longer, collaborative process
Trusted authority	Organizational representative
May break the rules to find solution	Establishes rules to prevent problems
The leader with high-visibility and authority	One of the leaders running the show behind the scenes
High confidence	Cautious

or other providers are always being watched by staff and their actions provide others with permission to do the same. The goal of the physician leader, and practice manager/administrator, is to create an understanding and supportive environment in which employees are respected, trusted, and held to the highest standard when providing patient care.

18.1.2 Practice Manager/Administrator Responsibilities

Practice management responsibilities are numerous and vary based upon the size and complexity of the practice and the availability of other resources. All practice managers and administrators, regardless of practice size, are directly responsible for the following functions:
- Personnel and human resources—hiring, firing, and performance management
- Employee benefit coordination
- Operations management, policies, and procedures
- Compliance with various agency requirements such as Health Insurance Portability and Accountability Act (HIPAA), Clinical Laboratory Improvement Amendments (CLIA), Americans with Disability Act (ADA), and Occupational Safety and Health Administration (OSHA)
- Billing and collections
- Facility maintenance
- Financial and expense management
- Patient experience and safety
- Marketing

More senior administrators of larger practices will most likely be more involved in, if not mostly responsible for, operations at an executive decision-making level for all of the above responsibilities as well as the following:
- Strategic planning and growth initiatives
- Human resource legal issues

- MD/provider recruitment and contract negotiations
- MD/provider compensation
- Negotiating and understanding complex financial agreements, facility leases, purchases, financing of equipment, and tax returns
- By-laws, shareholder agreements, and other important corporate documents
- Payor contract administration and negotiation
- Risk management and medical malpractice coverage and legal concerns
- Chairing or hosting multiple committees, including meetings of the governing body and physician staff meetings
- Supervising senior level staff, departments, managers, and other providers

18.1.3 Qualities of a Good Practice Manager/Administrator

Experience, education, and technical skills are certainly important, but, like the physician leader, the practice manager/administrator sets the tone, feel, and culture for the practice. What do you want the personality of your practice to be? Warm and kind? Efficient and fast-paced? Demanding and cutting-edge? Probably all of the above plus more. The practice manager/administrator must embody the personality traits and qualities of what you want the practice culture and patient experience to be. There exist many qualities and characteristics to consider when looking for the right management style and leadership for your practice. The important ones include being:
- An active listener
- A good communicator
- Interested in others
- Competent, responsible, accountable, and focused
- Humble, warm, empathetic

- Organized, detailed, and analytical
- Calm under pressure
- Patient and kind
- Resourceful
- A team builder, mentor, and mediator
- Knowledgeable about industry
- Curious and continuously learning
- Trustworthy, honest, appreciative, and respectful
- Likable
- Sense of humor

18.2 Conclusion

When it comes to the success of any physician practice, hiring a practice manager/administrator is one of the most important and significant investments you will ever make. The physician-administrator team should complement each other both in leadership style and business experience and skill. Hiring the right administrator should result in significant practice growth and success as well as many happy patients and staff for years to come.

19 A Primer on Employment Law for Dermatology Practices

David B. Chaffin JD

Abstract

Nearly every aspect of the employer/employee relationship is governed or colored by federal, state, and/or local law, and the body of employment law continues to grow. Hand in hand with this is a growth in the number and type of employer/employment disputes. Careful attention to the requirements of employment law is critical to avoid such disputes and to maintain a productive, stable, satisfied workforce. The law imposes limits on what can be said and done during the recruitment process. Documentation of offers of employment is strongly recommended; proposed terms and conditions of employment—especially that, if applicable, it is to be "at will"—should be specified. Minimum compensation is set by law, and varies from state to state. Employee benefits is a complex area of the law; where benefits are to be offered, expert guidance is recommended. Attempts to avoid the trouble and costs imposed by employer/employee law by classifying workers as independent contractors almost always fail. Employees must be paid (and withholdings made) regularly, and failure to do so can expose an employer (and the principals of a corporate employer) to substantial penalties. "Nonexempt" employees are entitled to overtime pay. Most states require meal breaks. Federal law requires retention of records related to hiring, promotion, demotion, and transfers, and wise employers keep detailed employment (and prospective employment) records. It is against the law everywhere to discriminate in the workplace based on race, national origin, sex, and other protected categories (which continue to be defined). Employees are entitled to workplace safety, but have no right to privacy with respect to employer computer systems. The legality of employee drug testing varies from place to place. It is critical to document termination decisions, which should be non emotional and must be based on non discriminatory reasons. There is no obligation to provide a reason for firing. Consideration should be given to a small severance payment in exchange for a release of claims.

Keywords: employment, discriminate, "at will," compensation, minimum wage, benefits, ERISA, independent contractor, constructive discharge, termination, severance

Top 10 Things You Need to Know

1. Elements of employment law vary from one location to the other, and employment law is evolving rapidly.
2. Hiring, firing, and all employment decisions in between must not be based on race, age, ethnicity, etc.
3. Offers should be in writing and contain basic terms, especially mentioning that employment is "at will," and should state conditions, for example, a noncompete must be signed.
4. The minimum wage varies from one location to the other.
5. Employee benefits issues implicate an especially complex area of the law and require expert assistance.
6. Authority to work must be verified, but background checks are optional.
7. Development of an employee handbook is worth the investment.
8. Retention of a payroll service is worth the investment.
9. It is virtually impossible to hire someone as an independent contractor.
10. Document, document, document: It can mean the difference between winning and losing a battle with a disgruntled former employee.

19.1 Introduction

Of the myriad types of business relationships, the employer–employee relationship may be, and probably is, the most regulated. Laws and rules govern everything from how to hire to how to fire. In the pages that follow, the core principles of employment law that are likely to arise in any business, including dermatology practices, are discussed, and a modicum of advice is provided. Avoidance of employment conflict and claims is a matter of high-priority for any well-run business, and this can be achieved by careful adherence to the dictates of the law and reliance on experts in the field.

First, a few disclaimers (the author is a lawyer, after all). An effort has been made to cover as many of the topics of concern as possible, but some, no doubt, have been missed. There is a lot that comes under the purview of employment law, and distilling it is challenging to put it mildly. Further, since the author is located in Massachusetts, this article emphasizes its law. The law varies from state to state, so readers elsewhere should not assume the law is the same for them. Finally, employment law is evolving rapidly. Readers must take care to consult current law. All of this is a long-winded way of saying that, if an issue arises, caution and expert consultation are recommended.

19.2 The Hiring Process

State and federal antidiscrimination statutes, and certain other laws, impose explicit and implicit limits on what can be said and done during the recruitment process. There cannot be the slightest suggestion of bias based on race, ethnicity, gender, gender identity, sexual orientation, pregnancy status or intentions, or age (among other protected categories) in help-wanted advertising or during interviews. Hiring efforts and hiring must be based on neutral criteria (unless the position objectively requires otherwise), although preference can be given to veterans and their spouses in certain circumstances. Notably, in Massachusetts it recently became the law that it is impermissible to ask a prospective employee how much he or she is being, or was being, paid in his or her current or past jobs. It is permissible to ask about compensation requirements, but not compensation history. Massachusetts law also forbids employers from requesting on initial job application forms any criminal offender record information.

While the law does not require offers of employment and employment contracts to be in writing, documenting them is strongly recommended. Oral offers and agreements can be binding and enforceable and prove to be a recipe for trouble: The last thing an employer wants is to face a disgruntled former employee's claim that he or she was orally promised employment for a particular term with particular, lavish benefits. While claims such as this typically fail, the transaction costs can be significant.[a]

The approach of most experienced employers is to use written offer letters that contain proposed terms and conditions of employment and that provide for acceptance by countersignature by the prospect. This is Contract Law 101: the letter is an offer to contract on the terms stated, the countersignature is an acceptance of the offer, and the acceptance forms a contract on the terms stated in the offer letter.

So, what should an offer letter say? Typically offer letters include the following:

- An introductory statement indicating that employment is being offered on the terms stated in the letter ("I am pleased to offer you a position as [ ] with [ ] on the following terms and conditions.");
- A description of the position including duties and responsibilities;
- A description of the compensation;
- A description of other benefits, for example, medical insurance, vacation, paid time off, and others;
- A statement that the employment is "at will";
- A statement that the offer is conditioned on verification of legal authority to work and perhaps a background check;
- A reference to other agreements that may be required as a condition to employment, for example, a confidentiality agreement, and other policies and rules; and
- Boilerplate (general terms and conditions).

A few words on some of these terms: The description of the position should leave room for expansion of the employee's duties and responsibilities. It frequently occurs that an employer will want to ask an employee to take on more, due to business needs or because the employee has become capable of handling more. Do not create a situation in

---

[a] Practitioners may want to consider employment practices liability insurance, which can provide coverage for employment-related liabilities, plus the costs associated with defending against such claims.

which the employee does and can refuse because the accepted offer letter—his or her employment contract—does not require him or her to do more.

Compensation, in the case of salary, is typically stated on an annual basis, but it should be made clear that the employment is not for a "term" or a specific period of time. The purpose is to avoid having a terminated employee claim that he or she was guaranteed a year of employment and is entitled to be paid for a year. This is done principally by stating the employment is at will (see below), but it does not hurt to state the compensation in terms of the periodic amount, and add the effective annual salary amount. In the case of hourly employment, the hourly rate should be stated, and it of course must equal or exceed the minimum wage applicable to the position. The minimum wage varies from one location to the other. The federal minimum wage, which is a floor, is currently $7.25 per hour. In the absence of a higher applicable minimum wage, this rate applies. In Massachusetts, the minimum wage for most jobs is $11.00 per hour. In New York State, the minimum wage currently varies from $10.40 to $13 per hour based on the size and location of the employer, and will increase to $15 per hour statewide by 2021.

The description of the benefits should reflect, naturally, the benefits that are provided to employees and that are being offered to the prospect. The types and character of benefits that must be provided vary from one location to the other. For example, in Massachusetts, specific types of parental leave are mandated by statute. However, the law does not require employers to provide a full suite of retirement and welfare (e.g., health, life, and disability benefits) benefits. The field of employee benefits—most of which are governed by the Employee Retirement Income Security Act ("ERISA")—is complex. A practitioner considering the establishment of employee benefits programs is strongly encouraged to consult an expert in the field.

It is critical that the offer letter state that the employment is "at will." "At-will" employment is employment that can be terminated at any time and for nearly any reason or no reason. In contrast, employment for a term ends only at the end of the term, meaning that earlier termination exposes the employer to compensation for the full term. Also, in contrast, an employment agreement can spell out the bases on which termination is permissible, meaning, similarly, that termination for other reasons exposes the employer to claims for breach of the contract. The exceptions to the "any reason" rule applicable to "at-will" employment fall into three categories. An "at-will" employee cannot be terminated (1) based on race, ethnicity, sexual-orientation, etc. (i.e., for discriminatory reasons), (2) based on a reason that violates public policy (e.g., to silence a whistleblower), or (3) to avoid paying the employee income earned pre-termination, for example, commissions.

The letter should reference, as well, that the prospective employee's legal authority to work will be verified. And it must be verified—but only after the prospect is hired. The antidiscrimination provisions of federal law prohibit checking this status in advance of hiring. Status can be checked readily utilizing the federal government's e-verify system.

Background checks are optional, but, depending on the position, advisable. Claims for negligent hiring are not unheard of, and prudence dictates that prospective employees, especially those charged with patient care or records, or with other sensitive duties, be carefully vetted. Under Massachusetts law, certain types of criminal records can be obtained by prospective employers. There exist services that conduct background checks.

The offer letter should also reference other and separate agreements that the employer wishes to have govern the prospect's employment. Many employers require confidentiality, noncompetition, and/or non-solicitation provisions. A full discussion of such agreements is beyond the scope of this article, and they seemingly are not critical for typical dermatology practices in any event. If a practice is engaged in proprietary research, however, or if there is a risk of practice members competing after departure, they may be worth considering. There are numerous variations on these themes, and the law governing them varies from one state to another; again, consulting an expert is recommended.

If the practice has an employee handbook, it should be referenced in the offer letter. If it has none, the practice should invest the relatively modest amount necessary to develop and implement a good one. Handbooks bring clarity, cut down on disputes about policies, and are useful tools when disciplinary issues arise. Topics typically covered include policy on illness, inclement weather, breaks, usage of technology, dispute resolution (e.g., mandatory arbitration), etc. A good employee handbook will also state unequivocally that it is not part of and does not form an employment contract, and does not convert the employment from employment "at will" to employment for a term or employment that can be terminated only for specific reasons. Any employment lawyer worth his or her salt can assist in preparing a handbook.

The offer letter should include some "boilerplate" language, including that, with the exception of any agreement and/or handbook referenced in the letter, it sets forth all the terms and conditions concerning the prospective employment. This will help avoid claims that additional promises were made. A provision that the prospect has had an opportunity to have his or her own counsel review the agreement also may be included, although this may be a bit too formal for many hires. It should also say that the prospect, by signing on a line provided below, has accepted the position on the terms set out in the offer letter and in any separate agreement and handbook.

Before concluding on the hiring process, a word about the recurrent issue of independent contractors is required. There are numerous burdens associated with having employees. Employers sometimes try to avoid some of these—for example, withholding and certain insurance obligations—by hiring people on an independent contractor basis, typically at higher hourly rates to make up for the lack of withholding and benefits. The law frowns on this. There are federal and state laws that establish very difficult tests for independent contractor status and create causes of action for wrongfully misclassifying employees as independent contractors. Thus, the courts and agencies have been flooded with claims, including class actions, and enforcement actions, involving so-called misclassification claims, and employers have been hit with large damages awards and penalties based on these claims. The penalties that can be imposed by taxing authorities vary based on whether the misclassification was unintentional. Unintentional misclassification penalties include, but are not limited to, $50 for each W-2 that the employer failed to file, plus payments and penalties with respect to income tax, Social Security, and Medicare, and failure to pay taxes. Additional fees and penalties, as well as criminal penalties, are possible where intentional conduct is involved. In short, it is inadvisable to attempt to avoid the burdens of being an employer by treating workers as independent contractors rather than employees.

19.3 The Day-to-Day of Employment

The law imposes multiple ongoing obligations on employers, some seemingly trivial, and others substantial. First, and obviously, employees must be paid, and with regular frequency. In Massachusetts, the law requires payment weekly or biweekly, with exceptions, of all wages earned within a fixed period of the payment date. Failure to pay wages and other amounts due when due can expose an employer to substantial penalties, including multiple damages and awards of attorneys' fees.

Employers must withhold and pay income taxes, Social Security, Medicare, and other amounts, including amounts, as designated by the employee, with respect to benefits. Employers must provide employees with reports of all such deductions. Amounts withheld must be put to the appropriate use: taxes withheld must be paid to the taxing authorities, and benefit payments must be paid to the relevant plan administrators. Given the complexity of the payment and withholding process, many employers outsource the payroll function to third-party payroll services. This is a wise step, as it minimizes the risk of running afoul of payroll laws.

"Nonexempt" employees are entitled to overtime pay—one and one-half times the employee's regular rate of pay—for hours worked over 40 in a given week. So who is exempt? Federal law creates categories of exempt employees, with revisions to those categories currently under consideration. In general, administrative, professional, and highly compensated employees are exempt, but there are specific criteria for each of these categories. The professional exemption, for example, applies only if the employee is compensated on a salary basis and principally performs work requiring advanced knowledge of a particular type.

In Massachusetts, and probably most other states, the law requires meal breaks. By statute, no person is required to work for more than six hours during a calendar day without an interval of at least 30 minutes for a meal.

Required and promised benefits must also be provided, and the law varies from one place to the other, and based on employer size, determining what benefits must be provided. For example, federal law requires only employers with 50 or more employees to offer adequate and affordable health insurance and leave under the Family and Medical Leave Act. In Massachusetts, smaller employers have this obligation. Employers must procure and keep in force workers' compensation insurance. Unemployment insurance is also required. In Massachusetts, an employer must provide paid time off, accruing at a rate reflective of time worked. If a nonmandatory benefit is promised as a term of employment, failure to provide it or provide it as promised or as required by the benefit plan or law can give rise to a claim for breach of the employment contract. If the benefit is one governed by ERISA, a comprehensive claim and claim resolution scheme comes into play, involving specialized duties, rights, remedies, and procedures.

Federal law requires retention of records related to hiring, promotion, demotion, and transfers. Adverse employment actions all too frequently precipitate meritless claims. To defend against such claims, detailed and accurate records are critical. Sophisticated employers have comprehensive systems of performance reviews and employee discipline, including provisions for how and when to document. The records generated allow good faith employers to fend off bad faith claims by disgruntled employees, which occur with depressing frequency. In short, document, document, document.

The law imposes some—not many—obligations relating to the workplace environment. There is no legal requirement that a place of work be rewarding, warm, inviting, or pleasant, nor is it against the law to be a difficult boss. The law rears its head only in select circumstances.

Massachusetts law recognizes the doctrine of "constructive discharge." Where working conditions are so poor that a reasonable person in the employee's shoes is compelled to resign, the resigning party may have a claim for breach of his or her employment contract. A claim for constructive discharge will not lie unless the conditions are objectively intolerable, that is, unusually aggravated or amounting to a continuous pattern of abuse. It is likely that other states also recognize claims for constructive discharges, but the successful claim is rare.

Much more significant, it is against the law everywhere to discriminate in the workplace based on race, national origin, sex, and other protected categories (which continue to be defined under state and federal law). This essentially means two things: adverse employment actions (failure to hire, termination, demotion, failure to promote, unequal raises, etc.) and other differential treatment based on an employee's membership in a protected class are forbidden. Likewise, environments that are hostile to a protected class, for example, an environment suffused with sexist comments or material are forbidden. It also is illegal to retaliate against an employee for complaining about discrimination or perceived discrimination (even if the complainant was not the victim of the discrimination). The law also imposes certain obligations with respect to disabled persons: Reasonable accommodations of an employee's disability may be required, for example, allowing a person with social phobia to work remotely, provided job performance is unaffected.[b]

We would be remiss if we did not say more about employment discrimination, as it undoubtedly is the single largest source of litigation arising out of the employer/employee relationship. There are comprehensive federal and state statutes prohibiting discrimination in the workplace. There are agencies that enforce these laws, such as the federal Equal Employment Opportunity Commission and state analogs like the Massachusetts Commission Against Discrimination. The statutes create specialized remedial schemes. An employee who believes he or she is the victim of discrimination in employment or retaliation may file a charge of discrimination with the federal and state agencies. The filing of a charge typically is a precondition to the pursuit of a claim under the statutes: A complaining employee cannot proceed directly to court. After a charge is filed, the accused employer (and perhaps manager) typically will respond to the charge, and the matter will proceed to investigation, conciliation efforts, and, if not dismissed, potentially a public hearing. At some point in the process, the employee may opt to pursue his or her claims in court. At the agency and in court, a specialized analytical approach developed by the United States Supreme Court is applied. Under it, the complaining employee or former employee, first, must make a relatively easy showing on certain points, for example, that he or she was qualified to do the job. After that,

---

[b] Some antidiscrimination statutes do not apply to small employers. For example, the core Massachusetts antidiscrimination statute, Chapter 151B, does not apply to an employer with fewer than six persons in its employ. That does not mean, however, that a small Massachusetts employer can discriminate with impunity: Other statutes come into play, although they are less targeted and arguably represent less exposure.

the employer (and perhaps manager) must show a legitimate, nondiscriminatory reason for the adverse action. If and when this is shown, the employee must prove that the reason is false and/or that the action was motivated by discriminatory animus.

Discrimination cases are common, and they can be quite expensive to defend, resolve, or otherwise conclude. It is critical, therefore, that employers be proactive and address potential claims of discrimination or retaliation promptly and appropriately. Consideration should be given to antidiscrimination training and the implementation of policies and programs to avoid problems and claims. If a problem is reported, the relevant records (e.g., personnel files) must be gathered and secured; records of the response to the report must be maintained. Employment professionals strongly recommend that managers and supervisors of the complaining party not investigate the complaint. The employer should designate a competent, knowledgeable neutral to investigate, and an appropriate, fair, and complete investigation must be conducted. Consulting with outside counsel on how to conduct the investigation—and what to do with the results—may be wise. If a claim ensues despite best efforts, counsel must be consulted.

Employees are entitled to a safe workplace, but an employee injured on the job may not assert a claim against his or her employer: Employees are barred from such claims under the exclusivity provisions of state workers' compensation acts.

Employees generally have no right to privacy with respect to employer computer systems. Thus, employees typically cannot cry foul if their work email is monitored, or if they are punished for improper usage of the Internet. At the same time, the law in some states, Massachusetts included, prohibits employers from secret taping of an employee's oral or wire communications; mechanical eavesdropping is forbidden. In some states, for example, Virginia, it is not forbidden.

Employee drug testing is not banned in Massachusetts, but an employer seeking to test must make a difficult showing of need.

19.4 Termination

Termination decisions usually are difficult. They represent a failure on someone's part, and emotions frequently run high. The terminated employee who accepts the correctness of the decision is rare. Human nature being what it is, many terminated employees will seek payback, or a payout. Proper handling of termination decisions can cut this risk.

- Except where termination is due to an egregious, undisputed event—such as an incident of workplace violence—the process should not be precipitous, and should not be emotional from the employer's perspective. The worst-case scenario must be considered: If an employee sues, the employer may be forced to justify the decision to an agency, judge, or jury. A hasty, angry firing will be viewed as unfair, and an adverse result may ensure. Progressive discipline should be the first resort, rather than termination.
- Everything should be documented. Again: Document, document, document.
- If termination is the decision, in most instances, the less said the better. "It's just not working out" is enough. There is no obligation, legal or otherwise, to reveal the reason(s) for the termination. Termination time is not the time to justify the decision; the temptation to do so should be resisted. But the truth is paramount. Little should be said, and the little that is said must be true.
- Terminated employees should be escorted out. It is not advisable to permit a terminated employee to finish out the day or week. Access to systems and premises should be cut off immediately. It should be assumed that the now former employee will not react well and that persons and property must be protected.
- Consideration should be given to a small severance payment in exchange for a release of claims.
- State unemployment agency inquiries should be responded to fully and truthfully.

19.5 Conclusion

A day rarely goes by that some new rule or regulation affecting the workplace does not come out. The body of employment law, already immense, continues to grow. This chapter only scratches the surface, but it is hoped that it will be adequate to stimulate thought and action, and point readers in the right direction when it comes to hiring (may it be frequent) and firing (may it be rare). The vast majority of employment relationships are mutually productive and rewarding. The suggestions provided above should enable readers to deal with the rest.

20 Essential Policies

Brooke A. Jackson MD

Abstract

Office policies are a critical component of an employee handbook and set the tone for your office culture and staff expectations. In this chapter, examples of these policies are given and include advice on how to create guidelines for your staff that allows for a clear and consistent workplace experience. Samples of such communications are outside employment policy, dress code and appearance policy, office safety and computer policy. It is important to have these policies in place and to review them at regular intervals so that they are current with changing workplace situations (e.g., cell phone use and electronic use). Having such policies in place from the start allows for ease of onboarding new staff and sets the tone for your workplace.

Keywords: staff policies, communication policy, outside employment policy, appearance and grooming, dress code, office safety, computer policy, voicemail policy, office gifts, policy on handling cash

Top 10 Things You Need to Know

1. Policies provide boundaries and structure for your practice.
2. Communicate your policies clearly and in writing to those who are affected by them and be sure to get their signature of understanding.
3. Review and revise policies annually or as situations arise.
4. Have policies available for review but schedule mandatory office meeting with staff to discuss updates/changes.
5. All communication between staff and vendors should take place on approved office devices/platforms (office email, phone, and fax) and not on personal devices.
6. All accounts must be opened with corporate emails and not personal ones. Management should maintain access with administrative capabilities to change, delete, and restrict accounts.
7. Gifts to patients and vendors require approval.
8. Restrict access to your patient care area and have a policy for limiting visitors in the examination room.
9. Inventory protocols are necessary to minimize risk of theft and embezzlement.
10. Be sure to have a policy for handling cash.

20.1 Introduction

Office policies are one of the most crucial components of your medical practice. Just as you have rules (policies) at home when raising your children, you must have policies in your office to provide structure, boundaries, and clarity for anyone interacting with your practice—employees, patients and vendors to prevent chaos. While some of these policies may seem like "common sense," it has been my experience that if the policy isn't in writing, it might as well not exist.

This chapter will set the framework with essential policies but you will need to review and revise these policies as your practice evolves. To this day, and after 14 years in private practice, I find the need to tweak my policy manual as the world of technology evolves and presents new challenges (e.g., patient devices in the examination room, staff social media, and the apple watch with staff).

It is crucial to communicate your policies to those who are affected by them. You cannot hold anyone accountable to a policy if they are unaware of its existence. Just as you have patients sign an informed consent prior to undergoing a procedure, your office policies provide similar information and guidance to employees, patients, and vendors: what is the policy (procedure), why it exists, how it is enforced, and what happens if there is a violation. I believe in transparency. No one wants to hear about a potential risk or side effect which they were unaware of after the fact. It is a given that your policy manual should be thick! On ounce of prevention…may result in your losing a potential hire or a patient but it has also been my experience that those who disagree with your policies and choose not to engage with your practice are those who would have been difficult employees or patients in the long run.

All policies should be in writing and accessible. Employee policies should be placed in the employee handbook or in the operations manual. Patient policies are included with our registration paperwork. Each new employee is required to read the employee handbook cover to cover on their first day of employment and acknowledge, with their signature, that they have read and understood it. This document is placed in their employment file. Any updates to the employee policies are discussed in a staff meeting with an updated signature required of each employee.

20.2 Essential Staff/Employee Policies

20.2.1 Sample Communication Policy

The Corporation encourages you to discuss any issue you may have with a coworker directly with that person. If a resolution is not reached, please arrange a meeting with the Practice Administrator to discuss any concern, problem, or issue that arises during the course of your employment. Any information discussed in an Open Communication meeting is considered confidential. Retaliation against any employee for appropriate usage of Open Communication channels is unacceptable. *Please remember it is counterproductive to a harmonious workplace for employees to create or repeat rumors or office gossip.* It is more constructive for an employee to consult his/her Practice Administrator immediately with any questions. The Corporation needs input from all employees and encourages everyone to communicate any suggestions. Good ideas are always welcome. Please share your ideas with management.

20.2.2 Sample Outside Employment Policy

Employees are allowed to accept other employment in addition to their employment with the practice, provided that it is approved in writing in advance by management and that such employment does not: (1) in any way conflict with the employee's employment with the practice; (2) that the outside employment demands do not compromise the employees' performance, and (3) employee's prospective employer does not in any way compete with the business of the Corporation.

20.3 Dress Code, Grooming, and Appearance

Your employees represent you, your brand, and they are often the first contact/impression a patient has with your business. Therefore, it is important that as a representative of your office your staff project professionalism at all times and complement your company's overall image. It is crucial that their attire is appropriate and do not pose as a distraction to other employees or patients. A dress code/uniform requirement for your staff will prevent misinterpretation of "office attire" and prevent staff wearing inappropriate or offensive attire. Wearing a uniform promotes team building for the staff and patient confidence in your practices.[1]

20.3.1 Sample Dress Code Policy

An employee's dress and grooming should be appropriate and professional. Employees shall wear their assigned uniform with soft-soled shoes. If you have doubt about appropriate clothing, please ask your office manager.

Attire

- Assigned laboratory coats may be worn as needed and when available.
- Name badges are to be pinned to the left-hand lapel.
- Clean, nonwrinkled scrubs are to be worn daily under laboratory coats. Consult the office manager for color choice (I recommend a solid muted color consistent with your brand/logo).
- Spandex or stretch clothing is not appropriate.
- Sports attire, including tee shirts, sweatshirts, sweat pants, shorts, and/or hiking boots are not acceptable.
- Footwear should be close toed and soft-soled; black shoes conducive to the workplace and not dangerous.

Appearance and Grooming

- Gum is not to be chewed in any public or patient contact area or while on the phone. Eating or drinking should take place only in the staff break room or private office space. A beverage in a closed container is permitted at work stations.
- Hair color and style should be neat, tidy, and natural in appearance. Bright colors (orange, red, purple, etc.) are not acceptable. Men's hair should not extend beyond or cover the ear or shirt collar. Extreme styles such as shaving or sculpting a design in the hair or allowing hair to fall into your eyes are not acceptable. Wearing artificial hair is acceptable as long as it appears natural. Women with long hair should wear it in a style that keeps it neat, tidy, and out of their face, and in a manner which will prevent hair coming in contact with patients.
- **Hair accessories:** Women may wear conservative combs, barrettes, and headbands that are no wider than one inch. Colors that are acceptable are silver, gold, pearl, tortoiseshell, clear, black, or a color that matches your wardrobe. Please limit the number of hair accessories worn, so that the hairstyle appears natural and in good taste.
- Tattoos and other body art and adornment should not be visible.
- Perfume and cologne should not be worn.
- Fingernails shall be no longer than ¼ inch, neatly filed, and appropriate for health care setting.[2]
- Nail polish should be neutral in color (transparent, light pink, peach, beige, and red). Bright (bright green, yellow, etc.) or overly dark colors (black, dark green, dark purple, etc.) are not acceptable. Decorations or decorative painting on nails is also unacceptable.
- **Rings**: Staff members may wear one ring per hand, with the exception of wedding bands. Rings must be of a style that cannot easily get caught on equipment or other objects and therefore constitute a safety hazard.
- **Watches/smart watches**: One watch may be worn, and should be worn in such a manner that it will not get caught on moving machinery or touch patients. Watches should not be a distraction from your duties; therefore, the use of apps on a smart watch during working hours is not allowed (texting, emailing, gaming, viewing of videos, recording, or photographing).

Use of smart watches to record, and photograph any patient, corporate information, or interaction is strictly forbidden and is grounds for immediate termination as this is a Health Insurance Portability and Accountability Act violation.

- **Makeup**: Makeup may be worn and should be used to enhance your natural appearance. Foundation should match your skin tone and blush should be used only to create a healthy glow. Eyeliner and eye shadow should be in neutral, natural tones to compliment the eye and should not extend beyond the natural eye area. Mascara may be worn only in shades of black or brown. Frosted or brightly colored eye shadows are not acceptable. Eyebrow pencil should be used only to enhance the natural shape of the brow. Lipstick should be in colors that create a natural look. Shades such as white, black, blue, or any very pale or very dark colors are not acceptable.
- **Jewelry:** Accessories and jewelry should be conservative, professional, and not dangling. Pierced body jewelry other than for pierced ears is not acceptable.
  - **Necklaces:** One simple necklace in gold or silver may be worn. All necklaces must be worn on the inside of the uniform top, and not as a decorative addition to the wardrobe, thereby preventing the necklace from interfering with job duties or constituting a safety or hygiene hazard.
  - **Bracelets:** Bracelets and ankle bracelets can constitute safety or hygiene risks and should not be worn. Medical alert bracelets are acceptable.
  - **Earrings**
    - Earrings must be those appropriate for business and that will not cause a safety hazard.
    - Long dangling or large hoop earrings are a safety hazard for most positions. Earrings should not be larger than an inch in diameter.
    - Earrings must be matched and be of a color like gold or silver that blends with the wardrobe.
    - A maximum of two earrings per ear, worn on the ear lobe, is permitted.
    - Ear lobe plugs are to be worn, and only skin color plates are acceptable.
    - Men may not wear earrings.

- **Personal hygiene:** Employees are in close contact with patients and fellow Staff members while at work and are expected to practice good hygiene. This includes showering daily, brushing teeth regularly, and using deodorant or antiperspirant and mouthwash.
- **Undergarments:** Employees are required to wear appropriate undergarments at all times. For those who perspire heavily, a tee shirt is recommended under their uniform top.
- Eating or drinking should take place only in the staff break room or private office space.

20.4 Safety

Patient and employee safety is everyone's responsibility. Safety is to be accorded primary importance in every aspect of planning and performing company activities.

20.4.1 Sample Office Safety Policy

The Corporation is committed to the safety and health of all employees and recognizes the need to comply with regulations governing injury, accident prevention, and employee safety. Maintaining a safe work environment, however, requires the continuous cooperation of all employees. If you are ever in doubt about how to safely perform a job, it is your responsibility to ask your supervisor and/or office manager for assistance. Any suspected unsafe conditions and all injuries that occur on the job must be reported immediately. Compliance with these safety rules is considered a condition of employment. Therefore, it is a requirement that each supervisor and/or office manager make the safety of employees an integral part of her/his regular management functions. It is the responsibility of each employee to accept and follow established safety regulations and procedures.

Reporting Safety Issues: All accidents, injuries, potential safety hazards, safety suggestions, and health- and safety-related issues must be reported immediately to your supervisor and/or office manager. An incident report must be completed and signed by reporting staff and office management.

If you or another employee is injured, you should contact outside emergency response agencies, if needed. If an injury does not require medical attention, a Supervisor and Employee Report of incident must be completed in case medical treatment is needed at a later point in time and to ensure that any existing safety hazards are corrected.

The Employee's Claim for Worker's Compensation Benefits Form must be completed in all cases in which an injury requiring medical attention has occurred. Federal law (Occupational Safety and Health Administration) requires that we keep records of all illnesses and accidents which occur during the workday.

In the case of a needle stick, you may wish to develop a relationship with an occupational medicine clinic or infectious disease office if referral is required.[3,4]

20.5 Computers, Electronic Mail, Electronic Record, and Voice Mail Usage Policy

The use of technology is now an integral part of medical practice. It is crucial to define the manner in which your business accounts are used by your staff. When setting up your various accounts, ensure that you have access to the master/administrator account and that all accounts are opened with a corporate credentials (email address). Management should maintain access to the master account with administrative capabilities to change passwords, restrict access, lock, delete, and review account usage as situations arise.

Recently, I have noticed a trend amongst pharmaceutical representatives, particularly those who sell aesthetic products and devices, asking staff to communicate with them through their cell phone. This practice should be discouraged as the relationship is with your business not your staff's personal cell phone.

20.5.1 Sample Policy

The Corporation makes every effort to provide the best available technology to those performing services for us. In this regard, the Corporation has installed, at substantial expense, equipment such as computers, electronic mail, and voice mail. This policy advises those who use our business equipment on the subject of access to and disclosure of computer-stored information, voicemail messages and electronic mail messages created, sent, or received by company employees with the use of company equipment.

This policy also sets forth policies on the proper use of the computer, voicemail, and electronic mail systems provided by the Corporation. Company property, including computers, electronic mail and voice mail, should only be used for conducting company business. Incidental and occasional personal use of company computers and our voice mail and electronic mail systems is permitted, but information and messages stored in these systems will be treated no differently from other business-related information and messages, as described below.

All communication between vendors, patients, and the corporation is to take place on office devices/platforms/apps. Use of personal cell phone, email, or other communication tools to conduct office business is prohibited. Communication between employees and vendors/patients regarding corporate matters on personal devices is grounds for disciplinary action up to and including termination.

The use of the electronic mail system may not be used to solicit for commercial ventures, religious or political causes, outside organizations, or other nonjob related solicitations. Furthermore, the electronic mail system is not to be used to create any offensive or disruptive messages. Among those which are considered offensive are any messages which contain sexual implications, racial slurs, gender-specific comments, or any other comments that offensively address someone's age, sexual orientation, religious or political beliefs, national origin, or disability. In addition, the electronic mail system shall not be used to send (upload) or receive (download) copyrighted materials, trade secrets, proprietary financial information, or similar materials, without prior authorization.

Although the Corporation provides certain codes to restrict access to computers, voice mail and electronic mail to protect these systems against external parties or entities obtaining unauthorized access, employees should understand that these systems are intended for business use, and all computer information, voice mail, and electronic mail messages are to be considered as company records.

The Corporation also needs to be able to respond to proper requests resulting from legal proceedings that call for electronically stored evidence. Therefore, the Corporation must, and does, maintain the right and the ability to enter into any of these systems and to inspect and review any and all data recorded in those systems. As the Corporation reserves the right to obtain access to all voice mail and electronic mail messages left on or transmitted over these systems, employees should not assume that such messages are private and confidential or that the Corporation or its designated representatives will not have a need to access and review this information. Individuals using the Corporation's business equipment should also have no expectation that any information stored on their computer—whether the information is contained on a computer hard drive, computer disks, or in any other manner—will be private.

The Corporation has the right to, but does not regularly monitor voice mail or electronic mail messages. The Corporation will, however, inspect the contents of computers, voice mail, or electronic mail in the course of an investigation triggered by indications of unacceptable behavior or as necessary to locate required information that is not more readily available by some other less intrusive means.

The contents of computers, voice mail, and electronic mail, properly obtained for some legitimate business purpose, may be disclosed by the Corporation if necessary, within or outside of the Corporation.

Given the Corporation's right to retrieve and read any electronic mail messages, such messages should be treated as confidential by other employees and accessed only by the intended recipient.

Any employee who violates this policy or uses the electronic communication systems for improper purposes may be subject to discipline up to, and including, immediate termination.

20.6 Gifts

20.6.1 Sample Policy on Gifts

Happy patients and vendors often want to express their gratitude with a gift. The availability of samples, products, injectables, and treatments are all of value and can be provided as gifts to patients and vendors unbeknownst to and at great cost to you. A policy on receiving and giving of gifts should be in place to maintain a team effort amongst your staff, avoid any direct/indirect pressure being placed on your patients and vendors, and minimize the risk of theft and of being embezzled.

This policy establishes the ethical conduct to be maintained by employees in relationships with patients and vendors. Unless approved in writing by the Corporation, employees of the Corporation may not offer to give or accept a gift, cash, or other item of value, including personal service, from an existing or prospective patient, supplier, or a representative of either in pursuance of business or in conjunction with negotiating business on behalf of the Corporation. This also includes any form of gratuity to or from employees of our suppliers or members of their families. Violation of this policy in any form will constitute grounds for immediate termination.

Samples and trade size samples are the property of the corporation and are to be given directly to _____ (I recommend an inventory system for these, particularly trade size injectables). Staff may not ask vendors for trade size samples for personal use.

20.7 Visitors

Consider the circumstances under which you will allow patient- or staff-related visitors in your office and restricted areas such as the examination room. It is not unusual for patients to bring another person with them to the office. Your patient has agreed to your office policies during registration, the visitor has not. Your staff has agreed to your office policies, their visitors have not.

Sample Policy on Visitors in Restricted Areas:

To provide for the safety and security of employees and patients, only authorized visitors (patients) are allowed past the reception area. Restricting unauthorized visitors helps maintain safety standards, protects against theft, ensures security of equipment, protects confidential information, safeguards employee welfare, and avoids potential distractions and disturbances.

Due to safety and security reasons, family and friends of employees are discouraged from visiting. All visitors should enter at the reception area. Authorized visitors will receive directions or be escorted to their destination. Employees are responsible for the conduct and safety of their visitors.

20.8 Arbitration Policy and Agreement

Your employee–employer relationship with each employee in your office will end at some point. While we all hope that the termination of this relationship ends amicably, it may not. An arbitration agreement defines how unresolved employment disputes will be handled.

20.8.1 Sample Arbitration Agreement

If an employment dispute arises while you are employed with our practice, the Corporation requires that you submit any such dispute arising out of your employment or the termination of your employment (including, but not limited to, claims of unlawful termination based on race, sex, age national origin, disability, breach of contract, or any other bias prohibited by law) exclusively to binding arbitration under the federal Arbitration Act, 9 U.S.C., Section 1. Similarly, any disputes arising during your employment involving claims of unlawful discrimination or harassment under federal or state statutes shall be submitted exclusively to binding arbitration under the above provisions. This arbitration shall be the exclusive means of resolving any dispute arising out of your employment or termination from employment by the Corporation or you, and no other action can be brought by employees in any court or any forum.

By simply accepting or continuing employment with the Corporation, you automatically agree that arbitration is the exclusive remedy for all disputes arising out of or related to your employment with the Corporation, and you agree to waive all rights to a civil court action regarding your employment and the termination of your employment with the Corporation; only the arbitrator, and not a judge nor a jury, will decide the dispute.

If you decide to dispute your termination or any other alleged incident during your employment, including but not limited to unlawful discrimination or harassment, you must deliver a written request for arbitration to the Corporation within one (1) year from the date of termination, or one (1) year from the date on which the alleged incident(s) or conduct occurred, and respond within fourteen (14) calendar days to each communication regarding the selection of an arbitrator and the scheduling of a hearing. If the Corporation does not receive a written request for arbitration from you within one (1) year, or if you do not respond to any communication from the Corporation about the arbitration proceedings within fourteen (14) calendar days, you will have waived any right to raise any claims arising out of the termination of your employment with the Corporation, or claims involving unlawful discrimination or harassment, in arbitration and in any court or other forum.

You and the Corporation shall each bear respective costs for legal representation at any such arbitration. The cost of the arbitrator and court reporter (if necessary) shall be shared equally by both parties.

20.9 Safety, Security, and Avoiding Theft

Invest in security cameras and an alarm system. The security cameras should be located over each point of transaction—front desk, office supplies, product, entrances to the office, staff lockers, and in-office safe. You must post a notice that security cameras are in use. An alarm system should not only notify you of an after hour intruder but should also have a panic button for an in-office use against an unwanted intruder or dangerous patient. Restrict staff after-hours access to your office.

Develop habits that ensure security as a matter of course and review them frequently. Know the location of all alarms, fire extinguishers, and AED device, and familiarize yourself with the proper procedure for using them should the need arise. Have regular meetings to review emergency procedures and equipment, including mock drills and CPR training.

- Make sure that all entrances are properly locked and secured. Rear entrances should be secured during the course of the day.
- Do not allow access to unauthorized persons in the office.
- Do not allow patients, vendors, or others to wander through the office.
- Only staff members are allowed in the restricted/staff-only areas.

20.10 Account Security

All accounts (email, vendor, banking, payroll, and financing) should be opened with restricted corporate emails and not personal ones. Management /practice owner should maintain access with administrative capabilities to change passwords and restrict access. Review practice management systems and consider restricting report access, particularly, to financial information. Restrict ability to alter, delete, and cancel financial transactions and invoice creation.

20.11 Policy on Handling Cash

Access to cash is a temptation. Consider whether your practice will allow cash. If you choose not to, please keep in mind the increased credit card fees you will incur as well as possible inconvenience to patients. If you do accept cash as a payment option, you must have a policy and procedure in place to handle cash.

20.11.1 Sample Policy Regarding Handling of Cash

- Allpatients who pay by cash are to be given a written receipt from the triplicate cash receipt book. Each receipt is to be signed by the staff who collected the cash.
- One copy to the patient.
- One copy attached to cash placed in the daily receipts.
- One copy stays in the receipt book.

20.11.2 Cash Box

- X amount in petty cash is on hand to make change for patients.
- Cash should be counted at the beginning of the day.
- If change is needed for patients, change can be made from the cash box with a completed receipt from the receipt book containing patient name, date, amount of change given, and staff signature.
- Cash should be counted at the end of the day and should total $150 or $150—any change given with the accompanying receipt.
- Write the amount of cash on the cash sheet in the box and sign.

References

[1] Wisestep. Available at: https://content.wisestep.com/top-pros-cons-wearing-uniforms-work/. Accessed November 7, 2019
[2] CDC. Available at: https://www.cdc.gov/healthywater/hygiene/hand/nail_hygiene.html. Accessed November 7, 2019
[3] CDC. Available at: https://www.cdc.gov/niosh/topics/bbp/emergnedl.html. Accessed November 7, 2019
[4] Clinician Consultation Center. Available at: http://nccc.ucsf.edu/clinical-resources/pep-resources/pep-quick-guide/. Accessed November 7, 2019

21 Questions to Ask When Bringing on a Physician

Kim Campbell MA

Abstract

Attracting a dermatologist to your practice can add significant value to your patients and your business. In order to ensure the process goes smoothly, plan a strategy ahead of time that details everything you require. Prior to meeting potential physicians, be sure to assess exactly what qualifications you are looking for which should compliment the practice. Check in with your colleagues and support staff and provide open communication among all parties. You want to find out why you should hire them while also showing the features and benefits of your dermatology practice. Set aside time to get to know each other and listen closely to what they are looking for, hearing what they say and how they say it is as important as their qualifications. It can be a bit of a balancing act managing expectations when adding a new physician to your dermatology practice. Preparing properly for the initial meeting and asking specific questions will allow you to find the right fit for exactly what you need.

Keywords: interviewing, hiring, retention, job posting

Top 10 Things You Need to Know

1. Start internally: Before you begin the search for a new physician, spend considerable time assessing what your needs are. Who is currently filling the position or duties and what dynamic are you looking for? Plan out, ahead of time, how you see the new physician fitting in and how s/he will support the entire team.

2. Share where you shine: After you know what your practice needs are, ask yourself what you have to offer the new physician. Focus here on the areas of your expertise and what your practice specializes in. How can they benefit from your expertise? Also, include how you encourage a work-life balance and the perks and benefits your new physician will receive.

3. Professional job posting: This might be one of the places where most practices can improve. It is not just a matter of putting a job description in publications anymore. There are different job boards specific to the industry and position you are hiring for. Also, an increasing number of people are finding career opportunities via social media or other websites. You need to find out where qualified dermatologists are looking for jobs. The next thing is to word your job posting in an enticing way. If you want a professional dermatologist, prepare a professional posting.

4. Reviewing applications: Plan ahead so you are able to provide adequate lead time to bring on a physician effectively. Although this might not always be possible, do your best not to rush the process. Plan the process thoroughly, so you can review applications thoroughly. Rushing to get a new physician in place can lead to costly mistakes.

5. Interview essentials: No matter how much or how little time you have, prepare your questions before the interview. We have suggested some of the basic things to cover but that might vary depending on your practice. To keep it simple, think of the interview process as an introduction to a working relationship. Treat all candidate dermatologists the way you would if it was their first day. If you can, have more than one person attend the interview to take notes or record, so you can review their answers afterward. Also, take a few minutes immediately after the interview to jot down your initial impressions.

6. Partner, employee, or contractor? How you structure the new physician position is critically important, depending on your business mission and model. There is no "one size fits all" and the first question you need to ask yourself when thinking about hiring a new physician is what you are looking for.

(Continued)

7. To negotiate or not, that is the question: When it comes to talking about compensation, bonuses and benefits, it can be difficult to know exactly what to say. Some practices prefer to simply state the salary in the posting and have everything in the open at the outset. For others, it is not as cut and dry. With partnerships and different payment strategies, this can be an area of negotiation. If this is the case, you best option is to be clear. Make sure, beforehand, you have an exact idea of what is acceptable and unacceptable, so you can convey that during negotiations.

8. Balanced expectations: Adding a physician to your practice can involve a considerable learning curve, especially if it is not something you have yet experienced. Make things go smoothly by being welcoming and patient. Balance your expectations with those of the incoming physician.

9. Physician retention: One part that is often overlooked in bringing on a physician is retention. Any preparation you do can affect how the physician adapts to the position and fits into the practice. Although you want the new hire to prove her/himself, you also want to set them up for success. Maintain an open, two-way communication channel with the entire team and check in with everyone after 30, 60, and 90 days to ensure everything is going well or to address any concerns. Remember, keeping a physician at your practice for the long term prevents the time and financial costs of repeatedly looking for new dermatologists. Be mindful of how you can retain a physician once they begin working with you.

10. Outsource it instead: The final thing you need to know is that you do not have to do it alone. There are agencies and services designed to help you find the best dermatologist for your practice. If there is any part in this process, from advertising the job posting to ascertaining what you are exactly looking for, that you are not comfortable with, look into who you can get to help you with that aspect. Outsourcing saves you time and weeds out the applicants that don't fit your practice, so you can focus on qualified physicians looking to join your team.

21.1 Introduction

Bringing on a new dermatologist can be either a tedious nightmare or a smooth transition depending on the questions you ask. Basically, you can make the process easier or more difficult on yourself and your practice depending on how well you are prepared and the details you put into the effort. Two practices I recently worked with did things very differently when they were bringing on a new physician, and their stories can shed light on why this is such an important area of focus.

The first practice was family-operated, with more than two decades of dermatology experience. They were experts in their field, had seemingly never-ending referrals, and were looking to expand outside of the family by bringing on a new physician to the professional practice they had built. At the outset, they asked each other what they wanted and created a job description to suit their purposes. They were sure to ask each candidate dermatologist about specific requirements and conducted a lengthy process of vetting candidates. In this way, they were certain to find the physician who would fit their practice exactly—or so they thought. And yet, months went on and they were not seeing a lot of interest in the position. What they didn't do was ask themselves all the right questions. They forgot to think about what they had to offer the new physician. They ignored the flip side of the process, where they had to showcase the benefits and features of working for their practice.

On the other end of the spectrum was another practice that had only been operational for a few years. From the outset, they had a team working on administration, communication, and marketing as much as the medical side of the practice. In this way, they quickly built an online following, which led to an overwhelming increase in patients. When looking to bring on a new physician they, too, looked at the practice and asked themselves who their ideal dermatologist would be. But they moved beyond that and focused on questions about how their ideal dermatologist would benefit from the position, practice, and location. Then, they tailored their search to highlight these advantages. They came from a position of showing what they had to offer, rather than demanding to see what new physicians could offer them. By simply framing the discussion and questions differently, they received an excess inflow of interested qualified dermatologists ready to move onto the interview stage.

21.2 Where Should You Start When Expanding Your Practice?

Proper preparation for expanding your practice is essential to further build your business. Although most practices are intimidated by the interview phase, that is just one aspect of the process. The process of finding a new physician actually begins before you know it, when the thoughts of requiring extra help begin to creep in, even before the actual decision is made. By the time you get to the interview stage, both parties usually have hopes for a particular outcome and certain expectations.

Adding a provider to your team can be a daunting task. The competition is fierce for new physicians, particularly ones with dermatology training. Before you hurry off to list your position, take a moment to plan and highlight your goals and ask the right questions. What does the practice need? How are you going to encourage potential candidates to join you? How will you know who is the right person for the job? You want to add someone who complements your practice and likes what you do.

Before you get too far ahead of yourself, it is best to set out a strategic plan that lays out everything you require, as well as what you can provide. When you begin the step-by-step process, always keep in mind the positives about your practice and how a physician might add to what you are already doing. Clearly list out all your must-haves and can't-stands for an incoming physician. If you list these clearly, you will be able to make the right choice for your practice. Ensure you know what positions you are looking to have filled, and you have adequate patients, staff, and space to support the new physician and fulfill your vision. A clear vision in your mind's eye as you begin will keep you on track as you work through each step.

Hiring a physician is a long-term investment. As such, a primary objective is to create a retentive and motivating environment. By following specific steps, you will not only ensure the process is structured and strategic but your success will also

be much more likely. What's more, your level of frustration will be much reduced. So, if you have not already done so, add these steps to the procedure your practice uses for bringing on a physician.

21.3 Step One: Plan Requirements for Onboarding a Physician

Keep the business side of things at the forefront by drawing up expected financial expenses and assets associated with adding a new physician. Make a detailed list of the financials you are expecting to provide, plus insurance, tax, supplies, or additional support staff.

A list delineating liabilities and assets of adding a physician makes sure there are no surprises, and that the return on investment makes sense for the amount of work and dedication required for the process.

These liabilities can then be compared with the assets of obtaining an additional service provider for your practice. At the top of the list should be improved quality of care, which may include new or different procedures, possibly extended locations and hours, or a reduced workload. Increased revenue ought to be calculated to ensure it offsets the expenses.

Since adding to your practice and recruiting a physician can be a rather personal endeavor, it is best to start with a business mindset, so you have a clear idea of the numbers and expectations before you find that perfect physician.

21.4 Step Two: Searching for a Physician

Before you begin the search, ask yourself what you are looking for. Preparing a job description and knowing how and where to search can be daunting, and can lead to disappointing results if not done right. That is why you need to start with the upper hand in relation to knowing exactly what you are looking for.

From thereon, do not advertise in publications and assume you are finished. Spend some time in this initial process to delve into where and how your ideal dermatologist is looking for new positions and then ask yourself "Why they would choose me?"

If you invest time beforehand to make the job description precise, laying out your expectations and other details, you will vet physicians immediately, thereby saving you time in the long run.

Once you have posted your job and begin to receive some responses, review the applicants in a strategic way. If the candidate dermatologist is local, an initial in-person meeting might be suitable, so they can get a feel of your practice's demographics. Before you get to know them or even arrange an interview, verify their credentials and ensure they are qualified. This might seem fairly obvious, but it is best to address this task early on rather than be sorry later. You want physicians who are ready to work now, not someone still trying to get their paperwork in order.

Depending on the location and the applicants, it also might be prudent to set up a screening phone call before an interview or in-practice visit is scheduled. This not only allows you both to get to know what you are looking for but also sets a foundation for the rest of the process.

21.5 Step Three: Getting to Know Potential Physicians

Once you have narrowed down your qualified applicants, set up a recruiting visit, so that questions can be addressed to both sides. Getting to know potential dermatologists is a pivotal step, as first impressions last. When you have set your visit/interview, spend some time planning out how it will go. Set aside one individual (yourself or another partner or manager) to lead the physician through the visit and establish interactions with everyone.

Make sure you have an agenda or timetable for everyone involved, so that you can accomplish showcasing your practice and interviewing your potential new physician.

Be sure to conduct a structured and formal interview, which is recommended to be carried out at the outset. If you wait, the physician might be on edge in anticipation of an interview and it can set an unnerving tone for the visit. Sitting down initially and asking formal questions can help ease the tension. Of course, you will want to also touch base at the end of the visit to ask any follow-up questions.

This offers an excellent chance to review your physician contracts, call, record keeping, policies, and procedure manual to ensure everything is clearly laid out. Allow the potential new provider to meet all partners, other physicians, administration staff, and anyone else involved in the practice.

We will delve a little deeper into the interview later in the chapter. For this step, it is all about meeting and greeting potential new physicians.

21.6 Step Four: Bringing on the Successful Physician

In order to successfully integrate a new physician into your practice, ensure you are diligent through the entire course of the process. Prepare a contract that covers all the required bases. Make a plan that lays out accountability, structure, and support before the physician starts. This will ensure the transition will be smooth for everyone involved in your practice.

Spend some time discussing policies, job description, and responsibilities, and go over concerns, staff expectations and other issues. Leave room for questions, paperwork, and adjustments. Advise everyone on the team to welcome the new physician and, if applicable, make an announcement to your patients highlighting the services and care the new dermatologist will offer, so that everyone is on the same page. Also, do not forget to check in with everyone in the practice in the first few weeks and periodically in order to touch base and see how everything is going.

21.7 Interview To-Do List

The interview is often the deciding factor in determining which physician will fit the requirements of your practice. It is also often the first meeting between you both, and it can prove to be an opportunity to see how the physician will fit in your practice. The questions you ask and that are asked of you form the basis of a working relationship and present an opportunity to gather as much information as possible about potential physicians.

Although every interview will be slightly different, proper preparation in this area is key. At the very least, come up with a list of questions you want to ask regarding the position and the physician's qualifications, experience, and expectations.

Ask yourself the following five questions in order to prepare for a successful interview that is both productive and informational in nature:

1. **What do you want to ask them?** Prior to the interview, make a list of important information you want to know and be sure to put those

questions at the beginning. This way you will not overlook them or run out of time.

2. **Who are you interviewing?** At the very least, review their CV and qualifications. If you have more time, do your homework and verify the information they provided to you. It can be beneficial to check with mutual colleagues about the candidate physician.

3. **Do you need help?** If your practice is busy and you are inundated or overwhelmed, don't be afraid to ask for help. Outsource the job search, or part of it, if time or resources are a concern.

4. **Why should they join your practice?** During your interview preparation and through the course of the entire process always keep this question in mind. Highlight the benefits you have to offer as well as the aspects of your practice that stand out.

5. **How will the office be affected?** Keep in mind during all of this that bringing on a new physician affects the entire office. Make sure you obtain feedback and suggestions from colleagues and other employees of the practice regarding specific details or questions in relation to how the dermatologist will fit the position.

This is also a great opportunity to cover the questions that current physicians and employees have and ensure the lines of communication are open. Providing a positive work environment involves every person in the office, so the interview and onboarding process should account for this as well.

21.8 Questions to Ask and Questions to Avoid

When bringing on a physician, certain questions that you ask can greatly influence the outcome. Properly planning out the right questions will set you off on the right foot. As you choose to word the questions, some version of the following topics should be included:

• Why are you interested in the position?
You want to get a feel of what makes the candidate a good physician. Their "why" should in a perfect world match yours. However, their answer will definitely shed light on how they will fit the position you are looking to fill.

• What expertise do you offer?
This question will allow the physician to open up about what areas or procedures they excel in

or are looking to specialize in. It also allows them to share some of their professional passions in a way that is similar to asking why they became a dermatologist, while encouraging a more complex answer.

• What is important to you as a physician?
The way they answer this question will shed light on how they will fit your practice. Ideally, patient care will be part of their answer.

• How would you describe your professional process?
Ask about how they interact with patients and coworkers. Sometimes more than one question might be better to cover multiple areas of their preferred work methods, depending on what you are looking for. This can include what their vision is for the potential position.

• Where do you see yourself in 5 and/or 10 years?
Adjust the number of years and the wording as you deem fit. The question is a good way to gauge where the candidate is going in her/his career. Without being discriminatory, you can find out if their career goals match what you are looking for.

• Do they match up with your practice's goals?
With respect to questions that you need to avoid, it is best to refrain from any questions that can be considered discriminatory. Age or lifestyle-based questions, as well as family planning, or things that might be perceived as too personal can make the new physician uncomfortable. It may also be against labor laws to make hiring decisions based on some of these answers.

Finally, make sure to ask if the candidate has any questions. This creates a great dialogue and gives you an idea about how much research they have conducted. Their questions and your discussion will begin to build the rapport that can support a great working environment.

21.9 Breaking Down the Benefits

Each individual practice will have a preference in relation to whether they want to have benefits laid out at the outset, or if they want to leave the discussion of salary until the negotiation stage or at the end of the interview. Cases exist for both options depending on how flexible you are in your financial offerings.

In some cases, with partnerships or contracted positions that offer physicians to have their own business under a cooperative agreement, some form of discussion must be carried out prior to breaking down the benefits. Choose the option that best fits your practice. By now you have taken the time to ask yourself the hard questions about what you have to offer.

Regardless of when and how you discuss salary, benefits and other terms, make sure you have it listed in detail, so it is easy to access when necessary. This way specifics on insurance, billing, bonuses, vacation, and moving expenses are well laid out, so you can easily answer any questions that arise.

21.10 Do You Feel a Connection?

While it is important to choose a physician whose experience, education, and qualifications fit the needs of your practice, you also want to get a personal feel of the dermatologist. For a successful working relationship to exist, there has to be mutual respect and level of comfort between both parties.

Planning ahead and asking the right questions will not only allow you to make a sound evaluation but also create time to get to know each other. What the dermatologist says and how they say it can be just as, if not more important, than their qualifications when it comes to ascertaining if they will be a good fit for your practice.

The question that is arguably more important than any other is "Do you feel a connection with the candidate? Do you want to work with her/him?"

21.11 Conclusion

While adding a new physician to your practice can be a complicated and time-consuming experience, having the right process in place will set you up for success. Spend a day or two in the practice with them, going through everything to see that they are off to a great start. Remember, time spent now prepares your new physician and your practice for a smooth transition. This prevents potential problems for your patient and practice.

Remember: Right match = Happy practice

Asking questions of your practice, yourself, and your team when you are bringing on a physician is a structured and comprehensive way to ensure the success of all involved. Also, with preparation, financial analysis, and overview of the needs of the practice, you will be able to factor in all aspects of the new position. Then, once you have found the person who fits what you are looking for, mentor her/him and provide the tools required to succeed. Be conscious about creating a culture of professionalism and support in order to attract promising candidates and build a productive and successful team.

22 Designing Your Cosmetic Dermatology Practice for Maximum Efficiency: A Case Study

Aleksandra Lindgren BA, Kathleen M. Welsh MD, FAAD

Abstract

Dermatology practice for most dermatologists continues to be a blend of cosmetic, surgical, and medical practice. The practice of Bay Area Cosmetic Dermatology (BACD) has been fully cosmetic for a period of 19 years and is recognized as a top practice in the country. During this time, there have been many lessons learned, resulting in a system of improved workplace efficiency and profitability. We hope the following insights will help physicians who are adding a cosmetic component to their practice or planning a cosmetically focused practice.

Keywords: cosmetic dermatology practice, medical office practice efficiency

---

Top 10 Things You Need to Know

1. Create and be true to your mission statement.
2. Build a dream team that has the right skill sets.
3. Pay attention to your office decor.
4. Identify your potential patients in order to meet demand.
5. Every patient should have a treatment plan.
6. Establish protocols for day-to-day operations.
7. Be creative with your appointment scheduling.
8. Internal marketing is one of the most cost-effective and efficient types of marketing.
9. Work to improve inventory control.
10. When things are not working, take the time to figure out why and how to fix it.

22.1 Your Vision, Your Mission

If you are providing cosmetic services, you should embrace it wholeheartedly, not just have a small sign in the corner that describes your willingness to do so. Create a meaningful mission statement that captures the goals and values that you want your practice to represent. How do you want to differentiate yourselves from other competing practices? What can you offer that is superior or has a better value? The most important part of this mission statement is that you and the other leaders of the practice model it daily.

Once you have your vision detailed, develop a business plan that is in line with your mission statement. If that means adding new services, consider your team's skill set and ensure adequate time and training to be successful. If your staff is confidently working in the right positions, your practice is more likely to become highly efficient. It is all about the people.

22.2 Building Your Dream Team

Traditional medical offices usually have receptionists, medical assistants, nurses, billing personnel, and office management staff. But the people seeking these traditional roles, as well as the typical descriptions for these roles, may not be the best fit for an efficient and profitable cosmetic or blended practice. Transform and vitalize your practice by rewriting your practice job descriptions. Write descriptions that are patient centered as this will reinforce your values of high patient satisfaction. Since it can take months to hire and train the right people for your positions, it is also important to constantly be on the lookout to recruit strong, new employees. It is more effective to be overstaffed than understaffed in a cosmetic practice as the lives of staff can be in constant flux with life events such as moving, marrying, falling ill, and returning to school. One unanswered phone call could mean thousands of dollars in missed opportunities.

For creating this dream team, let's first discuss the role of receptionists in your practice. Members of this team should answer calls, schedule appointments, greet people, and update their demographics. But a successful cosmetic practice should also have receptionists who will inform patients of your text message service for appointment reminders, encourage them to sign up for your email newsletter, and notify them of special offers. The receptionists should notice if a patient has not ordered products recently, and ask patients about refills or sign them up for a product auto-ship program. They should also suggest new procedures or products that are complementary to what each patient has just undergone in the office. Further, if team members find themselves in need of extra support, it is important that they are quickly able to summon other cross-trained staff to help.

Effectively, your receptionists could play many roles, including cosmetic coordinators and product specialists, in addition to their traditional role. Thus, as mentioned, this job description requires a different skill set than required by a traditional medical receptionist and should be advertised as much to attract people who are interested in a more business-oriented career, such as candidates with a background in sales and marketing. This does not mean that every receptionist has to play the exact same role. Some members belonging to this group could be dedicated to the phones, while others could face the public. There will be many staff and task variations that you could set up, but the goal is to have every team member invested in and capable of growing your practice. For some employees, this could mean matching salary to job expectation. There are many physicians who feel that they cannot afford the salary for someone with this skill set but consider that if this individual could encourage just one patient a day to undergo a simple laser procedure or restock their skin care products it would more than pay their salary.

Another important role in your practice is played by the cosmetic coordinator. Initially, this person can function as your cosmetic sales manager,

patient educator in all things cosmetic, and overseer of product ordering and inventory. With any down time, this person could also serve as a backup for the front desk staff, especially at times when duties become overdemanding at the front. A third suggestion for your dream team is to have a VIP patient coordinator who is the point person for frequent referrers, celebrities, and high utilizers. At BACD, these patients can bypass the front desk and communicate directly with the VIP concierge.

22.3 Office Design

Your office décor does not have to be excessively fancy, but it should definitely be clean and up-to-date. Common areas, like the waiting room, are best designed with neutral décor that is not too spa-like. Doctors and their medical practices are distinguished from spa franchises, and a professional waiting room should project that distinction. A sophisticated, modern, and gender-neutral waiting room will be welcoming to all of your patients including men. It is also important to sit in your own waiting room once a month to notice any excessive wear and tear that needs to be repaired or replaced. Further, displaying your skin care products around the office will give your patients a visual representation that you care about skin health and beauty. It is not necessary to have a separate waiting room for cosmetic patients as all of your patients are potential cosmetic patients. Welcoming all of them to try cosmetic products and procedures will be the best form of internal marketing.

22.4 Who Do You Serve?

If you have an existing practice it is important to know your patient demographics, such as average income and age. This information can help you tailor your offerings to meet the potential demand of your current patients. However, do not assume that younger patients or patients belonging to a lower income group are not interested in cosmetic procedures. Be sure to offer a range of products and services in order to capture both your untraditional patients and new ones.

Different age groups have different needs and desires. Millennials come to dermatology practices for preventive and enhancing cosmetic procedures, while older patients usually want services that can treat precancerous, sun-damaged skin as well as wrinkles. Acne patients in particular provide an entry to cosmetic procedures as they will often want treatments to repair scarring and uneven pigmentation after their acne is well controlled. Then, their mothers, fathers, and siblings may quickly become your patients once they get to know what other services you offer.

A simple questionnaire on every patient form should ask patients about any cosmetic procedures or skin care they are interested in. Similar to the retail setting, many people are wary of being sold to and will automatically reply that they are not interested in products when initially asked about them. Reframing the information about your services and products into a more educational format can help patients understand what you are offering. This information can also help create a physician–patient discussion regarding the best choice for the patient and his or her skin.

22.5 Day-to-Day Strategies

A protocol should be developed for the rooming of each patient. BACD's protocol is completed by medical assistants. It first involves reviewing allergies, medications, and past medical history. Then, the patients are asked about their satisfaction from their previous procedures, and prepped with consent and photos for any procedures to be conducted that day. Finally, an assessment of the patient's skin care routine and treatment plan is made and updated as required. In order to do so, all of the new hires have to undergo at least six months of training during which they are mentored as well as trained. Our staff utilizes product sales representatives and industry sponsored trainings to bring everyone up to speed on procedures and skin care products.

At BACD, we have experienced the most success by hiring aestheticians and training them to cofunction as medical assistants. Aestheticians usually have a passion for skin care, and new graduates in particular love the added clinical aspect. With this setup, they are able to both assist the cosmetic providers as well as schedule times to perform their own procedures such as chemical peels and facials.

22.6 The Treatment Plan

Patients need to know what procedures to perform next and when to repeat services.

Developing a treatment plan for each patient is key to patient retention and the growth of your practice.

Every patient is provided with a detailed annual treatment plan that focuses on their goals and needs. These treatment plans are both given to the patient and entered in the patient's medical record. The treatment plan can also be emailed with updates and reminders.

A sample plan for a 45-year-old woman might include the following points:
- Neuromodulators and fillers every four months as required.
- A significant collagen-building treatment such as a fractionated laser, radiofrequency, or high-frequency, focused ultrasound once a year tailored to her needs.
- Brightening treatments such as chemical peels every three months as required.
- A body treatment such as targeted fat reduction.
- Detailed instructions for her skin care.

The aesthetician/medical assistant take notes on each patient in the room and then enter these notes into a template in the patient's electronic medical record (EMR). This allows the providers to spend more face-to-face time with the patients. Then, in between patients or at the end of the day, the notes can be quickly reviewed for accuracy.

22.7 Scheduling

BACD uses block scheduling for the first few patients of the day and traditional scheduling during the rest of the day. Block scheduling means that four patients are booked at the same time for the first appointment of the day with the next appointment scheduled 40 minutes later. The patients are informed of the group scheduling at booking and informed that they will be out within the hour. Usually there are one to two straightforward appointments that can be seen first, while the other patients numb for their procedures. This type of scheduling in the morning makes use of all the appointment slots without any lag time for numbing. It also minimizes getting behind early in the day due to a late arrival first thing in the morning. Patients scheduled for procedures later in the day are also booked without extra time allotted for numbing. Instead, numbing cream is applied when the patient is first brought into the examination room; providers rely on cold air, ice, instant freeze spray, nitrous oxide, distractions, and vibration to achieve additional anesthesia as required. This type of scheduling eliminates much of the waiting time in the examination rooms.

If the provider is running more than 15 minutes behind, an attempt is made to call the next few patients to keep them informed of the delay. Service recovery may include a small gift or discount if wait times are excessive. Patients usually do not mind waiting as they understand that medicine is not always predictable, but they always appreciate the courtesy of knowing what is going on, so that they can make plans for the rest of the day.

To aid with scheduling, we attempt to have all providers schedule the same amount of time for all procedures and visits. Two days ahead of time, a staff member checks each providers' schedule for accuracy of booking and then again on the day of the appointment. Patients receive an automated text or phone call 48 hours ahead of scheduling. Deposits are taken on a credit card at the time of booking appointments that are more than 30 minutes long, and our cancellation policy is explained at the time of booking. Deposits are also required for new patients who book appointments. This policy has significantly reduced no shows. Patients who miss appointments are called the same day, and if a patient no shows more than two appointments, a deposit is required to book further appointments. Patients who get upset or angry at this policy are probably not patients you want in your practice. A missed appointment is a missed opportunity for everybody. In addition, the office has all examination rooms set up identically, so that the usage of rooms can be flexible when certain providers are busier than others or when providers are on vacation. Each room includes a small back stock of the most used supplies in order to minimize lost time looking for a missing item in the larger back stock outside of the examination room. This set up also helps save time when restocking and ordering supplies. If you sell skin care products, we recommend that you have testers available of all of the products you regularly recommend in a convenient place just outside of the examination rooms, so your staff can easily demonstrate their use at the time of recommendation.

22.8 Efficient Marketing

Marketing is and should be an essential part of your business plan. You should attempt to develop an in-house marketing team and lay out an annual template for all of your marketing programs. If you do not possess this expertise, it can be outsourced quite easily. Internal marketing remains the most efficient way to let your patients know what services you offer and promote them. The core of our internal marketing is a biannual newsletter that we produce in-house that focuses more on new services than on educational material. In addition, we have a quarterly email newsletter on current topics. When trying to add a cosmetic component to an existing practice, use demographic information to identify patients who would be interested and market with directed email campaigns, pamphlets and posters, and in-person during medical appointments. The use of wall-mounted lightboxes in the hallways and closed-circuit televisions with looped service information and before and after pictures, in the waiting room and each examination room, are other effective forms of marketing. Practice brochures explaining service offerings are also kept in each examination room and in the reception room. Internal marketing also means educating patients about procedures that are complementary to procedures that they are performing that day and noticing possible issues that they may be interested in correcting. It is a form of service extended to patient to notice that they have a large "age spot" on their cheek, determine if they are interested in removing it, and inform them that your staff can carry it out the same day. Another efficient way of letting your patients know what services you offer is to make a simple menu of services and give it to every patient as they leave or enter the office. This information can be linked to more extensive data on your website. Efficient internal marketing also means asking patients to refer their friends and family members to the practice. Patients usually assume you are as busy as you would like to be, so it is important to ask them point blank for referrals.

Marketing budgets can be maximized by comarketing with the industries you work with. Even if your suppliers do not have a formal program, they may be willing to invest in this type of marketing with you. Also, make sure you are on all the industry website physician locator pages. Other options include using the industry sales representatives to engage in marketing for you in your waiting room. We have them come into the office during peak hours to explain their procedures and products to patients who are interested. Representatives who bring coffee and light snacks tend to further encourage your patients to interact with them. As these representatives have received extensive training in sales and education from their respective industries, they also act as role models for the staff by advising on how to explain and sell their product or procedure.

External marketing can also include reaching out to other practices that do not offer your services and letting them know that you are available for referrals. Honor these referrals with a thank you note and by not poaching their patients. Unfortunately, marketing with ratio, television, and traditional media may only raise awareness about the procedure, rather than yield new patients, unless you have an extraordinarily large budget to spend on these marketing avenues. In a crowded market, you will be essentially advertising for your competitors as much as you are for yourself. A better use of dollars involves investing in Google ads, thereby boosting your social media presence.

22.9 Efficient Ordering and Inventory

Nothing is more frustrating than realizing that you ran out of laser tips before a large scheduled procedure or ran out of a product that you have just enthusiastically recommended to a patient. These problems can be avoided by using an inventory control system that flags items when they are low, and then having one or two staff members responsible for managing inventory. It is also important to know the shipping schedules of your suppliers, so that you can save valuable storage space and not have more back stock then you require.

Inventory control programs can help you with loss control, but they cannot substitute for physical counts. Physical inventory counts are time-consuming in nature and often placed on the back burner behind other office projects. An easier way to get it done is to use bar coding on all of your supplies and products, and stagger the number of counts during the year. You should inventory your top selling and most expensive products more frequently, because the rapid turnover may result in more missing products. If the physical inventory yields discrepancies, you can also inventory those products more frequently until you figure out why the product is missing. In the retail setting, cosmetic items tend to have a shrinkage of 3 to 4%, but in an office where the public does not have access to the products, you should aim for 1 to 2%.

A sample schedule might include:

Group	Inventory in terms of cost or turnover	Number of inventory counts per year
1	Top 20%	8
2	Middle 60%	6
3	Bottom 20%	4

Even with tight inventory control, inevitably, once in a while, you will run out of a needed supply, or a piece of equipment will break down when it is desperately needed. Thus, forging good relationships with other local cosmetic practitioners as well as local sales representatives is important, so that loaner inventory or use of demo equipment may be arranged.

22.10 Improving Systems

Few days ever go perfectly, but if you find yourself getting frustrated by the same things over and over, take some time to dissect the problems into manageable pieces. An example from our practice was variable staffing during different parts of the day. Our staff seemed to disappear at midday and at the end of the day. Some staff were taking required breaks and others could not stay late if we were behind schedule due to childcare demands. The following solution was tabled: An additional staff member was hired to provide relief for breaks and lunch and start later in the day to cover the end of the day.

This was an extremely simple solution, but it took months of frustration to actually figure out what was going on. Adding a staff member increased sale in the last few hours of clinic time and turned out to be cost-effective in terms of decreasing overtime. When problems arise, ask everyone involved both where they think things are going wrong and recommendations for a system that could be put in place to improve the issue. Involving your staff in problem solving encourages them to take ownership of their possible roles in the problem as well as the solution. Encourage your staff to participate in ongoing, patient-centered quality improvement. If you cannot figure out how to improve or fix a problem, reach out to your colleagues, consultants, and even patients. There is always an answer and it is extremely satisfying to be able to find it and implement it.

An attitude of "it can always be better" guarantees maximum efficiency, continued quality improvement, and good patient experience.

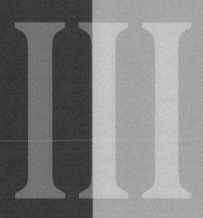

23 "It Depends": No-show Fees, Cancellation Policies, and Deposits for Procedures

Sara Hogan MD, Omer Ibrahim MD, Jeffrey S. Dover MD, FRCPC

Abstract

No-show appointments and cancellations result in wasted resources, suboptimal utilization of staff, decreased physician productivity, and, most importantly, missed opportunities for patient care. Efforts must be made to minimize these occurrences and subsequent disruptions to a practice. No-show and cancellation fees, prepayments, and procedure deposits are effective tools in addressing these issues, but they should be implemented to influence patient behavior, and not to recover lost revenue. When and how these policies are employed depends on numerous factors, not limited to the patient–physician dynamic, practice culture, and personal style and preference.

Keywords: no-show appointments, cancellation, prepayment, patient compliance, patient attendance

Top 10 Things You Need to Know

1. Communicate clearly: Effective communication allows for establishment of a patient–physician relationship and establishes the significance of keeping appointments. Practice policies on no-show fees, cancellations, and deposits on procedures should be clearly displayed for patients throughout the patient registration and scheduling process, and printed on appointment cards and billing statements.
2. Keep messaging consistent: Although there may be variances in individual patient circumstances and physician preferences, messages must be consistent. Administrative staff, nursing staff, and physicians should all be well versed in practice policies.
3. Engage patients in the scheduling process: Patients who feel involved in the scheduling process are more likely to keep their appointments. Ask patients when they would like to come in for their follow-up appointment, rather than offer the next first available appointment.
4. Optimize scheduling templates: Research shows that patients are less likely to keep their appointments if they experience prolonged scheduling lead times and extended waits in the waiting room. Keeping wait lists to a minimum and strategically building overbook appointment slots can improve patient access.
5. Remind patients in advance: Patients should be contacted at least once in 48 hours but preferably twice before their appointments and given an opportunity to reschedule, if necessary. Have staff make personal phone calls or utilize automated text and/or email reminder services regarding upcoming appointments.
6. Follow-up with patients who no-show: Contact patients after they missed their appointments and offer them an opportunity to reschedule. Ask specific questions to uncover why they did not keep their appointment. This can help identify trends (e.g., a particularly susceptible day and time slot) and areas of opportunity to decrease no-show appointments.
7. Document everything: All contact with patients regarding no-shows, cancellations, and deposits on procedures should be documented in a section of the patient chart that can be accessed by administrative staff and physicians. This allows for everyone to be on the same page and patterns in patient behavior to be easily identified.
8. Know your patient population: Take time to understand who comes to visit you. Patients in rural areas may travel hours and long miles to make their appointment. Patients in urban areas may rely on public transit lines that are not always predictable. Patients with disabilities may require extra assistance to arrive at your practice.
9. Be judicious with fees: Life happens. Make exceptions for medical emergencies, car accidents, extenuating family circumstances, etc. Give patients one or two grace warnings before implementing a no-show or cancellation fee. When a fee is applied, it should be priced adequately high to influence patient behavior, but not so high that it drives a patient away.
10. Show appreciation: Thank the patients who always keep their appointments. Let them know that they are valued by you and your practice. Maximizing the patient–physician relationship will increase the chance that patients will continue to keep their appointments.

Opening Vignette

Patient X is a 49-year-old female patient with severe psoriasis (> 50% BSA [body surface area]) and psoriatic arthritis that you are treating with bi-monthly adalimumab injections and topical corticosteroids. From your previous appointments, you have learned that although she adheres to her treatment regimen, she has a chaotic personal life. In the past 12 months, she has missed two appointments. She called the day after her first missed appointment to apologize and reschedule. She made her rescheduled appointment but then missed her second appointment and was lost to follow-up for a few months. Yesterday, she was scheduled to be seen, but again missed her appointment. She is calling today to reschedule. As her dermatologist, what is your next step?

- Tell your front desk to reschedule the patient and mail her an order form for laboratory monitoring
- Tell your front desk to reschedule the patient and charge her a $75 no-show fee
- Charge her a $75 no-show fee and discharge her from your practice
- Discharge her from your practice

How would the situation change if any of the following details were different?

A. Patient X is a cosmetic patient and the aforementioned appointments are earmarked for botulinum injections?

B. Patient X has a 1.2 cm well-differentiated invasive squamous cell carcinoma on her left forearm, and the aforementioned appointments are allotted for a surgical excision?

C. Patient X has visiting your practice for over 15 years and before the past 12 months, had no history of missed appointments?

D. Patient X and you share several mutual friends and are acquaintances outside of the office?

23.1 Introduction

A no-show appointment is defined as a patient missing an appointment with little or no communication. An appointment cancellation, in comparison, is when a patient cancels or reschedules less than 24 hours before the appointment. Both no-show appointments and cancellations can negatively impact a medical practice. There exists some data to suggest that dermatology patients continue to use dermatology services after no-show appointments, often in the form of emergency department visits and hospitalizations, and subsequently incur increased costs to an entire health system.[1] Resources are wasted, staff is not fully utilized, physician productivity is decreased and, most importantly, patients do not receive the medical care that they require. This last point is of particular relevance to dermatology, given how widespread access issues are throughout the specialty. A dermatology no-show or cancellation is also a missed opportunity for another patient who desires care.

There are different ways to calculate a no-show rate. A practice may include only patients who fail to present themselves for an appointment, or also factor in same-day cancellations since either scenario results in an appointment slot not being filled. It may be helpful for practices to determine no-show rates for individual physicians as well as for the entire practice.

No-show appointment rates depend, perhaps, most strongly on medical practice setting. Academic medical centers, community health centers, and inner city clinics have an estimated 10 to 30% no-show rate compared to 2 to 15% in private practices.[2] The rate of no-show appointments varies among specialties, with higher rates in neurology, psychiatry, and general surgery, and with most specialties reporting a median patient no-show rate between 5 and 20%.[3,4] An accurate no-show rate for dermatology is not readily available in the literature. The most commonly cited dermatology no-show appointment rate range is 17 to 31%, based on a study of one Canadian dermatology practice.[5] More recent studies of nonattendance at academic dermatology departments found a comparable rate, that is, between 13.3 and 21.9%.[1,6,7] Our private practices have no-show rates—which include same-day cancellations—of 8.58 and 18% respectively, which suggest actual values are lower than what is documented in the literature.

23.2 Why Do Patients No-show for Appointments?

The literature on no-show appointments is wide-ranging across specialties, practice models, and countries, making it difficult to draw consistent conclusions on why they occur. The majority of studies focus on identifying factors that predict the likelihood of missed appointments. Dermatology is a specialty, that in much of the US, is characterized by limited availability of physicians and extended wait lists for new patients. The likelihood of a missed appointment is higher with longer patient wait times, which increases the risk of a patient forgetting they made an appointment or the medical problem resolving on its own.[4,8] One case study found that appointments made with a lead time of more than three weeks corresponded with a 53% no-show or cancellation rate.[4] This places dermatology practices at particular risk of no-show appointments.

Dermatology appointment no-show risk differs according to the type of appointment. New dermatology patient appointments are, as expected, more likely to be missed than established patient appointments.[6,10,11] Monday morning is an especially vulnerable workday for no-show appointments.[8] Tuesdays after a long weekend and Mondays are even worse. Urgent care dermatology clinics exhibit higher no-show and cancellation rates than urban academic general dermatology outpatient clinics.[5,7] Appointments with resident physicians have a significantly higher percentage of missed appointments than those with attending physicians.[12] As an increasing number of dermatology practices utilize website scheduling services, online appointments appear to have lower no-show rates compared to appointments made through traditional methods.[13]

The picture is textured when it comes to understanding the type of patient who misses his or her appointment and his/her perception of the consequences of no-shows (▶ Table 23.1). Patients may not understand the effect of their failure to be present for appointments. In one study, 41% of patients who no-showed for outpatient appointments believed that their missed appointment actually had a *positive* effect on clinic operations.[14] Those patients also reported feeling anxious about

an appointment outcome, decreased perception of disease severity, and feeling disrespected by long wait times as reasons that they were less likely to keep appointments.[14] Recurrent patient characteristics associated with missed appointments include lower health literacy and lower income level, being publicly insured, having unreliable transportation, or inability to miss work.[11–19] Patients who self-pay or who have private insurance with a copayment are more likely to keep an appointment. One study found that dermatology patients with coinsurance were 20% more likely to miss than appointment than those with copayments, due to greater potential financial burden.[8] Patient age and gender are less reliably associated with missed appointments. Some studies suggest that younger patients are more likely to forget appointments, while older patients are more likely to keep appointments, and that very old patients are at high risk of missing appointments.[8,10,16] Other studies have demonstrated neither a male or female predilection to missing appointments, and a few studies suggest that ethnic minorities may be more likely to break appointments.[3,8,10,14,16] Overall, the most consistent finding in the literature, and in our experience, is that patients with a history of no-show appointments are most likely to no-show to future appointments.

23.3 The Anatomy of a No-show Fee

The exact cost of no-show appointments and cancellations is not well described, although one study estimated that a medical practice loses up to $200 for each missed appointment.[9] This is a significant underestimate for surgical, cosmetic, and procedural practices. The financial impact is rarely balanced by revenue from same-day appointments.[20] As such, a medical practice may opt to charge patients a no-show or cancellation fee. A Medical Group Management Association survey found that only one-fourth of responding medical practices charged patients with a no-show fee.[4] The percentage of dermatology practices that utilize no-show or cancellation fees is not known.

This fee does not recoup the cost of a missed appointment; rather, it is designed to shape patient behavior. The decision of whether to institute fees is complex in nature. Will patient behavior be altered or will the negative connotation of the fee outweigh the benefit? Before instituting a

Table 23.1 Factors predicting a no-show appointment

Patient	Practice
History of no-shows	Access to appointments
Forgetfulness	Long lead times
Perceived severity of health issue	Prolonged wait room times
New patient status	
Poor health literacy	

no-show or cancellation fee policy, a few variables must be considered. First, should your practice adopt no-show fees, cancellation fees, or both? Cancellation fees are less frequently employed, but are reasonable given the difficulty of filling a same-day appointment. The incidence of patient no-shows and cancellations must be determined early in the process of adopting no-show fees. A practice should decide if the time spent by staff to enforce no-show fees is worth the effort. If staff exerts great energy to collect fees from no-show patients (e.g., making telephone calls and following up on billed charges), the practice will likely regain minimal to no revenue lost from missed appointments. Next, the mixture of payers for a practice should be taken into account. Medicaid and certain private insurers strictly prohibit such fees. If the practice enters into a contract with insurance payers who do not allow no-show fees, the practice will likely not be able to collect them. Alternatively, practices can have a written contract detailing an exception to insurance policies signed by patients at the time of patient registration. In addition, physicians in the practice must consider their feelings regarding no-show fees. If some dermatologists within a practice do not feel strongly about charging patients who miss their appointments, there will be challenges encountered in consistently collecting fees.

Once the decision is made within a practice to implement no-show or cancellation fees, a secondary set of factors must be evaluated (▶Table 23.2). Foremost is when to enforce the fees– should patients be charged after the first, second, or third offense? Grace warnings are appreciated by patients, but how many should they be allowed? Special considerations may be made depending on the physician or the patient. A physician may not want to enforce fees readily with certain patients, for example, in the setting of a friendly relationship,

shared acquaintanceship outside of work (i.e., dermatologists who live and practice in small towns), or other extenuating circumstances (e.g., a loyal cosmetic dermatology patient, a complex medical dermatology patient with several comorbidities or a disability, a patient who travels a far distance to get to an appointment, or a patient who relies on a government-sponsored ride-share service). There is no perfect way to go about enforcing no-show fees as it depends on the circumstance.

Next, a practice must determine how much to charge patients. A typical no-show fee for a follow-up appointment, depending on the specialty, is between $25 and $75.[4] For larger pricier procedures that require larger chunks of provider time, staff involvement, procedure room, and possibly expensive consumables, the no-show fee may be larger ($500–1000). It is important to remember that these fees serve to influence patient behavior, not recoup lost revenue. Fees should be priced to deter no-show appointments, not drive patients away. Moreover, all dermatologists in a practice should charge the same amount for a no-show or cancellation fee. A study from Spain found that female dermatologists charged consistently lower no-show fees, even after adjusting for other variables.[21] Having a set fee schedule decreases confusion. In addition, a practice should determine how to optimize fee collection, whether through registering credit cards on files at time of scheduling or generating bills after an appointment is missed. If credit card numbers are kept in files, the practice must have a secure method for storing patient personal information.

A practice that opts to implement no-show and cancellation fees must communicate this clearly with patients. Practice policies on no-show fees, cancellations, and deposits on procedures should be clearly displayed for patients through the patient registration and scheduling process, and

Table 23.2 Considerations regarding no-show and cancellation fees

Patient	Interpersonal	Practice
What kind of appointment access do your patients want?	What is your relationship with the patient?	Do your physicians reschedule frequently?
Does this patient no-show/cancel frequently?	What is your vision for your practice of medicine?	Do schedules frequently run behind?
Is there a patient credit card held on file?	How often are you communicating with your patients?	Are there long delays before appointments are made?
Are there any extenuating circumstances?	What is your target patient volume?	What is your payer mix?

printed on appointment cards and billing statements. This clear communication establishes the importance of patients keeping appointments. Although patient circumstances and physician preferences vary, messaging must be consistent in nature—administrative staff, nursing staff, and physicians should all be well versed in practice policies. Internal communication regarding the events leading to a fee charge should also be well documented. All contact with patients regarding no-shows, cancellations, and deposits on procedures should be documented in a section of the patient chart that can be accessed by administrative staff and physicians. This allows for everyone to be on the same page, and patterns in no-shows, cancellations, and patient behavior (e.g., so-called "repeat offenders") to be more easily identified.

23.4 Prepayments and Deposits on Procedures

One limitation in research on no-shows and cancellations is that patients who did not show for appointments in a single instance are not distinguished from those who did not show in multiple instances. When a patient does not show more than once, he or she is considered a chronic no-show-er. If no-show fees are not an option in this case, there exist alternatives to influence patient behavior. Patients could be scheduled at specific times (e.g., double booked during a busy time of the clinic workday). They could also be asked to make a deposit at the time of scheduling an appointment (i.e., prepayment). They could also provide a credit card with the understanding that it will be charged if they do not show up for an appointment. If a patient then keeps his or her appointment, this prepayment or deposit could be applied to costs associated with appointment or kept on file for future appointments. Certain appointments or procedures may require a large block of time, devoted support staff, expensive consumables, or reservation of an operating room. Given that a no-show or cancellation for these appointments has considerable financial impact, a deposit should be collected at the time of scheduling. Deposits for these larger procedures can range from 50 to 100% of the cost of the procedure.

23.5 Reducing No-shows

The best way to avoid collecting a no-show fee is to minimize no-show appointments. Central to this is reminding patients at least once but preferably twice in the days leading up to their appointments by phone call, email, or text message. Ideally, patients would receive two reminders: one that is 5 days before the appointment, followed by a second reminder 1 to 2 days before the appointment. Surveys of patients who fail to show for appointments reveal that a surprising number of patients are not reminded of appointments or forget their appointments altogether.[11,18] Allowing patients the opportunity to reschedule in a timely manner gives the practice an opportunity to fill the appointment vacancy. Moreover, engaging patients through the scheduling process increases the likelihood of kept appointments. Research shows that long lead times correspond with missed appointments. To the extent possible, query patients about their next availability to follow-up and schedule them at that date, instead of offering the first next available appointment several months away.

Make scheduling adjustments to reduce risks of no-shows or the financial impact if no-shows do occur. Clinic schedules ideally take into account each patient's no-show probability.[22] For example, a known last-minute cancellation patient should be scheduled as a double-booked appointment before lunch. If this patient missed his or her appointment, the time allocated for the appointment can be spent attending to another patient and then completing charting. A practice may also adopt a policy where only two members of a family can be scheduled together at a time, so as to minimize the likelihood of a block of no-show appointments.

Maintaining open communication and a structured approach in dealing with patients who miss their appointments is crucial. No-show patients should be contacted after their first missed appointment, and given a chance to reschedule. Reasons as to why patients did not show can be elucidated, which provides an opportunity for improvement. Calling no-show patients is also important for patients with complex dermatology conditions, and ensures that they are not lost to follow-up entirely.[17] It is our recommendation that a patient receive a written communication and a no-show fee after a second no-show appointment and be dismissed from the practice after a third consecutive missed appointment.

Maximizing the patient–physician relationship will increase the chance that patients will continue to keep their appointments. Impressing upon patients that we care about them and that their dermatologic care is an important part of their well-being helps patients feel valued.

The opening vignette highlights the nuances of the dermatology patient–physician relationship in the context of no-show appointments. The most appropriate answer for all scenarios depends on so many factors. For some it is (B), charge her a $75 no show fee and reschedule her, while for others, it is option (C), charge her a $75 no-show fee and discharge her from your practice. Patient X was afforded several opportunities to reschedule after not showing up to previous appointments, yet she continues to no-show. The vignette assumes that practice policies were communicated, queries were made into the patient's previous absences (e.g., to identify any extenuating circumstances), and proper documentation of patient noncompliance was made. Should you decide to discharge her, patient X should be sent a certified letter that gives 30-days' notice of her dismissal, states practice no-show and cancellation policies, lists specific examples of patient noncompliance, and provides recommendations for future treatment (i.e., in the case of poorly managed psoriasis or unmanaged squamous cell carcinoma) with another dermatologist. If applicable, the patient's insurance provider should be informed of dismissal from the practice to help with transition of his or her care to another dermatologist.

Whether option (C) is, in fact, pursued for your real-life patient X is ultimately up to you. The "correct" answer for a clinical vignette does not always translate to the correct answer for a patient, dermatologist, or practice, as it truly depends on the circumstance.

23.6 Conclusion

No-show appointments and cancellations are a reality of all dermatology practices. Efforts must be made to minimize these occurrences and subsequent disruptions to the practice. No-show fees and cancellation fees should be implemented to influence patient behavior, not to recoup lost revenue from missed appointments. If, when, and how these policies are employed depends on numerous factors, not limited to the patient–physician dynamic and practice culture.

References

[1] Halim K, Weng QY, Kuye I, Joyce C, Mostaghimi A. Use of health care resources and costs after patient nonattendance in dermatology. JAMA Dermatol 2016;152(2):220–221

[2] Petaschnick J. Missed appointments cause multiple problems. Health Care Collector 2018;31(8):10–11

[3] Dantas LF, Fleck JL, Cyrino Oliveira FL, Hamacher S. No-shows in appointment scheduling—a systematic literature review. Health Policy 2018;122(4):412–421

[4] Medical Group Management Association. Maximizing Patient Access and Scheduling: An MGMA Research and Analysis Report. August 2017. Available at: https://www.mgma.com/getattachment/Products/Products/Maximizing-Patient-Access-and-Scheduling/PatientAccessSchedulingResearchReport-INTER_FINAL.PDF.aspx. Accessed January 30, 2019

[5] Canizares MJ, Penneys NS. The incidence of nonattendance at an urgent care dermatology clinic. J Am Acad Dermatol 2002;46(3):457–459

[6] Pehr K. No show: incidence of nonattendance at a dermatology practice in a single universal payer model. J Cutan Med Surg 2007;11(2):53–56

[7] Penneys NS, Glaser DA. The incidence of cancellation and nonattendance at a dermatology clinic. J Am Acad Dermatol 1999;40(5 Pt 1):714–718

[8] Cronin PR, DeCoste L, Kimball AB. A multivariate analysis of dermatology missed appointment predictors. JAMA Dermatol 2013; 149(12):1435–1437

[9] Perez FD, Xie J, Sin A, et al. Characteristics and direct costs of academic pediatric subspecialty outpatient no-show events. J Healthc Qual 2014;36(4):32–42

[10] Cohen AD, Dreiher J, Vardy DA, Weitzman D. Nonattendance in a dermatology clinic—a large sample analysis. J Eur Acad Dermatol Venereol 2008;22(10):1178–1183

[11] Bottomley WW, Cotterill JA. An audit of the factors involved in new patient non-attendance in a dermatology out-patient department. Clin Exp Dermatol 1994;19(5):399–400

[12] Frankel S, Farrow A, West R. Non-attendance or non-invitation? A case-control study of failed outpatient appointments. BMJ 1989;298 (6684):1343–1345

[13] Siddiqui Z, Rashid R. Cancellations and patient access to physicians: ZocDoc and the evolution of e-medicine. Dermatol Online J 2013;19(4):14

[14] Lacy NL, Paulman A, Reuter MD, Lovejoy B. Why we don't come: patient perceptions on no-shows. Ann Fam Med 2004;2(6):541–545

[15] Verbov J. Why 100 patients failed to keep an outpatient appointment—audit in a dermatology department. J R Soc Med 1992;85(5): 277–278

[16] Burkhart CG. Improving the rate of kept appointments at dermatology clinics. J Am Acad Dermatol 2001;44(2):313–314

[17] Nasseri E, Bertrand J, Brassard D, Fortier-Riberdy G, Marcil I. Physician survey regarding patient nonattendance at follow-up appointments at a university-affiliated medical dermatology clinic. J Cutan Med Surg 2012;16(2):92–96

[18] Moustafa FA, Ramsey L. Case letter: factors associated with missed dermatology. Cutis 2015;96(5):E20–E23

[19] Hon KL, Leung TF, Ma KC. Issues regarding non-attendance at a paediatric dermatology centre. Clin Exp Dermatol 2002;27(8):711–713

[20] Moore CG, Wilson-Witherspoon P, Probst JC. Time and money: effects of no-shows at a family practice residency clinic. Fam Med 2001;33(7):522–527

[21] Martin-Gorgojo A, García-Doval I, Del Río de la Torre E. Survey on private dermatology practice characteristics and fees in Spain in 2018. Actas Dermosifiliogr 2018

[22] Daggy J, Lawley M, Willis D, et al. Using no-show modeling to improve clinic performance. Health Informatics J 2010;16(4):246–259

24 Reminder Calls/Texts: Implementing an Effective Appointment Reminder System

Reena Jogi MD

Abstract

Appointment reminders are a critical part of any dermatology practice. They serve to reduce no-shows, manage cancellations, and encourage patient engagement. Although a variety of methods exist for appointment reminders, some are clearly superior to others, and the goal of this chapter is to outline the advantages of these various methods. Ultimately, choosing a system that helps save valuable staff time, while significantly increasing appointment attendance and patient engagement, can make a world of difference for a busy dermatology practice.

Keywords: appointment reminders, texts, no-shows, cancellations, automation, SMS

Top 10 Things You Need to Know

1. Sending patients appointment reminders is a critical service that benefits the patient experience, including access to care, continuity of care, and satisfaction.
2. Appointment reminders serve an important business function by reducing no-shows and managing cancellations, ultimately increasing topline revenue for your practice.
3. Providers are allowed under Health Insurance Portability and Accountability Act (HIPAA) to send appointment reminders without a specific "opt-in" on behalf of the patient—it's considered a part of patient treatment.
4. A wide range of studies have found that appointment reminders are effective at reducing no-shows and increasing attendance.
5. Appointment reminders can be sent via text message, phone call, snail mail, and email. Each medium possesses varying effectiveness.
6. Texting is the most widely used and frequently used smartphone functionality. It also has the highest and fastest read rate.
7. Automation of appointment reminders can save valuable staff time.
8. Ensure your reminder provides your patient with adequate time to reschedule if necessary but not too much time that the reminder is not at the top of his or her mind.
9. To boost effectiveness of appointment reminders, include additional information in the reminder in the form of preprocedure instructions or intake information.
10. The most effective appointment reminders are two-way; they allow patients to engage with the reminder in some capacity.

24.1 The Cost of Missed Appointments

24.1.1 The Patient Experience

When patients miss an appointment, the results can be detrimental to both your patients and practice alike. As dermatologists running busy practices, we know that new patient wait times can be lengthy. In fact, across midsized markets nationally, patients are waiting an average of over 35 days for a dermatology appointment—9% longer than the average medical wait times in a given area.[1] It is in the best interest of both your practice and your patients that once patients are able to secure an appointment, they actually show up. Yet there are countless situations that can lead patients to miss a long-awaited appointment, including transportation challenges, forgetting the appointment or being confused over the date and time of the appointment, and normal life challenges like being unable to leave work or school.[2]

As physicians, we know that when patients miss an appointment, it has an impact on relationship, continuity of care, satisfaction, and health outcomes.[3,4] We also know that patient experience is critical to a successful dermatology practice. When a patient misses an appointment because he or she forgot, or was confused about the date, time, or location, and then must wait to secure a new appointment, that particular patient's continuity of care is disrupted. He or she is also likely to have a suboptimalplethora of studies out experience, placing serious strain on the relationship between the patient and his or her loyalty to your practice.

24.1.2 The Business of Your Practice

Beyond the impact on your patients' health and experiences, missed appointments can put a massive dent in your practice's revenue. Appointment cancellations, no-shows, and incomplete referrals combined with long wait times all contribute to an estimated $650,000 annual lost revenue.[5] The true cost of those gaps in your practice's schedule goes beyond lost reimbursement. Studies show that those gaps can add up to an enormous social cost which includes "unused or misused personnel time, equipment and ward capacity," etc.[6] In other words, there is an opportunity cost created by missed appointments, as your staff time, equipment, office space, and other resources are not being fully utilized.

Prior to owning my own practice, I had worked primarily at practices that used phone calls for appointment reminders. While this was used with varying success and efficiency at each practice, overall, it carried the cost of large number of hours of staff time as well as a high number of no-shows and missed appointments. Phone call reminders tend to involve clunky processes that can be both inefficient and ineffective inevitably resulting in holes in the schedule. This wastes staff's time in two ways: first by taking their time away from other duties to make phone call reminders and second by not allowing them to stay busy during the clinic day as a result of missed appointments.

24.2 Increasing Attendance with Appointment Reminders

24.2.1 Combating Forgetfulness

Among all of the possible reasons for missing an appointment, forgetting about the appointment is one of the most common. In fact, a national study of missed appointments found that forgetfulness and or confusion over the date, time, or location of the appointment were the reasons behind 40%

of missed appointments.[2] The good news from this study is that dermatologists can be proactive in addressing a large portion of these barriers by simply sending clear and targeted appointment reminders to their patients.

24.2.2 The Effectiveness of Reminders

There exists a plethora of studies out there showcasing just how effective appointment reminders can be at increasing appointment attendance in health care settings. One massive meta-analysis found "consistent evidence that all types of reminder systems are effective at improving appointment attendance across a range of health care settings and patient populations."[7] Another study even showed that patients receiving appointment reminders were 25% less likely to miss an appointment.[8] Appointment reminders also make it more likely that the patient will show up on time. Busy dermatology practices like my own cannot afford to have patients show up late, as it throws off the whole schedule and can increase wait times for other patients. Sending an appointment reminder makes it more likely that the patient will show up and show up on time. The evidence is incontrovertible; implementing an appointment reminder system in your practice is an effective way to reduce missed appointments, ultimately improving the patient experience and your practice's business.

24.2.3 A Part of Patient Treatment

According to the marketing rules in the Health Insurance Portability and Accountability Act (HIPAA), dermatologists and other physicians cannot use a patient's contact information to send marketing messages without specific consent to do so. So if you plan on sending your patients notices about cosmetic specials, make sure to ask your patients to specifically "opt-in" for promotional content from your practice. Marketing, however, does not include appointment reminders. HIPAA specifies that anything relevant to patient treatment, such as appointment reminders, is not considered "marketing" and therefore does not require a patient "opt-in."[9]

The requirement to receive a patient's prior authorization in order to share marketing announcements is not only a legal requirement but also an ethical one. Keeping appointment reminders and other messages specific to patient care (prescription pick-up reminders, referral information, newly available services, etc.) separate from marketing communications makes it more likely that the patient will pay attention and or respond to the care-related messaging, thereby improving attendance and patient engagement.

Generally, appointment reminders contribute to an improved patient experience by generating positive interactions between the patient and your practice from the very beginning. They make sure your patients can access desired or necessary treatment, reduce confusion throughout the process, and offer a polished and warm welcome to your patients before they even walk through your practice's doors.

24.3 Not All Reminders Are Created Equal

Huge variation exists in reminder systems, including how, when, and with what information you are contacting your patients. As mentioned earlier, there have been a wide range of studies conducted around appointment reminders and missed appointments, and many have looked at the relative effectiveness of different reminder system designs. Below are a few ways you can vary the design of your reminder system as well as some notes on the effectiveness of those variations.

24.3.1 Medium: Phone, Text, Email, and Mail

There are four primary mediums practices used to communicate with patients—phone, text, email, and regular mail. Text messages boast the highest contact rate (meaning how often did the patient actually look at the text) at around 97 to 99% in health care.[7] In comparison, phone contact rates hover between 30 and 60%, and email open rates are closer to 20%.[10,11] One study comparing phone, email, and text appointment reminders found that the text reminders resulted in the lowest no-show rate.[12] And what about snail mail? A study from 1994, back when texting and email were less ubiquitous, showed little to no difference between using postcard reminders and no reminders at all.[13]

It is becoming easier and more effective to use text messaging over other communication mediums. Text messaging is the most frequently used smartphone feature, and people of all ages and backgrounds are texting—even the over

55 population sends nearly 250 texts a month.[14] Patient satisfaction rates with physician–patient texting is also high, somewhere between 77 and 96%.[15]

Ultimately, the most effective appointment reminder medium is the one your patients prefer. In a perfect world, you would contact each individual patient via his or her medium of choice. Unfortunately, that would not result in an efficient workflow for your practice. Regardless, patients are open to receiving reminders of varying mediums, although they prefer an electronic medium (i.e., not phone or snail mail), so they can respond at the most convenient time for them.[10] As we all become more and more inundated with information, getting real-time reminders that are quick and easy to digest and respond to is critical. And, when given a choice, evidence suggests patients prefer text message reminders.[16]

24.3.2 Automation: Saving Staff Time

With the technology available today, it seems wasteful of your practice's staff time to implement a reminder system that is not automated to some degree. Certainly, messages should be personalized for the concerned patient, including the patient's name as well as specific details and instructions relevant to his or her appointment. Those details, however, can be automatically generated by an advanced system. Ideally, your appointment reminder system will integrate with your practice management system, electronic health record (EHR), and other software your practice uses to create a singular system that works to seamlessly push and pull relevant information. This will allow you to automatically send personalized appointment reminders at the intervals you choose, resulting in better use of staff time and happier staff overall.

24.3.3 The Timing: Allowing Your Patients Time to Plan

A systematic review comparing various appointment reminder systems looked at the optimal timing of reminders. It found that the optimal timing of an appointment reminder is somewhere between 1 and 7 days.[9] Earlier reminders allow your patients time to rearrange their schedules or contact your office to reschedule or cancel if necessary. This is especially important if the patient made the appointment over a month prior. Earlier reminders also allow your practice time to fill empty appointment slots if your patient does decide to reschedule or cancel. Too early, and the patient may not feel a sufficient sense of urgency, and may not be able to predict their schedule with adequate accuracy to act. Try to schedule your reminders to go out twice—once around the 7-day mark, and a second time around the 2-day mark. This will increase the likelihood your patients will respond if their schedule changes.

24.3.4 The Content: What to Include in Your Reminders

At a minimum, an effective appointment reminder should include the date, time, and location of the appointment. It should also include the provider's name as well as any pertinent appointment-specific information (i.e., take all medications as usual the day of Mohs surgery, or hold nonessential blood thinners prior to filler appointments or other preprocedure instructions). An identical systematic review referenced in regard to reminder timing also looked at "reminder only" messages (with appointment details only) and compared to "reminder plus" messages. Reminder plus messages could include supporting clinical information (i.e., the Mohs surgery preprocedure instructions), intake instructions, health education information, or some sort of confirmation requirement. The review found that the "reminder plus" messages were generally more effective at improving attendance. When implementing your reminder system, consider how you can use the opportunity to connect with your patients in meaningful ways. Health education information and intake instructions to save the patient's time in the office can both help make your appointments more meaningful. Two-way communication channels that allow your patients to confirm their appointments or request to reschedule are a must-have. Patients have begun expecting the ability to engage in two-way mobile communications, and this functionality will greatly improve patient satisfaction while providing you with the information you need to better manage your practice's schedule.

24.3.5 The Cost: Ensuring a Return on Investment

Appointment reminder systems should improve the patient experience and drive an increase in revenue for your practice. Any effective reminder system will be able to demonstrate a clear return on investment while providing the elements of a reminder system you have deemed most important. A key consideration when looking at cost is the investment in staff time to learn and manage the new system versus the time spent previously sending reminders. An effective system will be simple and easy to implement so that staff can spend valuable time providing a greater level of customer service or performing other needed duties as opposed to manually generating reminders or troubleshooting a clunky reminder system.

24.4 Conclusion

I get text reminders for just about everything these days, and it's been a huge convenience for me because, like most people, when I'm at work I can't easily answer the phone. A text allows me to respond at my own leisure. Technology now allows my practice to offer my patients this same convenience in an automated way that actually saves staff time.

When the practice first opened, we initially used a service that sounded good in theory; however, we quickly found that it lacked much of the functionality that we required. It required loading a program on one front desk computer, and that computer had to remain turned on during the evening when reminders were sent out. If the staff member forgot to leave the computer on, the process would fail. In addition, the reminders that were sent out were only one-way, and we had to rely on a staff member who had to run a report each morning to remove cancellations from the schedule.

We quickly discovered Luma Health (www.lumahealth.io), and we have been using them for appointment reminders for over 2 years. This company offers all of the features outlined in the previous sections such as automation, engagement, texts, and practice management system integration. It also offers solutions to many other issues facing busy practices, such as feedback and reputation management, self-scheduling, referral management, and clinical messaging.

There are a lot of factors to consider when implementing an appointment reminder system. Keep in mind that the ultimate goal of improving patient experience supports your practice's business. Implementing a system that can save valuable staff time, significantly increase appointment attendance, and engage patients can be a game changer for your practice.

Do's and Don'ts for Appointment Reminders

Do's:

- **Consider your patients' preference:** When in doubt, send a text. It's affordable, easy to automate, and people of all ages read and respond to texts.
- **Automate whenever possible:** It saves valuable staff time that could be spent providing a higher quality of customer service along with other important duties.
- **Include relevant information in your reminders:** This could include intake instructions, directions to your practice, background information about a procedure, and more.
- **Choose a system that integrates with your EHR and practice management systems:** This will make the previous items—automating and personalizing your communications—seamless.
- **Give your patients the ability to respond and engage:** This can include the ability to confirm their appointment, reschedule, watch a health education video, etc. More two-way communication produces more engaged patients, ultimately improving the overall patient experience.

Don'ts:

- **Try to do everything manually:** Investing in technology and automated workflows will save you time, money, and headaches.
- **Send your reminders too early or too close to the appointment:** Too early and the appointment may not be at the top of the patient's mind. Too close to the appointment and your patients may not have time to contact you in order to reschedule if necessary.
- **Be generic:** Technology makes it easy to personalize your reminders, and customization means your patients get relevant, engaging, and actionable information.
- **Leave it up to the patient:** Be proactive about confirming appointments to provide your patients with a better experience and increase the likelihood of being notified if the patient needs to reschedule.

Checklist

- ☐ **Evaluate your current reminder system.** How well is it working? Is your no-show rate above 10%? Is staff spending a significant amount of time making manual phone calls or mailers? How much is your system costing you in terms of technology, lost revenue, and staff time?
- ☐ **Consider a system that would work better.** Think about what you are looking for in a new system—it could be increased automation, a built-in rescheduling method, etc.—and decide what your budget for that system looks like. From my point of view, an effective system is one that includes the following points:
  - Automates and runs without constant monitoring
  - Knows the difference between a mobile and a landline number, for example, and works with your existing patient data
  - Can be easily tweaked and adjusted through an intuitive interface
  - Integrates with your practice management system
  - Allows infinite SMS messaging without extra charges.
  - Does more than just reminders—can also follow-up with patients to give feedback, drive them to post positive reviews, and automatically fill from a digital waitlist.
- ☐ **Identify a technology partner that can implement your desired system.** Your technology partner should be able to help you implement an easy-to-use system that can allow you to customize your reminders to your patients.
- ☐ **Design messages that are engaging.** Think about what your patients need to know before they come in for an appointment. If possible, segment your reminders to provide relevant information based on the patient's appointment type.
- ☐ **Watch your patients become happier and your practice more successful.**

References

[1] Merritt Hawkins. 2017 Survey of Physician Appointment Wait Times and Medicare and Medicaid Acceptance Rates. Available at: https://www.merritthawkins.com/uploadedFiles/MerrittHawkins/Content/Pdf/mha2017wait-timesurveyPDF.pdf. Accessed October 18, 2019

[2] Crutchfield TM, Kistler CE. Getting Patients in the Door: Medical Appointment Reminder Preferences. Available at: https://www.ncbi.nlm.nih.gov/pubmed/28182131. Accessed October 18, 2019

[3] Saultz JW, Lochner J. Interpersonal Continuity of Care and Care Outcomes: A Critical Review. Available at: https://www.aafpfoundation.org/content/dam/foundation/documents/who-we-are/cfhm/classicsfamilymedicine/InterpersonalContinuityofCareSaultz.pdf

[4] Martin C, Perfect T, Mantle G. Non-Attendance in Primary Care. Available at: https://academic.oup.com/fampra/article/22/6/638/497972. Accessed October 18, 2019

[5] Luma Health. Available at: www.lumahealth.io. Accessed October 18, 2019

[6] Mbada E, Nonvignon J, Ajayi O, et al. Impact of Missed Appointments for Out-Patient Physiotherapy on Cost, Efficiency, and Patients' Recovery. Available at: https://www.sciencedirect.com/science/article/pii/S1013702512000462. Accessed October 18, 2019

[7] McLean SM, Booth A, Gee M, et al. Appointment Reminder Systems Are Effective but Not Optimal. Available at: https://www.ncbi.nlm.nih.gov/pubmed/27110102. Accessed October 18, 2019

[8] Lin C, et al. Text Message Reminders Increase Appointment Adherence in a Pediatric Clinic. https://www.hindawi.com/journals/ijpedi/2016/8487378/

[9] U.S. Department of Health & Human Services. 45 CFR 164.501, 164.508(a)(3). Available at: https://www.hhs.gov/hipaa/for-professionals/privacy/guidance/marketing/index.html. Accessed October 18, 2019

[10] Mclean S, Booth A, Gee M, et al. Appointment Reminder Systems Are Effective but Not Optimal: Results of a Systematic Review and Evidence Synthesis Employing Realist Principles. Available at: https://pdfs.semanticscholar.org/aaa1/728c-77299477c3ec1a32952826fabb0a159b.pdf. Accessed October 18, 2019

[11] txtsignal. SMS Marketing vs. Email Marketing: The 2017 Comparison. Available at: https://txtsignal.com/sms-marketing-vs-email-2017/. Accessed October 18, 2019

[12] Wegrzyniak LM, Hedderly D, Chaudry K, et al. Measuring the Effectiveness of Patient-Chosen Reminder Methods in a Private Orthodontic Practice. Available at: http://www.angle.org/doi/pdf/10.2319/090517-597.1?code=angf-site. Accessed October 18, 2019

[13] Moser SE. Effectiveness of Post Card Appointment Reminders. Available at: https://www.ncbi.nlm.nih.gov/pubmed/7976479. Accessed October 18, 2019

[14] Experian Marketing Services' Simmons Connect. 18–24-Year-Old Smartphone Owners Send and Receive Almost 4K Texts per xiv Month. Available at: https://www.marketingcharts.com/industries/telecom-industries-27993/attachment/experian-text-message-activity-byage-mar2013. Accessed October 18, 2019

[15] Fischer HH, Moore SL, Johnson TL, Everhart RM, Batal H, Davidsoni AJ. Appointment Reminders by Text Message in a Safety Net Health Care System. Available at: https://www.ncbi.nlm.nih.gov/pmc/articles/PMC5983071/. Accessed October 18, 2019

[16] Perron NJ, Dao MD, Righini MC, et al. Text-Messaging versus Telephone Reminders to Reduce Missed Appointments in an Academic Primary Care Clinic. Available at: https://www.ncbi.nlm.nih.gov/pmc/articles/PMC3623700/. Accessed October 18, 2019

25 Is There a Better Way to Answer Calls?

Amy Derick MD

Abstract

On-demand answering of phone calls presents organizational challenges due to fluctuations in call volume, variety of call purpose, and agents who are known for high turnover. Management of this complex process is an important part of running an efficient dermatology practice. The purpose of this chapter is to review suggested methods for minimizing the volume of inbound phone calls and maximizing the success of phone calls received.

Methods discussed for minimizing the volume of inbound calls include the following:

1. Allow patients to schedule appointments online. Integrate these requests with practice management software if possible.
2. Anticipate common patient questions. Make answers available on the practice's website or on education documents distributed to patients.
3. Consider writing for generic medications. These prescriptions reduce the volume of calls from the pharmacy related to prior authorizations. Patients will be less likely to call with concerns regarding the price of medications.
4. Survey patients to measure satisfaction after each appointment. Surveys provide a mechanism for patients to voice concerns without a phone call.

Methods discussed for maximizing the success of phone calls received include the following:

1. Sort inbound phone calls by purpose to ensure the answering agent is the most appropriate person to assist the patient.
2. Staff answering agents adequately for the volume of inbound calls. Reducing time on hold will increase patient satisfaction and minimize call abandonment rate.
3. Train answering agents with best practices for style and phone etiquette. Consider using scripts for common patient interactions.
4. Provide effective management of the inbound call team. Use data analytics and call audits to ensure the quality of agents. Ensure that agents are comfortable and have access to appropriate equipment.

Keywords: call center, phone system, IVR, SLA, abandon rate, call scripting, auditing

Top 10 Things You Need to Know

1. Minimize scheduling call volume by offering online scheduling tools.
2. Better education in the office means fewer patients calling with questions.
3. Writing generic medications will yield fewer pharmacy-related calls.
4. Decide what features you need, and select a phone system appropriate for your practice.
5. Know the laws in your state related to call recording.
6. Decide what hold times are acceptable for your patients and staff accordingly.
7. Write scripts for your most common patient interactions.
8. Train your staff to accept accountability for first-call resolution.
9. Audit calls regularly to ensure quality.
10. Use data to ensure the efficiency of your call center operations.

25.1 Introduction

A phone call to a dermatology practice can represent an opportunity to generate revenue (e.g., new patient appointment) or address a patient issue (e.g., staff managing a patient complaint). Calls can also range from urgent (e.g., acute full-body rash) to not urgent (e.g., medical records requests). Since all calls consume valuable staff time, managing this process well is an important part of running an efficient practice.

An efficient dermatology practice should focus on two things: (1) minimizing the number of inbound phone calls that consume the practice's resources, and (2) maximizing the instances of patients calling the office, and the call center agents delivering excellent customer service and solving their patients' issues on the first call.

25.2 Minimizing Calls

25.2.1 On-line Scheduling

Scheduling appointments online can reduce the volume of inbound calls. Some online scheduling tools may be fully integrated with the practice's management software. These tools may allow a patient to select a specific appointment date, time, purpose, and provider, and reserve them in the practice's software without any phone-based communication. Other online scheduling tools are not fully integrated (e.g., a web-based form that simply indicates an appointment preference to your scheduling department). While this type of solution may still require an outbound phone call to confirm the details of the appointment, these outbound calls can be made during off-peak times, when they are less likely to cause delays for other inbound callers.

25.2.2 Patient Questions

Anticipating patient questions and handling them in the office will decrease future calls concerning questions to the office. This is particularly true in the case of postsurgical patients. Instructions should be given to the patient in writing and by voice, and preferably ahead of a planned procedure. If you give the patient both the pre and postoperative instructions ahead of the surgery, the patient might see something on the postoperative instructions that could pose an issue. For example, no golfing for 2 weeks after the surgery.

Install a mechanism where patients can send questions (with photos) securely through your website or patient portal. Having this capacity allows your staff to answer questions in a less time-sensitive manner. In addition, the messages can be forwarded directly to the person who can resolve the issue. The patient can then be contacted by phone or a secure electronic mechanism.

Try to have information for commonly asked questions on your website in a visible location. For example, the insurances that your practice accepts, locations of your practice(s) with photo(s) of the exterior of the building, and snip of a map. If your building is difficult to find, tell your patients how to locate the practice on their first call.

25.2.3 Pharmacy-Related Calls

The number of calls from either the pharmacy or the patient related to prescriptions can be significant. These calls may include questions about how to take a prescription (which can be managed through education in the office), prior authorization issues, or issues related to the cost of prescriptions. Writing for mostly generic medications (when indicated) will decrease the number of phone calls to your office. As most practices do not have the ability to predict the cost of prescription medications at the time of the appointment, writing for generic medications ensures the best probability of prescription coverage, without a prior authorization, at the lowest cost to the patient.

25.2.4 Complaints

Providing patients with an excellent experience is the best way of minimizing complaints. In addition, sending every patient an electronic survey after each appointment provides the patient with a mechanism to voice concerns in writing. These concerns may require a follow-up phone call, but they can be triaged and handled by appropriate staff.

When you do get an inbound phone call, you want to give the caller a great experience as well as get first contact resolution, when possible.

25.2.5 Sorting

If you have multiple practice locations, having one phone number is helpful when dealing with patient calls. This is especially true if certain functions (e.g., billing or scheduling) are handled centrally.

Depending on your call volume, a phone system may be required. There are two types: basic and advanced. A basic system is one in which an inbound call rings simultaneously on all phones connected to that line. With enough calls, a basic system may not be adequate. You will not be able to measure key metrics on a basic phone system, so you will not know if your demand is being met, if you are staffed correctly, or how long patients are waiting on the phone. Employees can become frustrated because there is less accountability for who should answer the phone. A lack of certain features (e.g., call back feature) on basic systems leads to suboptimal patient experience.

Advanced phone systems have an ability to view a dashboard of active calls, collect and analyze data, and record and store calls for retrieval. If an advanced system is used, typically a phone tree (IVR) is implemented.

There are many different advanced phone systems to choose from. However, know that all advanced phone system options fall into two general categories: cloud-based and on-premise solutions.

Cloud-based phone systems are good for small- to medium-sized practices as they have flexibility with most features. They use competitively priced voice over Internet protocol (VOIP) phone lines that are more flexible than T1 or regular phone line. As the "lines" dedicated to the practice are flexible (meaning the number of active "lines" can quickly scale up and down), the system can accommodate large swings in call volume. In addition, cloud-based phone solutions allow you to grow smoothly over time as your call volume increases. These cloud-based systems are usually sold using a subscription model, allowing for quick addition of call capacity, new extensions, and re-routing of calls. However, there are some potential drawbacks to cloud-based phone systems. As they are managed by a third-party service provider, you must make sure that you engage a vendor with a proven track record. Have your attorney review your contract before you sign, so that you know what to expect if you decide to switch vendors in the future. Also, if you use a cloud-based phone system, when your Internet is out, your phones are down too. When the Internet is down, many practices elect not to see patients. With a cloud-based system, you'd be unable to call the patients to tell them not to come. You also need to make sure you have adequate bandwidth with low latency (less than 100 ms). If you do not have adequate bandwidth or reliable latency, there could be an audible delay between the voice of the caller and practice which is uncomfortable. Finally, you'll need to consider whether a Business Associate Agreement (BAA) is required. Normally, telecommunications providers would be considered "conduits" and would therefore not necessitate a BAA. However, with a cloud-based phone system, the vendor may be storing information that contains PHI such as voicemail, call logs, etc. Discuss the contract and the requirement for a BAA with your legal team prior to executing the contract.

On-premise phone systems may be more cost-effective for medium- to large-size practices. Although the initial cost may be higher, if set up correctly, the cost of the system may be less in the long run. In addition, you are not exposed to a subscription fee that may increase over time. There is no need for a BAA since the system is contained within your practice. Modern on-premise systems require very little hardware and can be installed on a robust computer workstation or small server. These systems are not connected to the Internet and therefore provide phone service in the face of an Internet outage. The downsides to having an on-premise system is that it is more complicated to set up and maintain, and you'll need to have confidence in your IT team to be able to manage it. There are also many choices related to the setup of the system, which may frustrate many dermatologists. Also, you'll have to choose your own phone line vendor including VOIP or traditional phone lines.

If an advanced solution is chosen, using a phone tree (IVR) is helpful. The greeting at the beginning of the call may contain a disclosure that the call is being recorded for quality and training, depending on your state's "wiretapping" laws. Make sure you know the laws in your state related to the recording of phone calls. Disclosures that are automatically played at the beginning of every call ensure the disclosure is heard. You should verify that the patient cannot skip that portion of the call by entering an extension. When you have a well-designed phone tree, the patient is less likely to require a handoff between agents. For example, if the patient has a billing call, he or she should be routed directly to the billing department and not be forced into the queue of people scheduling appointments. Careful phone tree planning will hopefully sort callers into appropriate queues where their request or question can be handled by the person who answers the phone. You may choose to send certain phone calls directly into voicemail, so they can be handled at off-peak times or in batches. If this is done, you should record a message on the voicemail, explaining the expected time frame when the patient will hear back. Some systems allow the patient to elect to go to VM when they are waiting in a queue by pushing a button. A newer phone feature is the ability for the caller to request a callback when waiting in queue. When the caller pushes this button, they are prompted to hang up after their call back number is verified. When the next available agent assigned to that queue is idle, the agent's phone rings and the system calls the patient back automatically. One key metric for a call center is abandonment rate, when the caller just hangs up while waiting. Since instituting the callback feature in our call center one year ago, our abandonment rate has decreased by approximately 70%. Of note is the fact that if the outbound phone call generated from using the callback feature is not answered, it is counted as an abandoned call.

25.2.6 Answering the Phone as Quickly as Possible

In call centers, one key metric is the Service Level Agreement (SLA). The SLA is defined as the percentage of calls answered in a certain amount of time that is acceptable for your callers to wait. If the hold time is longer than the defined SLA time, it is considered a breach.

Answering the phone quickly is a complicated process. It requires an available agent to answer the phone when the patient calls the practice. If you do not have any available agents at the time of the call, the call will be first placed in queue, and then the caller will be placed on hold. Staffing plays a key role in increasing the percentage of phone calls answered within the SLA. Calls to dermatology practices tend to cluster around certain times of the day. Some common peaks include the 9:00 am hour and lunch time. The peak of calls around the lunch hour may make it difficult for your call center agents to take breaks at regular times. You do not want to have your phone lines turned off during the lunch hour. Although this gives your team a break, you will be missing calls. In a small office, this sometimes leaves one to two people with different lunch times than the rest of the team.

You'll have to make a choice whether to staff the bare minimum of agents, staff for the maximum call volumes that you see, or staff somewhere in between. Be mindful that call center agents are a difficult group to keep happy, and turnover and no-show rates can be high. It puts pressure on the remaining agents to answer calls nonstop if the phones are staffed with minimal people.

If patients are waiting in queue, many offices choose to have pleasant music playing with occasional reminders that the caller is still in queue. Some phone systems allow for the caller to be informed about their place in the queue and estimate wait times.

Medicare binds all of Medicare prescription health plans (PHPs) to provide a service level where 80% of phone calls are answered within 30 seconds, and requires an average speed of answer to be less than 30 seconds with a 5% or less abandonment rate. Dermatology practices are, however, not required to meet this standard.

There are many ways to sort the calls among the agents once they are in queue. The Ring All or Round Robin methods are popular. Many call center agents appreciate the Round Robin method because they know when the phone rings at their stations, and it also means that it is their turn to answer it. Having accountability for each call that rings improves the individual agent time to pick up the phone.

Once the call is answered, make sure your agents are trained to tell the difference between urgent and nonurgent calls and how to escalate a call. For nonurgent calls, create policies on the range of acceptable times for completion of the task related to the call. Develop a system of tracking open and closed tickets if possible.

25.2.7 Interaction between Agent and Caller

It is important to have a standardized greeting. This will create a consistent presentation of your brand. Preferably, the person answering the phones should not be distracted from this duty by other time-sensitive tasks. For example, it is not ideal to have a receptionist answering phones, because that person is also responsible for timely face-to-face interactions with patients in the office. If an employee must choose between a responsibility to answer a ringing phone or help a waiting patient, clearly one or the other will be disappointed.

When talking to a caller, it is important to establish their identity immediately. If he or she is calling on behalf of someone else, ensure the patient has authorized the caller to speak on his or her behalf. With every interaction, there will be a set of steps that need to be taken to satisfy the patient's request (e.g., new patient calling to book an appointment). It is important to formalize these procedures and provide scripting, where applicable. This allows for consistency and decreased likelihood for errors.

Callers value "First Contact Resolution," which means they got what they needed from that call. Set a culture where each agent takes responsibility for solving patients' problems rather than passing the buck. Most callers are willing to be placed on hold if they know they will have their issue resolved at that time. In some practices, two levels of agents may be required. In this scenario, the first level mostly handles scheduling calls: booking, rescheduling, and canceling appointments. The second level handles calls that require advanced clinical skills such as giving patients advice on wound care.

When talking on the phone, especially when booking an appointment, the agents should minimize "dead air." Dead air is the quiet when someone is typing in information into the computer. It is important to repeat back information as you are entering it to keep the patient engaged in the process. You also want to cultivate a group of agents who are even-keeled and professional. For example, you never want an agent to lose their temper and yell at a patient. You also don't want an agent to become too familiar and unprofessional, as idle conversation takes time and might not be appreciated by the patient.

25.2.8 Building an Effective Team

Hiring happy, productive, and reliable people is always ideal. However, even the most promising agents require training. Training will help agents learn the procedures and scripts for your call center, and how to have a good tone when fielding a call. If you have call recording software, periodically audit with a numerical score for script consistency and tone. Use these recordings as coaching tools. If there is a particularly good or bad call, consider adding it to the curriculum of your training program.

Use data. The data that is collected from the phone system can be used to evaluate and, if shared transparently, motivate call center agents. High-performing agents appreciate the fact that they are on top. Agents who fare poorly on key metrics may require additional training, or they may self-select out. Also, data allows agents to quantify their work in order to know how many phone calls they took that day, etc. A strong manager who is willing to get into a queue helps improve morale on busy days.

Make your agents comfortable. Ergonomic chairs, monitor mounts, and padded keyboards provide comfort. Wireless headsets allow agents to type more easily without cradling their phone in their necks.

25.3 Conclusion

On-demand answering of phone calls presents organizational challenges due to fluctuations in call volume, variety of call purpose, and agents who are known for high turnover.

Minimize the number of on-demand calls by working to decrease call volume. For the phone calls that you do receive, consider sorting them in an efficient way, collecting data, and servicing these calls with friendly and trained staff who are accountable for the calls that they receive.

26 Critical Components of Consents and Documentation

Misha Zarbafian MD, David J. Goldberg MD, JD

Abstract

Understanding the components of consent and documentation has become increasingly critical for dermatologists, as the continued expansion of procedural options has opened the door for legal ramifications. Plaintiffs, who are pursuing causes of action in negligence, must prove that the dermatologist's failure to meet the reasonable standard of care directly caused damages. While this standard can be challenging to define, dermatologists can generally protect themselves by practicing in a fashion that is both consistent across patients and similar to their peers. We recommend approaching informed consent as an educational discussion which includes patients in the decision-making process. This discussion must occur before performing the procedure, be sufficiently informative, permit a voluntary decision, and be undertaken with a patient or legal representative who has the capacity to make such a decision. Each discussion must contain certain minimum elements such as the nature of the proposed procedure and its potential risks. However, the dermatologist must consider additional elements such as deciding which risks the patient should be warned about. Dermatologists will often be unable to recall specific discussions with patients, so informed consent discussions, in addition to other notable discussions, should always be documented in the patient chart. Other strategies, such as the prioritization of effective communication and patient satisfaction, can also help reduce litigation. Complications and lawsuits cannot be prevented; however, dermatologists can help protect themselves from the consequences of a malpractice suit by understanding the importance of informed consent, written documentation, and the basic principles of a cause of action in negligence.

Keywords: medico-legal, informed consent, negligence, standard of care, medical malpractice, documentation

Top 10 Things You Need to Know

1. Procedural dermatology continues to show impressive growth in the variety of treatments available to patients. As this growth continues, the potential for lawsuits will also rise.
2. Dermatologists can help protect themselves from malpractice suits by understanding the importance of proper informed consent, written documentation, and the basic principles of a cause of action in negligence.
3. In order to obtain proper informed consent, the patient or legal representative must be adequately informed, make a voluntary decision, and have the capacity to comprehend and communicate the decision.
4. The standard of care is often determined on a case-by-case basis with many medical and legal influences, but can be described as the way the majority of physicians, within a scope of medicine, would practice.
5. Neither the standard of care, nor the contents of an informed consent discussion, should change depending on the training background or experience of the dermatologist.
6. The occurrence of a complication is not synonymous with an instance of medical malpractice. To successfully claim a cause of action in negligence, a plaintiff must show the presence of the following four required elements: duty of care, breach of duty, causation, and damages.
7. Habit evidence can be used to testify to a dermatologist's behavior that is sufficiently uniform and repetitive in practice. However, this may not always be sufficient in court, so written documentation in the patient's chart is of paramount importance.
8. When considering whether to suggest a procedure, the dermatologist should evaluate the psychological profile of the patient for the presence of factors that may indicate a greater likelihood of patient dissatisfaction.

(Continued)

26.1 The Legal Landscape in Dermatology

The market for procedural dermatology continues to expand, as exciting advancements have revolutionized the field with enhanced quality and a nearly endless variety of therapeutic options. This progress resulted in a 120.2% increase (from 3.4 to 7.6 million) in the number of dermatologic surgical procedures performed between 2001 and 2007, with soft tissue augmentation and neurotoxin injections showing the greatest growth.[1] According to the American Society of Plastic Surgeons (2017),[2] there were approximately 17.5 million cosmetic procedures performed in the United States in 2017, which represented a 2% growth from 2016. A staggering number (15.7 million) of these procedures were minimally invasive, with botulinum toxin type A, soft tissue augmentation, and chemical peels being the most commonly performed.[2] As the number of both physicians and nonphysicians performing dermatologic procedures increases, the potential for legal ramifications also inevitably rises. In fact, facing a medical malpractice suit at some point may be almost inevitable for a cosmetic dermatologist in today's litigious landscape. Dermatologists can help protect themselves from the consequences of a malpractice suit by understanding the importance of informed consent, written documentation, and the basic principles of a cause of action in negligence.

26.2 Informed Consent

26.2.1 The Difference between Informed and Implied Consent

It is generally accepted that a dermatologist may perform routine history-taking and physical examination to arrive at a diagnosis. The dermatologist would be considered to have implied consent to provide this basic care for a patient in his or her clinic. Any intervention or procedure that extends beyond routine care requires that the dermatologist obtains informed consent.

26.2.2 What Is Informed Consent?

The importance of obtaining proper and documented informed consent cannot be overstated. It is the responsibility of the dermatologist to obtain informed consent prior to performing a procedure on a patient. It is prudent for the dermatologist to obtain informed consent in both verbal and written forms. Informed consent actually refers to a discussion which includes patients in the decision-making process, and requires the following three criteria to be met:[3] First, the patients must possess the capacity to comprehend and assess the benefits and risks of both the procedure and its alternatives, and to communicate their decision. To accomplish this, the information must be communicated with using language the patient can comfortably understand. Second, patients must be adequately informed regarding their diagnosis and therapeutic options. This should include answering any questions the patient may have. A more detailed discussion regarding what information dermatologists should include in the discussion can be found below (see Section 26.2.3). Finally, patients must be making their own voluntary decision, without any coercion. All these of these criteria must be met in order for a patient to provide informed consent for a particular procedure or intervention.

26.2.3 Art of Communication: Things to Include When Obtaining Informed Consent

There is a fine balance between disclosing enough information to adequately educate the patient, and bombarding them with so much information that they become overwhelmed by minutiae. The discussion to obtain informed consent must include the reasonable standard; unfortunately, this is

Table 26.1 Federal government mandate on contents for proper informed consent[3,4]

Minimum elements	Additional elements
Name of the hospital where the procedure is to take place	Name of the practitioner who conducted the informed consent discussion with the patient or the patient's representative
Name of the specific procedure	Date, time, and signature of the person witnessing the patient or the patient's legal representative signing the consent form
Name of the responsible practitioner who is performing the procedure	Indication or listing of the material risks of the procedure or treatment that were discussed with the patient or the patient's representative
Statement that the procedure (including anticipated benefits, material risks,[a] and alternative therapies) was explained to the patient or the patient's legal representative	Statement, if relevant, that physicians other than the operative practitioner, including but not limited to residents, will be performing important tasks related to the surgery
Date and time the informed consent form is signed by the patient or the patient's legal representative	Statement, if relevant, that qualified medical practitioners, who are not physicians, will only operate within their scope of practice
Signature of the patient or legal representative	
Other considerations if there is an applicable State law governing the content of the form	

[a]Material risks could include risks with a high degree of likelihood but a low degree of severity, as well as those with a very low degree of likelihood but high degree of severity.
Data from: Federal Code Title 42 Tag A-0238 §482.24(2)(v).

a vague concept which is determined on a case-by-case basis (see section 26.5). The federal government has published guidelines on what written informed consent should include, which have been listed in ▶ Table 26.1.[3,4] These minimum elements should be encompassed in every informed consent discussion, and must be individualized for each particular procedure. The dermatologist must use their clinical acumen and knowledge of the current medical literature to determine the pertinent benefits, material risks, and alternative therapies (including not undergoing treatment) for disclosure.

Clinicians may be at higher risk of litigation when failing to determine patient preferences.[5] Prioritizing open communication and setting realistic expectations at the outset enhance patient satisfaction, and can help reduce the risk of future litigation (see Section 26.5). The experience level or training history of the dermatologist should not have an impact on what is included in the discussion; a dermatologist and family physician performing the same soft tissue augmentation procedure should provide the patient with the same reasonable

standard of information. Two examples of reasonable informed consent forms can be seen in ▶ Fig. 26.1a and ▶ Fig. 26.1b.

26.3 Negligence and the Standard of Care

26.3.1 Negligence

Analysis of over 1,000 closed claims against dermatologists from 1991 to 2015 revealed that the top medical errors resulting in liability claims were the improper performance of procedures, errors in diagnosis, and medication errors, and in that order.[6] However, the occurrence of a complication from a procedure is not synonymous with medical malpractice. For example, the local recurrence of a squamous cell carcinoma may occur even if the initial surgery was performed exceptionally well. There are four required elements to prove negligence. These are as follows: (1) Duty of care, meaning that the dermatologist owed a legal duty to the plaintiff to perform a particular procedure or intervention; (2) Breach of duty, meaning the physician allegedly failed to perform the procedure or intervention at the reasonable standard of care; (3) Causation, meaning that the breach of duty was the direct cause of the plaintiff's suffered damages; and (4) Damages, whether economic or noneconomic (such as psychological harm), suffered by the plaintiff. In order to be successful in a cause of action in negligence claim, the suing plaintiff must show the presence of all four required elements.[7]

26.3.2 The Standard of Care

By virtue of providing dermatological services to patients, dermatologists owe a duty of care. In order to identify a breach of that duty, the standard of care must be defined. This standard is typically defined by courts as the presence and use of skills ordinarily possessed by a physician performing a particular intervention within a scope of practice. It can also be said that the standard of care represents the fashion in which the majority of physicians practice within a similar field of medicine. It is important to note that this definition does not require that a physician performs at the highest level amongst his peers; rather, the physician needs only to adhere to the reasonable standard. Furthermore, similar to the concept of informed consent, the standard of care for a specific procedure should be identical regardless of the previous experience or training of the physician performing the procedure. A physician falling short of this reasonable standard of care would be prone to medical malpractice litigation, and would be at risk of a court holding them negligent if the other required elements were also substantiated by the plaintiff.

Fig. 26.1 (a) Example of reasonable informed consent form for treatment with filler agents.

NAME_____   DATE_____

PATIENT CONSENT FOR TREATMENT WITH FILLER AGENTS

The use of and indications for filler agents have been explained to me by my physician. I have had the opportunity to have all questions answered to my satisfaction. I have been specifically informed that the following may occur after the injections: Swelling, redness, pain, itching, discoloration and tenderness at the implant site. They typically resolve spontaneously within several days after injection into the skin. There are extremely rare isolated reports of blindness resulting from filler injection in the area of the forehead. In Dr. Goldberg's over 30 years of treating thousands of patients and performing multiple FDA studies, he has never seen this complication. Other types of reactions are very rare, but rare patients may experience localized reactions thought to be of a hypersensitivity nature. These have usually consisted of swelling at the implant site, sometimes affecting the surrounding tissues. Redness, tenderness and rarely acne-like formations have also been reported. These reactions have either started a few days after injection or after a delay of 2-4 weeks and have been described as mild to moderate. In most instances, such reactions are self-limiting.

I also understand that the duration of filler agent enhancement may depend on the chosen agent, injection site and my own personal skin. Touch-up and follow-up treatment helps sustain the desired degree of correction. My doctor has explained to me the unique characteristics of each filler agent. I also understand that some products are FDA approved for wrinkles. Others have FDA approval for other uses. For those, the treatment of wrinkles is considered off-label use.

I agree that Dr. David Goldberg and/or designated associates may take photographs and/or videotapes of me during and/or immediately after my procedure, as well as subsequent office visits. I understand that these photographs may be published in a variety of sources including all forms of social media. In such an event, I will not be identified by name. I expect no compensation for these photographs and/or videotapes and waive all rights to any claims for payments or royalties. I also release Skin Laser and Surgery Specialists of NY & NJ, and its associated staff, from any liability in connection with the use of such photographs and/or videos.

I consent to being treated with the chosen filler agent (Belotero, Restylane, Radiesse, Sculptra, Voluma, Juvederm, Bellafil, or Perlane).

_____   _____
Patient Signature   Date

_____   _____
Witness   Date

212.7508900 115 E.57ᵗʰ Street, Suite 400, New York, NY 10022   210.441.9890 20 Prospect Avenue, Suite 702, Hackensack, NJ 07061
908.359.8980 105 Raider Boulevard, Suite 203 Hillsborough, NJ 08844

a

(Continued)

Skin Laser & Surgery Specialists of NY & NJ

OPERATIVE CONSENT: LASER/LIGHT
SOURCE/RADIOFREQUENCY SURGERY

Patient _____ Date_____

I am aware that laser/light source and radiofrequency surgeries are relatively new procedures. My doctor has explained to me that much of what has been written about these methods in newspapers, magazines, television, etc. has been sensationalized. I understand the nature, goals, limitations, and possible complications of this procedure, and I have discussed alternative forms of treatment. I have had the opportunity to ask questions about the procedure, its limitations and possible complications (see below).

I clearly understand and accept the following:

1. The goal of these surgeries, as in any cosmetic procedure, is improvement, not perfection.
2. The final result may not be apparent for months postoperatively.
3. In order to achieve the best possible result, more than one procedure may be required. There will be a charge for any further operation performed.
4. Strict adherence to the postoperative regimen (i.e. appropriate wound care and sun avoidance) is necessary in order to achieve the best possible result.
5. The surgical fee is paid for the operation itself and subsequent postoperative office visits. There is no guarantee that the expected or anticipated results will be achieved.

Although complications following laser/light source/radiofrequency surgery are infrequent, I understand that the following may occur:

1. Bleeding which in rare instances could require hospitalization.
2. Infection is rare but should it occur, treatment with antibiotics may be required.
3. Objectionable scarring is rare, but various kinds of scars are possible.
4. Alterations of skin pigmentation may occur in the areas of laser surgery. These are usually temporary, but rarely can be permanent.

In addition to these possible complications, I am aware of the general risk inherent in all surgical procedures and anesthetic administration.

I agree that Dr. David Goldberg and/or designated associates may take photographs and/or videotapes of me during and/or immediately after my procedure, as well as subsequent office visits. I understand that these photographs may be published in a variety of sources including all forms of social media. In such an event, I will not be identified by name. I expect no compensation for these photographs and/or videotapes and waive all rights to any claims for payments or royalties. I also release Skin Laser and Surgery Specialists of NY & NJ, and its associated staff, from any liability in connection with the use of such photographs and/or videos.

This authorization is given for the purpose of facilitating my care and shall supersede all previous authorizations and/or agreements executed by me. My signature certifies that I understand the goals, limitations and possible complications of laser surgery, and that I wish to proceed with the operation.

_____   _____
Patient Signature   Date

_____   _____
Witness   Date

212.750.8900   115 E. 57th Street, Suite 400, New York, NY 10022   201.441.9890   20 Prospect Avenue, Suite 702, Hackensack, NJ 07601
908.359.8980   89 Valley Road, Montclair, NJ 07042   908.359.8980   105 Raider Boulevard, Suite 203, Hillsborough, NJ 08844

b

Fig. 26.1 (*Continued*) (b) Example of reasonable informed consent form for laser or radiofrequency surgery.

The abundance of innovation and experimental concepts that make procedural dermatology so exciting may also leave its providers susceptible to litigation. Many treatments may fall into regulatory gaps or be used off-label, without clearance by the Food and Drugs Administration (FDA). Some cosmetic dermatologists may not view themselves as experimenters, but as innovators who are customizing a treatment for a unique patient concern. This approach can lead to variable legal outcomes. For example, a dermatologist who uses a standard hair-removal system around the eyelashes resulting in damage to the iris will have a difficult time defending their practice, even if informed consent was obtained. However, a dermatologist using a laser instead of a scalpel to excise a nevus with no resultant scar may be considered an innovator. Neither of these examples show a dermatologist practicing in a similar fashion to his/her peers, but the former would be much more prone to litigation. It follows that most clinical innovation treads a fine line between standard practice and experimental research. As recommended by The National Commission for the Protection of Human Subjects of Biomedical and Behavioral Research, any "radically new" procedure should be formally researched at an early stage to determine its clinical efficacy and safety.[8] When considering innovative procedures, dermatologists would be prudent to assess the evidence in the literature, consult with colleagues, document proper informed consent, and err on the side of being conservative.

Defining the standard of care is a critical component of any cause of action in negligence; unfortunately, this standard is not clearly definable and is frequently determined on a case-by-case basis.

There have been significant efforts within both the medical and legal professions to achieve a clearer definition of the standard of care, or, at the very least, enhance the ability to define it with greater ease and uniformity. Unfortunately, inconsistencies both within and across these two professions have actually clouded the definition further.

Medical Influences on the Standard of Care Definition

Nationally recognized societies, boards, and commissions, such as the American Academy of Dermatology, have become increasingly active in producing clinical practice guidelines (CPGs) to enhance and promote evidence-based patient care. These CPGs are intended to transparently assess and summarize the evidence behind current medical literature and expert opinions, and to also remain free from bias or conflicts of interest.[9] Naturally, dermatologists must also employ their clinical acumen when considering CPGs to identify situations where patient management should deviate from these standardized recommendations. While such documents are not intended to serve as legal evidence for the standard of care, they inevitably play a role in informing this discussion, given their authoritative nature and evidence-based statements.[10] Some may attempt to argue that CPGs should represent the manner in which the majority of physicians within a particular scope of practice should operate, thus equating CPGs to the standard of care. This line of thinking has certain flaws. CPGs from various societies may conflict with one another for the management of the same condition in some instances, making it challenging to discern which set of recommendations to use as the standard. For example, a dermatologist using one of many equally acceptable treatment methods for a particular condition should not have to explain why his or her practice deviates from the recommendations of a specific set of CPGs. In addition, the process of creating CPGs is complex and time-consuming, so some recommendations may become outdated soon after they are published. While some organizations may attach disclaimers to their CPGs, stating that they are not intended to replace physician discretion, dermatologists should be aware that CPGs may be used to approximate the standard of care in a medical malpractice claim.[9]

Legal Influences on the Standard of Care Definition

From a legal perspective, the standard of care is often defined by the testimony of an expert witness, or as what the justice system determines. The basis of the expert witness testimony may stem from any of the expert's personal practice, the practices of other experts that he/she has observed, relevant evidence-based literature, pertinent legislation, and/or recognized courses where the subject in question is taught. Expert witness testimony can be brought forward by both the plaintiff and the defendant, with both sides contributing to the court's definition of the standard of care for the allegation in question.

In summary, the standard of care is a pragmatic concept that is determined on a case-by-case basis. Dermatologists must use their own clinical acumen supported by evidence-based medical literature, CPGs, previous legal precedents, and observations of fellow experts in their field, to meet the reasonable standard of care. Dermatologists may protect themselves against a cause of action in negligence by conducting appropriate informed consent discussions, maintaining written documentation and records, and practicing in a manner that is similar to their peers in the same field.

In the end, in order for a plaintiff to win his/her case against a defendant dermatologist, it must be shown that the breach of duty caused damages. Most commonly these are economic damages, although emotional damages are considered. In the aesthetic dermatology arena, any scar caused by treatment will be said to incur economic damages.

26.4 Habit Evidence and the Importance of Written Documentation

Rule 406 of the Federal Rules of Evidence defines habit evidence, stating "evidence of a person's habit or an organization's routine practice may be admitted to prove that on a particular occasion the person or organization acted in accordance with the habit or routine practice."[11] This must be differentiated from character evidence, or using "evidence of a person's character or character trait" to "prove that on a particular occasion the person acted in accordance with the character or trait."[11]

Consider a scenario where Dr. A, like many other dermatologists, performs a myriad of skin biopsies over the course of each clinic day. She obtains proper informed consent prior to performing each biopsy, including detailing the purpose of the biopsy, possible course of disease if the biopsy is not performed, possibility of further required treatment depending on the results, and potential risks such as a scar at the biopsy site. She conducts this same discussion and obtains informed consent prior to performing a biopsy on the face of a 25-year-old actress, and notes in the chart that the "biopsy was discussed in detail with the patient." She does not obtain written informed consent, and does not document in the patient chart about specific side effects that were discussed. Unfortunately, the biopsy does leave a scar behind. Dr. A is served notice of litigation months later, as the patient claims the scar has ended her acting career. Dr. A does not recall the specific conversation with this patient and has no written evidence either, but feels confident that she warned about potential scarring as she does this with every patient prior to performing a biopsy. Will such habit evidence suffice in a court of law?

One of the first reported medical malpractice cases in which habit evidence was accepted was *Meyer v. United States*.[12] In this case, the plaintiff sued her dentist after experiencing numbness on the right side of her gum line and tongue following extraction of her wisdom teeth. She claimed that she had not been counselled about the potential risk of nerve damage, and that she may not have consented to the procedure if she had known this risk existed. While the dentist could not recall treating this specific patient, he testified his defense based on his chart documentation and his general habits in daily practice. The court ruled that the dentist demonstrated sufficient evidence of routinely informing patients about the potential risks of surgery. This has since set a legal precedent for the rulings of numerous other medical malpractice cases.

In order for habit evidence to be admissible, there must be a adequately large sample size to show that the habit is sufficiently uniform and repetitive. It is unlikely that the average dermatologist, such as Dr. A, would be able to recall the details of specific discussions with patients. As a result, they may often try to rely upon evidence of routinely providing patients with certain pieces of information. Proof of such a habit must be demonstrated, and though not always required, having witnesses testify to prior specific instances of conduct may be beneficial. If a dermatologist performs a particular procedure less commonly, such as laser hair removal, that dermatologist would have a much harder time employing habit evidence as proof for discussion of a potential complication. It should also be noted that courts have previously recognized that patients too may not recall specific details of interactions with their physicians, particularly in the case of patient amnesia secondary to an anxiety-provoking or stressful encounter. This form of evidence could be used in an attempt to counter habit evidence in a medical malpractice claim.

Referring to our previous example, the habit evidence rule would generally allow Dr. A to testify to her habit of routinely counselling patients about the risk of scarring prior to a biopsy. However, this type of evidence may not always be sufficient, and should not be relied upon exclusively. Written documentation in the patient's chart, particularly for informed consent prior to a procedure, is of paramount importance.

26.5 Patient Factors

26.5.1 Determining the Psychological Profile and Enhancing Patient Satisfaction

When considering whether to suggest a procedure, dermatologists should evaluate the psychological profile of the patient to identify any factors that may indicate a greater likelihood of patient dissatisfaction. Examples of such risk factors may include very negative self-image or self-esteem, suspicion of mental health issues such as body dysmorphic disorder,[13] unrealistic patient expectations, or a history of frequent dissatisfaction with procedure outcomes, among others. It is favorable for the dermatologist to always, but particularly in these situations, err on the side of being conservative, encourage questions from the patient, and establish clear and realistic expectations. Of course, written informed consent should also be documented in the patient chart.

Patients may sue physicians for a variety of reasons, including poor communication, retribution, economic motives, and negligence. Simply taking additional time to interact well with patients, and enhance their understanding of what outcomes can be achieved through various procedures, can help reduce accusations of negligence. Using clear language, being honest, and ensuring that patients feel heard keeps patients involved and content, and happy patients pursue litigation less often.

26.5.2 Once a Patient Sues

When you receive "the letter" from a patient or attorney, you may have multiple thoughts racing through your mind all at once. The first step involves taking a deep breath and relax; complications and lawsuits cannot be entirely prevented. That being said, there are some "Dos and Don'ts" to consider when you receive notice of medical malpractice litigation.

What to Do

- Immediately:
  - Notify your medical malpractice carrier and the National Practitioner Data Bank of the impending litigation.
  - Review the patient chart and your own memory of the incident in question.
- In the near future:
  - Evaluate your own physical and mental constitution, and think about the pros and cons of settling versus going to trial.
  - If you decide to settle, you may consider offering either a partial or full refund.
  - If offering a refund, it is required that the patient sign a Release to eliminate liability.
  - Hire a lawyer that you trust to draft the Release very carefully. For example, ensure that it prevents both current or future litigation pertaining to the incident in question, state that the consideration was accepted voluntarily by the patient for a full compromise, and avoid an admission of negligence. Any mistakes, such as incorrect, broad, or vague word selection, could create future issues upholding the Release in court.
- In the longer term:
  - Use this experience to identify potential flaws in your routine practice of maintaining written documentation and obtaining informed consent.

What Not to Do

- Never, ever, ever, change medical records.
- Do not admit negligence. Providing a refund is not an admission of fault, and this should be clearly stated in the Release.
- Avoid a doom and gloom approach, as this will prevent you from thinking logically about the best course of action. Lawsuits and complications cannot be prevented.

Medical Malpractice Case Study

The senior author experienced a medical malpractice case against himself over 2 decades ago that illustrates many of the principles of this chapter. The patient was a world-renowned US economist who presented with a large recurrent basal cell carcinoma of his left cheek. He underwent Mohs surgery, saw a local plastic surgeon for the repair, and never returned to the Mohs office. Three years later, he had a massive recurrence of the skin cancer. A lawsuit was filed. The plaintiff contended that the breach in duty was that the skin cancer recurred, and the damages were related to the large hole in his cheek which led to a loss in income of millions of dollars. But was there really a breach? The Mohs slides were reviewed by an outside pathologist who reported observing no evidence of skin tumor. The mere evidence of a recurrence is not, per se, a breach in duty. Ultimately, the involved judge threw the case out of court.

References

[1] Lolis M, Dunbar SW, Goldberg DJ, Hansen TJ, MacFarlane DF. Patient safety in procedural dermatology: part II. Safety related to cosmetic procedures. J Am Acad Dermatol 2015;73(1):15–24, quiz 25–26

[2] 2017 Plastic Surgery Statistics. American Society of Plastic Surgeons. Available at: https://www.plasticsurgery.org/news/plastic-surgery-statistics. Published 2018. Accessed December 6, 2018

[3] Cocanour CS. Informed consent—it's more than a signature on a piece of paper. Am J Surg 2017;214(6):993–997

[4] 42 Code of Federal Regulations 482.24 - Condition of participation: Medical record services.

Legal Information Institute. Available at: https://www.law.cornell.edu/cfr/text/42/482.24. Published 2012. Accessed December 6, 2018

[5] Durand MA, Moulton B, Cockle E, Mann M, Elwyn G. Can shared decision-making reduce medical malpractice litigation? A systematic review. BMC Health Serv Res 2015; 15(1):167

[6] Kornmehl H, Singh S, Adler BL, Wolf AE, Bochner DA, Armstrong AW. Characteristics of medical liability claims against dermatologists from 1991 through 2015. JAMA Dermatol 2018;154(2):160–166

[7] The treatment relationship: confidentiality, consent, and conflicts of interest. In: Hall MA, Orentlicher D, Bobinski MA, Bagley N, Cohen IG, eds. Health Care Law and Ethics. New York, NY: Wolters Kluwer; 2018:201–202

[8] National Research Act, Pub L 93:348

[9] Introduction. In: Steinberg E, Greenfield S, Wolman DM, Mancher M, Graham R, eds. Clinical Practice Guidelines We Can Trust. Washington, D.C.: National Academies Press; 2011:18–19

[10] Ruhl DS, Siegal G. Medical malpractice implications of clinical practice guidelines. Otolaryngol Head Neck Surg 2017;157(2):175–177

[11] Rule 406 – Habit; Routine Practice. Federal Rules of Evidence. Available at: https://www.rulesofevidence.org/article-iv/rule-406/. Published 2018. Accessed December 10, 2018

[12] Meyer v. United States, 638 F.2d 155 (10th Cir. 1980)

[13] Sweis IE, Spitz J, Barry DR Jr, Cohen M. A review of body dysmorphic disorder in aesthetic surgery patients and the legal implications. Aesthetic Plast Surg 2017;41(4):949–954

27 Patient Portals and Communication in the Age of EMR

Girish S. Munavalli MD, MHS, FACMS

Abstract

Patient portals are an Internet-based gateway for one-way and two-way communication between the patient and the dermatology practice. If utilized to the fullest extent, patients can perform such routine tasks as pre-populating all relevant information required for new and established visits. Patients can complete data entry and update such items as insurance plan information, current medications, and review of systems. Portals can also facilitate secure, HIPAA-compliant communication between the patient and physician, to answer questions about their visit. Most of the most popular Dermatology EMR applications are utilizing portals as part of the patient electronic health care experience; however, most patients do not utilize these functions. That is likely to change in the future. MIPS and MACRA both list the use of patient exchange as a requirement for meaningful use, which provides even more impetus for practice and patient adoption.

Keywords: EMR, patient portals, MPS, MACRA

Top 10 Things You Need to Know

1. In a 2014 report, only 32% of US patients surveyed had access to a patient portal.
   Fifty-two percent of patients were offered access to their medical records in 2017, which is up from 20% of patients in 2014, the data showed.
2. Interestingly, over half of the patients offered patient portal access viewed their own medical records, which translates to 28% of the total survey population.
3. A patient portal is a secure online website which allows for convenient 24-hour access to your personal Electronic Health Record (EHR) from any device with an Internet connection.
4. Typically, every institution has its own portal, with some interconnection with in-network providers.
5. Portals put the onus on the patient to input and update their information, but it should always be verified.
6. Portals can also contain links to relevant, patient-specific information, for example, information on skin diseases or posttreatment protocols.
7. Portals can foster better patient–physician interaction and diminish patient frustration over lack of access.
8. As of January 2020, most commercially available Dermatology-specific EMR/practice management (PM) applications have patient portals.
9. Although patient portals provided patients with an expanded view of their own health, patients still only used a handful of those functions.
10. Patient portals add significantly to a patient's ability to communicate with your office. While to the uninitiated the portal may seem like an unnecessary encumbrance, once it's installed and functional both you and the patients will find it tremendously advantageous for communication.

27.1 Introduction

In theory, widespread and frequent use of a secure, online, mobile-friendly patient portal is an ideal way to facilitate nonurgent communication between physicians and their patients. In this chapter, the rationale for creation of a patient portal, as well as utilization of portals to optimize patient–physician interaction in dermatology, will be discussed.

A patient portal is a gateway, principally a secure website on the Internet, where patients can go to visualize information regarding their medical visits to a dermatologist (or nonphysician provider), as well as update their own specific information such as demographics, medication lists, and complete medical history. As the demand for dermatological treatments grows in the US, more women and men are seeking the care dermatologists provide. The shortage of dermatologists in some regions of the US can make it difficult for some clinics to keep up with the demand for services and information requests. These circumstances can create challenging conditions for the office staff of the dermatology practice. Portal options, via ones' own EHR, or via HIPAA-compliant third-party patient portal vendors are available to help relieve the pressure and simultaneously ensure an exceptional patient experience.

Good communication is a key to all successful professional relationships. With the pressure of such high demand for treatment, and the constraints of time, communicating with patients more than the most basic information may seem impossible to do. A patient portal can function as a useful tool to facilitate more effective communication. In addition, accessing personal medical records through a patient portal can help patients to be more actively involved in their own health care. Accessing family members' health information can help family members take care of them more easily. On a more practical level, portals can eliminate phone tag with the doctor and sometimes even save a trip to the doctor's office.

The features of patient portals may vary, but typically allow one to securely view and print portions of their medical record, including recent doctor visits, discharge summaries, medications, immunizations, allergies, and most laboratory results anytime and from anywhere with Internet access.

Other features can include the following:

- Requesting prescription refills
- Scheduling nonurgent appointments
- Updating demographics
- Making secure payments
- Downloading or completing intake forms before the actual visit

How did the mandatory use of patient portals evolve in the current medical environment? Under the Medicare Access and CHIP Reauthorization Act (MACRA), which was passed and signed into law in April 2015, eligible physicians participate in either the merit-based incentive payment system (MIPS) or an advanced alternative payment model (AAPM). MIPS and AAPMs are collectively referred to as the quality payment program (QPP). With the MIPS track, a final score is calculated based on performance across four performance categories. As detailed below, the patient portal is part of this scoring system.

The MIPS point/scoring system was government designed and implemented and affects an eligible provider's ultimate monetary reimbursement (QPP) for services rendered to Medicare patients, based on participation. MIPS is made up of four performance categories, essentially representing several previously offered Medicare reporting programs, which are renovated and combined into one. The MIPS performance categories in order of potential for patient portal impact (highest to lowest) are as follows:

1. **Advancing care information**: Focuses on information exchange and interoperability, replacing the Medicare and Medicaid EHR incentive program, which were also known as meaningful use (stages 1 and 2).
2. **Quality**: Measures a provider's delivery of quality care, replacing the physician quality reporting system (PQRS), which expired in 2016, and incorporating the value-based payment modifier system.
3. **Improvement activities**: A new category created to measure a provider's focus on care coordination, beneficiary engagement, and patient safety.
4. **Cost**: Relates to resource use, replacing the value-based payment modifier.

Previously, in order to successfully attest to stages 1 or 2 of meaningful use, eligible dermatologists were required to fulfill the patient portal requirement at each stage. A pathway was provided for each stage, with regard to specific levels of patient portal utilization by the patients.

Stage 1 Requirements:

As a core measure of stage 1 meaningful use, eligible dermatologists were to provide patients with the ability to view online, download, and transmit their health information. Specifically, more than 50% of all unique patients attended to by the eligible professional during the EHR reporting period were to be provided timely online access to their health information subject to the eligible professional's discretion to withhold certain information.

Eligible dermatologists were excluded from this measure if they neither order nor create any of the information listed for inclusion, as part of the measure, except for "patient name" and "providers' name and contact information."

Stage 2 Requirements:

As a core measure of stage 2 meaningful use, eligible dermatologists were required to provide patients with an electronic copy of their health information (diagnostic test results, problem lists, medication lists, and allergies) upon request. Specifically, 50% of patients must have had access to an electronic copy of their health information and 5% of patients must have used the capability to access and download their information. Eligible

Dermatologists were excluded from this measure if they do not order or create any of the information listed for inclusion as part of this measure.

For both stage 1 and stage 2 measures, patient health information was to be available within 4 business days of when the information is available to the eligible Dermatologist.

27.2 Portals and Communication

As occurred commonly with the sunsetted meaningful use stage 2 program, incentive payments were paid (or overpaid) to providers with patient portals that provided at least 50% of their patients with access to their medical records online, and at least one patient per eligible provider was required to view, transmit, and download their health summary. Advancing Care Information (ACI) essentially replaces the meaningful use program and further raises the bar.

The updated performance category, ACI, is highly dependent on patient portal technology, with about half of its subcategory measures achievable through patient portal features. With the use of certified patient portal technology, physicians can accumulate MIPS points with relative ease (▶ Fig. 27.1). Detailed calculation of MIPS performance score is beyond the scope of this chapter. Suffice to say that attestation, calculation, and submission of interoperability measure data can be a confusing process. Thankfully, CMS allows for third-party intermediary support. A third-party intermediary is an entity that collects and submits data on behalf of MIPS eligible clinicians. Intermediaries can be a qualified registry, qualified clinical data registry (QCDR), health IT vendor who obtains data from a MIPS eligible clinician's certified electronic health record technology (CEHRT), or a Centers for Medicare & Medicaid Service (CMS)-approved survey vendor. For most of us that utilize a certified EHR, that company can submit on our behalf.[1]

Because Dermatology is still primarily a small, outpatient, private practice-based specialty, adoption of portals has been slower to occur compared to other large specialties with access to in-patient EHRs, and motivation for interoperability between the clinic and hospital/institutions. More extensive published surveys of the patient base of other specialties can help dermatologists to predict trends in patient portal utilization. One particularly useful survey data set can be found in the national cancer

Objective	Weight	Maximum points
e-prescribing	e-prescribing**	10 points
	Bouns: Query of prescription drug monitoring program (PDMP)	5 bonus points
	Bouns: Verify opiod treatment agreement*	5 bonus points
Health information exchange	Support electronic referral loops by sending health information**	20 points
	Support electronic referral loops by receiving and incorporating health information**	20 points
Provide to patient exchange	Provide patients electronic access to their health information	40 points
Public health and clinical data exchange	Report to two different public health agencies o clinical data registries for any of the following:	10 points
	Immunization registry reporting**	
	Electronic case reporting**	
	Public health registry reporting**	
	Clinical data retgistry reporting**	
	Syndromic surveillance reporting**	

*Required beginning in 2020
**Exclusions available

Please note: CMS has changed the name and combined some of the measures. however, the requirements for the measures remain similar. detailed measure specifications and exclusions can be found on the CMS QPP website (qpp.cms.qov).   ↑ Top

Fig. 27.1 Portal as a part of the MIPS points scoring scale.

institute's 2017 health information trends survey. Oncology researchers looked at patient EHR use trends, patient portal uptake, digital health, and mobile health adoption technology.[2]

Fifty-two percent of patients were offered access to their medical records in 2017, which was up from 42% of patients in 2014, the data showed. Over half of the patients offered patient portal access viewed their own medical records, which translates to 28% of the total survey population. Twenty four percent of patients did not view their online medical records, even after being granted access to them. The reasons for not viewing patient health records included the following:

- Wanting to speak with providers in person (76%).
- Limited perceived need to view medical records (59%).
- Privacy concerns (25%).
- No avenue to access the website (20%).
- No longer having an online medical record (19%).

Providers played a big role in prompting a patient to view his or her own medical record. Sixty-three percent of patients who viewed their medical records were encouraged to do so by their providers. Only 38% of patients who viewed their medical records took the initiative on their own.

Patient portals incorporated a number of patient-facing functions that could assist patients to manage their own health. Nearly all (92%) of patient portals allowed patients to view laboratory results, while 79% offered updated medication lists, 76% showed visit summaries, and 70% display problem lists. Sixty percent of patient portals offered access to allergy lists, 55% showed immunization or vaccination history, and 51% showed clinician notes. Although patient portals provided patients with an expanded view of their own health, patients still only used a handful of those functions.

Overwhelmingly, patients used the portal to view their laboratory results (85%). This may have value in dermatology, for example, in isotretinoin follow-up visits. Sixty-two percent of patients used portals for more clinical tasks, such as scheduling appointments, completing paperwork, and refilling prescriptions. Only 14% of patients used their portal to transmit medical records to another provider, despite federal calls for patients to be in charge of health data sharing. Patient caregivers also saw utility in patient portals. Eighteen percent of individuals accessing a digital medical record functioned as some sort of medical caregiver for a patient. Twenty-five percent of all caregivers viewed a medical record for a client, child, or other family member.

The oncology survey data correlates well with prior observations from industry that mirror patient use of portals.

The following graphs summarize the previous findings from a survey study conducted in 2014 (https://www.softwareadvice.com/medical/industryview/patient-portals-2014/) (see ▶Table 27.1 and. ▶Table 27.2).

More recently, the same website (https://www. softwareadvice.com) asked 385 patients what their top frustrations with portals were.[3] The responses were similar but included a category of image management, which is more pertinent to Dermatology (▶Table 27.3).

As of January 2020, most commercially available Dermatology-specific EMR/practice management (PM) applications have portals (▶Table 27.4).[3] Most are customizable within the software itself, or through the use of standard web programming or techniques (HTML, JAVA, Frames). Portals are designed to allow quick access to demographics, laboratory results, request scheduling, inquire about billing, request prescription refills, and secure messaging with providers/triage nurses.[4]

Table 27.1 Survey study showing most requested patient portal features

Most-requested patient portal features	%
Schedule appointments	24
View test/lab results	22
View bills/make payments	21
Check prescriptions/refills	19
Exchange emails with staff	10
None of the above	5

Source: Data based on Software Advice. https://www.softwareadvice.com/medical/industryview/patient-portals-2014/

Table 27.2 Survey study showing patients' top frustrations with patient portals

Patients' top frustrations with patient portals	%
Unresponsive staff	34
Confusing interface	33
Automatic emails	22
Notes in medical jargon	11

Source: Data based on Software Advice. https://www.softwareadvice.com/medical/industryview/patient-portals-2014/

Mobile alerts and notifications are more commonly being used on mobile-optimized versions and apps.

Table 27.3 Survey study showing patients' top frustrations with portals

Patients' top frustrations with portals	%
A confusing website interface	69
Not receiving a response to a query	64
Clinical info not being posted in a timely manner	54
Regularly receiving automated emails	33
Seeing clinical notes that use medical jargon	21
Inability to upload images for doctors to see	15
Not being shown how to use it	14

Source: Data based on Software Advice. Data based on https://www.softwareadvice.com/resources/patient-portals-top-benefits-features/

Newer portal features in dermatology include the ability to check insurance benefits and upload images for telemedicine and surgical follow-up. Social media updates can also be incorporated into portals, so patients can get updated on practice happenings (▶Fig. 27.2). With the popularity of cosmetics procedures and in-office products, coupon codes and discounts can be exclusively be delivered in a targeted fashion via the portal.

27.3 Conclusion

Portals have opened up new avenues for communication between patients and practices in this era of the increasingly demanding health care environment. Day-to-day challenges of higher patient volume and more documentation-intensive

Table 27.4 Dermatology-specific medical software features

Software	PORTAL	EMR	PM
Advanced MD	✓	✓	✓
DrChrono EHR	✓	✓	✓
AthenaHealth EHR	✓	✓	✓
Kareo Clinical EHR		✓	✓
PrognoCIS	✓	✓	✓
Compulink Healthcare Solutions		✓	✓
Azalea	✓	✓	✓
CureMD	✓	✓	✓
MDConnection	✓		✓
NovoClinical	✓		
eClinicalWorks		✓	✓
ChARM EHR	✓	✓	✓
Modernizing Medicine	✓	✓	✓
TotalMD		✓	✓
Harmony e/Notes		✓	✓
patientNOW	✓	✓	✓
Centricity		✓	
Aesthetics Pro Online		✓	✓
Nextech	✓	✓	✓
ChartPerfect			
EZDERM	✓	✓	✓
Allscripts		✓	✓
NueMD		✓	✓

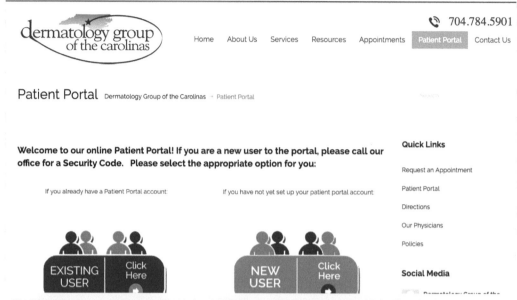

Fig. 27.2 Example of patient portal from a large multi-site, multi-physician dermatology practice.

records threaten to fracture the patient–physician relationship. Portals can help to strengthen this relationship by boosting access and communication.

References

[1] Quality Payment Program. Available at: https://qpp.cms.gov/. Accessed November 7, 2019

[2] The Office of the National Coordinator. Available at: https://www.healthit.gov/sites/default/files/page/2018–03/HINTS-2017-Consumer-Data-Brief-3.21.18.pdf. Accessed November 7, 2019

[3] Software Advice. Available at: www.softwareadvice.com. Accessed November 7, 2019

[4] HIMSS. Available at: https://www.himss.org/library/electronic-patient-portals-patient-and-provider-perceptions. Accessed November 7, 2019

28 Teledermatology Ground Rules

Curtis Asbury MD, FAAD

Abstract

Telemedicine is becoming more mainstream in dermatology. Teledermatology could be a paradigm shift in how patients receive dermatology care and can greatly increase access. At the moment, there are many different platforms with different models of reimbursement and patient populations. It can be used in consultation with other physicians or as direct care to the patient. Though the field is relatively new and is ripe with potential pitfalls, dermatologists would be wise to lead the charge into teledermatology or else be left behind.

Keywords: teledermatology, telederm, store and forward, telemedicine, technology, Internet

Top 10 Things You Need to Know

1. Adding teledermatology to your practice should add value to your practice and not be done simply because the technology is available.
2. Follow-up visits via teledermatology is an easy way to get your toes wet and can prove to be the best of both worlds.
3. Consider various platforms before deciding on what to offer: with electronic medical records (EMRs), it is not always easy getting your data out of each platform, so changing platforms is not something to be considered lightly.
4. You can use multiple platforms as a way of tapping into different markets, just as some people use Instagram, while others use Facebook.
5. Do not consider to offer teledermatology as a way to simply bring in easy revenue, as it is often more time consuming than attending to the patient in person.
6. Reimbursement is currently in flux—it may be the easiest to have your patients pay for it out of their pocket rather than trying to obtain insurance to reimburse.
7. While store and forward is far more convenient and efficient for the busy dermatologist (and busy patient), most states and payers only pay for live, two-way video and audio teledermatology.
8. While many dermatologists are moving away from inpatient consultation, teledermatology can be used as a way for you to get back involved with your local hospitals/emergency rooms (ERs).
9. Liability is a concern, as you will be held to the same standard of care as in-person dermatology.
10. Even if you don't use teledermatology, become knowledgeable about it because it is not going away!

28.1 Introduction

What could be better than sitting with your feet in the sand, sipping a piña colada, while treating patients from your cell phone? Teledermatology is here and it is sure to get bigger and better every year. As we rely more and more on the all-powerful computer in our pocket—the smartphone—patients will expect to be able to use their iPhone to have their skin questions answered. The busy dermatologist may simply choose to ignore these patients and keep treating patients in their office, but you would be best to not forget recent history: taxis versus Uber and Lyft.

Taxi drivers used to be in a situation similar to dermatologists. They had a near monopoly on local ride hailing due to regulations that limited the number of taxi medallions in a city. Taxi medallions rose in price because of their scarcity, with medallions being sold for over one million dollars in New York City in 2013. Technology stepped in with Uber, creating a platform using which riders could hail a car by simply using their cellphone. Riders, especially younger, more tech savvy riders, found this process to be an easier and more efficient way of getting from point A to point B. Taxi companies attempted many tactics including legislation, regulation, and even bullying, to limit Uber and other ride sharing apps from gaining market share; but in the end, technology is here to stay. In 2018, the price of a taxi medallion dipped to under $200,000.

Dermatologists are like taxi drivers! There is a near monopoly on dermatology care due to the difficulty of getting through medical school, obtaining one of a few residency spots, and the limited number of dermatologists in many areas of the country. Technology can change this scenario just like what happened with taxi drivers. Teledermatology stands to increase the ease of which patients can get their skin lesions and rashes diagnosed—it can happen all from their cellphone. If dermatologists don't want to end up like the taxi drivers and their rapidly devaluing medallions, then we need to be on the front lines embracing technology rather than letting others take over this part of the field.

28.2 Rule One: Add Teledermatology to Add Value

The real question for your business is why are you adding teledermatology? Don't add teledermatology simply because you can, as there are real legal liabilities present and it is not always easy to switch teledermatology platforms after you start. There are many valid reasons for offering teledermatology as part of your practice, but they should all add value to your practice.

- Do you want to make it easier for new patients to find you?
- Do you want an online presence to drive patients into your office or simply be a part of your practice that only exists online?
- Do you want to make it easier for your current patients to follow-up with you?
- Do you want to increase access to patients who live in an underserved area, too far for them to drive to your office?
- Do you want to leverage teledermatology as a way to efficiently triage patients from the ER or consult inpatients in the hospital?
- Do you want to provide a way for our increasingly mobile population (e.g., college students and snowbirds) to maintain continuity of care with you?

Answers to these questions can help you better assess whether teledermatology is a good fit for your practice, and more importantly, which type of teledermatology you should use, and how you should market it. If this seems overwhelming, consider simply adding a teledermatology follow-up option for your current patients as a conservative way to enter the teledermatology market.

28.3 Rule Two: Pick the Right Platform(s) to Use

If it seems like there are a lot of choices when it comes to teledermatology platforms, it's because there is! Competition is high right now and there are no obvious choices as to which platform is superior to others. Technology is constantly changing and evolving, and as such, it behooves you to be flexible in what you choose. However, this is easier said than done! Anyone who has ever migrated from one EMR to another knows that the companies do not make it easy for you to switch. teledermatology platforms are not as complicated as EMRs but there is no universal format for how the data can be downloaded and moved from one service to another and to your EMR. There are some general categories to think about when choosing a platform:

- **Built-in:** There are some EMRs that come with teledermatology visits built into the EMR. The advantage is that your virtual visits are in the same system as your office visits, but you will have to market this yourself, and it would be best used by the current patients in your practice.
- **App:** There are many smartphone apps for both Android and iPhone that will drive new patients to you, but you also cede control to these apps and will share the revenue with the app developer.
- **Insurance:** Some commercial insurances have their own telemedicine platforms and will often cover these virtual visits through their platform but they are usually not derm-specific platforms.
- **Texting and email:** Most likely to be used for curbside consults with other physicians; some dermatologists will communicate minimally with their patients via text and email, although there are Health Insurance Portability and Accountability Act concerns and appropriate boundaries that need to be set.

Consider using multiple platforms as a way of increasing your access. Use your EMRs in-built teledermatology for existing follow-up visits while you use an iPhone app to gain patients from outside your practice. There are even condition-specific teledermatology apps to increase exposure to a specific patient, for example, there are apps specific to acne, hair loss, and even genital herpes!

28.4 Rule Three: You Gotta Get Paid

You can't offer a new service to your business if it's not good for your bottom line. That said, it is unlikely that teledermatology will be a primary revenue generating service line for most practices, as it does not pay as much for the time as attending to a patient in person. Reimbursement from third-party payors is complex, state-dependent, and often not feasible. There is wider acceptance from federal and state programs (Medicare, Medicaid, etc.) to reimburse for live, two-way audio–video teledermatology (think: Facetime or Skype) than for store-and-forward (think: texting or iMessage), and even then, there are a lot of rules and regulations that must be met.

So how do you get paid? The easiest way by far is to simply go outside the world of insurance and offer teledermatology as a cash service for your practice. The majority of apps work this way—the patient usually pays a set fee via credit card for the virtual visit. With some platforms, the dermatologist sets the fee, while others are set by the teledermatology company. Some platforms don't charge the patient if the dermatologist requests that the patient come in for a visit IRL (in real life).

Questions to Ask

- Can I set the fee or is it set by the company?
- How is the fee split between the dermatologist and the teledermatology company?
- How are refund requests handled?
- Is there a monthly fee that the practice must pay to be on the platform?

28.5 Rule Four: Teledermatology Can Work Well …

With the right patient selection and the right clinical problem, teledermatology can be more effective for both you and the patient.

Personal Anecdote

Recently, a hospitalist sent me a text message from the ER with a picture of a patient's legs. They were bilaterally red, with some scaling and itching present. It is likely no surprise to you that this patient was being admitted for "bilateral lower extremity cellulitis" with IV antibiotics on order. What was surprising to me was that the hospitalist took the time to text me and then listened when I told him that his pictures looked like stasis dermatitis instead of cellulitis. The patient was discharged and followed-up with me the next day where I prescribed topical steroids and compression stockings. This was not fancy teledermatology but it was effective.

28.6 Rule Five: …But Not Always

Look out for the landmines in teledermatology! Payment is not the only concern. Liability is another—you must check with your malpractice carrier to make sure you are covered for telemedicine. Standard of care is currently based on in-person visits, so if you make an incorrect diagnosis because of a poor picture, you will still be held responsible. As teledermatology is still in its infancy, we do not have a lot of precedent for malpractice and only time will tell how this will shake out. Are you legally responsible if a patient sends you a picture of a seborrheic keratosis which you correctly diagnose, but you fail to see the melanoma that is slightly out of focus at the edge of the picture? We don't know.

You'll also need to manage patients differently. Patients need guidance on how to take proper photos for diagnosis. Some teledermatology apps give guidance on appropriate photos while others are woefully lacking in documentation. It may also be difficult to feel comfortable diagnosing without viewing in three-dimensional with all your tools. I like using dermoscopy to diagnose skin lesions but the majority of teledermatology apps do not support dermoscopy, and the majority of patients will not be buying a dermatoscope for home use regardless. The inability to palpate or use side lighting can also be problematic. In the end, you can bring the patient to the office if the image quality is not satisfactory, but if this is too common, then you will end up with dissatisfied patients who were looking for an iPhone diagnosis.

28.7 Conclusion

Even if you think that your practice doesn't need teledermatology to be successful, teledermatology is here and it isn't going away. While there are many patients who will only want to be seen in person, this number will decline as the patients become savvier and the technology becomes easier to use. Some dermatologists think that teledermatology will help devalue our field by allowing any "provider" with a smartphone to become a dermatologist. It's easier online than in person to obfuscate credentials, making it easier for nondermatologists to provide teledermatology services. There are already commercial teledermatology apps that charge less than $30 a visit—many copays are more than this. As competition increases in the teledermatology space, we may see a race to the bottom and prices for patients will decrease further.

This does not mean that dermatologists should avoid teledermatology, but quite the opposite. If dermatologists fail to take part in these technological advances, then others will take our place. Rather than racing to the bottom, we can set the standard for what teledermatology can be. Teledermatology can greatly increase access to your practice and your expertise—if you allow it.

29 Risk Management

Abel Torres MD, JD, MBA; Colton Nielson MD

Abstract

The practice of dermatology involves science, the art of medicine, and business. Like any business, it needs appropriate risk management such as managing adverse events and resultant medico-legal claims. Dermatologists are fortunate in that they are sued less than many other specialists but may be falling behind other specialists in reduction of claims. Thus, it is important for dermatologists to practice appropriate risk management since common occurrences in dermatology are responsible for many claims. The causes for suits are varied but a common thread centers around communication.

Similarly, techniques for risk management such as informed consent, checklists, apologies, root cause analysis, and use of tools such as mnemonics involve the proper use or means of communication. Despite preventive measures, things can still go wrong, in which case physicians should be knowledgeable in the proper selection of malpractice insurance, limits on liability, and arbitration.

Keywords: risk management, communication, informed consent, checklists, root cause analysis, malpractice insurance, limits on liability, arbitration

Top 10 Things You Need to Know

1. Most physicians can expect to be sued at least once during their career.
2. Claims against physicians are falling, with dermatologists ranking low but dermatologists falling behind other physicians.
3. For dermatologists, the most common reasons for a claim are errors during operative or diagnostic skin procedures and the most common outcome resulting in a claim is dyschromia.
4. When you analyze the reasons for claims, the common thread is poor communication, either written or verbal.
5. Remember the refrain "speed kills" to remind you to slow down and look at informed consent and/or documentation as an opportunity to slow down.
6. Checklists and protocols such as time-outs are a good way to minimize errors and maximize good care.
7. A root cause analysis (RCA) peer review program in your practice is a good way to improve care, minimize errors, and deal with adverse events. If done properly, they provide protections from legal discovery.
8. When an adverse event occurs, the triple AAA mnemonic can guide you and your staff with regard to the best steps to take in order to handle the situation.
9. Minimizing conversation between you and your staff with others, other than your attorney or through the RCA, when an adverse event occurs helps avoid misunderstandings and protect all of you.
10. Malpractice insurance, especially occurrence type, will provide peace of mind and is part of prevention preparation and aftermath protection.

29.1 Introduction

Risk management/medical malpractice discussions among dermatologists often either elicit a "fright and flight" response or one of indifference. Fright because the consensus is high that most physicians (75% in low risk specialties and 99% in high-risk specialties) can expect to be sued at least once during their career by age 65.[1] For dermatologists, indifference results because some studies report an annual rate of claims of less than 6% among all specialists.[1] A 2008 study by Moshell et al reported a rate of claims of 1.1% against dermatologists.[2] A more recent study by Kornmehl and colleagues at USC, which looked at trends in liability claims against dermatologists from 1991 to 2015 on patients with closed claims (claims that formally enter the legal process in the United States and reach resolution with or without payment), confirmed a similar rate of 1.2% of closed claims against dermatologists.[3] Add to this a backdrop of falling claims against physicians,

183

with dermatologists ranking very low (21 out of 28 specialties) in the incidence of reported claims versus other specialists, and it's easy to see why some dermatologists are increasingly indifferent to the issue of malpractice.[3,4] Yet, if one analyzes the data a little closer, we notice the following: First, physicians are still being sued and our rate of awards has been inching upward.[5] Second, dermatologists are falling behind other specialists in that, while dermatologists have seen a reduction of 29.2% for paid claims, the net reduction for dermatologists is only 2.5% compared to 17.9% for other specialties.[3] Furthermore, although our rate of claims is 1.2%, we also only account for 1.4% of all physicians. Thus, if we were to compare the percentage of claims for dermatologists to our percentage of the physician pool, we would find a ratio of 1.2 / 1.4 = 0.86 which could be interpreted as meaning that we are reporting claims in numbers that are proportionate to our numbers in the physician population.[3] Thus, previous statistics may have created a false sense of security.

Consider that some dermatology closed claims, involving melanoma care, have had astronomical awards in the millions.[5] Consider also that a common cause for closed claims is dyspigmentation, which is a common occurrence in dermatology care and over which the physician may have little control.[3] While we do not need to live in fear, indifference may lead to unnecessary economic and personal pain. Economic pain also includes unplanned costs and lost time. In a 2017 Medscape survey of 4,000 physicians across 25 specialties, 67% of sued physicians spent at least 1 or more hours in trial-related meetings and 47% spent more than 10 hours.[4] Several studies have documented that both physical and emotional pain occurs when physicians react to lawsuits.[6] The end result can be increasing frustration and job dissatisfaction among physicians. The above-mentioned Medscape survey revealed that 26% of responders feel they can no longer trust patients and 6% left the practice of medicine altogether.[4]

So, what is a dermatologist to do? First, acknowledge that a malpractice suit can occur and that a claim regarding an adverse event does not necessarily mean you failed. Second, take steps to minimize adverse events and associated suits. Third, have a system in place, so that when an adverse event occurs, it gets handled to help the patient and minimize the risk of a suit. Fourth, have a process in place to deal with the actual lawsuit and

the aftermath of a lawsuit. These steps will be addressed individually below.

29.2 Techniques for Risk Management

Addressing the first and second steps requires understanding why doctors are sued. According to a 2017 Medscape survey, the top reasons physicians are sued include claims of: (1) failure to diagnose (31%); (2) complications (27%); (3) poor outcome (24%); and (4) failure to properly treat (17%). Interestingly, poor documentation (3%) and lack of informed consent (2%) accounted for a small percentage of the claims.[4] Yet, reliance on numbers alone can be misleading, especially as they relate to documentation and informed consent. Kornmehl et al found that errors that occurred during an operative or diagnostic skin procedure as well as misdiagnoses were the first and second highest reason for claims, respectively, and that the most common outcome resulting in claims for dermatologists was dyschromia, a not uncommon or unexpected outcome in dealing with skin disease. So, why then should dyschromia lead to a claim? Lack of appropriate and clear communication may be a key factor in this regard. Thus, documenting (written) and informed consent (verbal), communication, both have more meaning than how often they are reasons for independent formal claims. Dr. Lee S. Goldsmith, a physician attorney who claims to represent plaintiffs and defendants, notes he gets 40 calls a month which result in him filing one claim per month. He describes his top five reasons for lawsuits as being[1]: patients seek answers that physicians don't give,[2] patients have billing disputes,[5] patients feel that details are missing,[3] patients sue out of desperation, and[4] patients react to the physicians actions.[7] The majority, if not all of these reasons, revolve around poor communication. Recently, I came upon an article where the author, John P. McGahan, made the analogy between malpractice management and auto accidents. He said, "speed kills."[8] In the current medical landscape, physicians are asked to do more and attend to more patients in less time. Similarly, records must be completed ever more quickly. This "speed" can "kill" written or verbal communication with patients or providers lead to errors. The informed consent process and the documentation process can be viewed as an opportunity to slow down and build rapport and communication with the patient and other providers. Thus, just as with motor vehicles where slowing down can reduce "traffic tickets," "car crashes," and "bystander injury," so too may slowing down and properly communicating reduce adverse events and subsequent claims. This may even ultimately increase physician's productivity by reducing lost time dealing with claims.

Atul A. Gawande made the concept of checklists key to prevent medical errors.[9] Checklists can help prevent wrong site surgeries, help assure completeness of care, and are very useful for follow-up. Consider that written protocols and checklists are just a different form of communication and thus in line with the previous discussion on the importance of communication. Checklists can easily be incorporated into electronic medical records, into the informed consent process, and for the process of communicating with other health care providers. It is advisable for physicians to take the time to develop or adopt existing checklists as much as possible.

Although slowing down and use of checklists can be of great benefit, to err is human and inevitable. The important thing is to catch the error as soon as possible and prevent it from recurring. Root cause analysis is a problem-solving technique by which root causes of faults or problems are identified when an adverse event occurs. The facts and circumstances are evaluated to assess what went wrong and how it can be prevented in the future.[10] In the interest of public safety, laws and regulations allow for this kind of activity in the form of morbidity and mortality peer review activity, with protection from legal discovery, in order to encourage this type of self-evaluation.[11] Discovery is the process including depositions, interrogatories, and admissions, where lawyers seek information to determine if a claim is justified or support that claim. Protection from discovery helps the public good by encouraging health care providers to be as honest and open as possible without repercussions. Thus, patient care can be improved and future patients can benefit. Yet, it is important to remember that these legal protections or immunity from discovery require adherence to specific rules such as: (a) it must be part of a formal process that has a formal resolution/plan of action, (b) the discussions and associated materials must be kept confidential, and (c) only those individuals that need to be a part of the process must be involved. Only then is the information discussed in a root cause/peer review analysis granted a limited immunity from legal discovery. Unfortunately, some attorneys wrongfully try to access this information to bolster their case or obtain insight as to other possible claims. Some go so far as to have the patients complain to the medical boards, so that the boards undertake an investigation of the physician. The records so obtained are then public records that can be legally obtained and afford plaintiff lawyers a peak into the tent of protected information. Thus, it is important when conducting a RCA to be well-versed in the state and local regulations, and it is wiser to keep as much of the discussions oral rather than create a paper record that may be misconstrued. Furthermore, the principle of confidentiality/preservation of attorney client privilege is something that should be observed from the beginning of the occurrence of any adverse event. Having a protocol already in place for a peer review RCA is very helpful to remind physicians and staff that there are legal protections available and that the time to discuss any adverse event that occurs should be during the RCA process and not at any other time. This benefits both the patients and the health care providers. Remember that, as a physician, only the discussions with your attorney or designated malpractice insurance representative have the same privilege of immunity from discovery. Any discussions with your spouse or clergy may have limited discovery protections and although "misery loves company" and sharing can be good, it's best not to discuss the adverse event with anyone until you have consulted with your attorney.

Apologizing to a patient is an ethical and personal decision each physician must make and there is no right or wrong answer. Certainly, we ourselves would like an apology if we were wronged. The problem is that until all of the facts are evaluated you will not know if you did "wrong" the patient. Medical malpractice requires that there be a duty with and a deviation from that duty/standard of care that proximately causes damage to the patient. Four components (duty, breach of the duty, proximate causation, and actual damage) must exist for malpractice to be found and therefore it's possible that a physician who is responsible for even three of the components, but not all four, would be found not to have committed malpractice/professional negligence. However, there is a movement called "Sorry Works" proposing physicians apologize when an adverse event occurs under their control.[12,13] The proponents explain that individuals have to be properly trained and protocols have to be followed for this to be an effective course of action. They claim that ultimately the health care providers and patients benefit. There is no doubt that some of the steps described for an apology, such as disclosing to the patient while not prematurely admitting guilt, empathizing with the patient, and following a RCA type process, are valuable. What is less clear is whether patients and physicians benefit as much as health care institutions do.[14] In one study by James Patterson at Vanderbilt University, there did not appear to be much benefit to physicians in terms of a lower incidence of claims. The data for patient benefit is just as unclear. This is supported by a Medscape survey which found that 83% of responders did not believe that apologizing would have changed the outcome of the lawsuit based on their experience during the lawsuit. Thus, as stated earlier, whether or not to apologize is a personal decision, but any apology should be well thought out and performed through a formal process rather than an impulsive act. The survey further supports this contention in that when asked what they would have done differently, physicians answered: document better = 22%, ordered tests (10%), phrased discussion differently = 8%, spent more time with patient (8%), referred to another physician or gotten second opinion (15%), read chart better = 6% and nothing = 38%.[4] Thus, an apology alone may not necessarily change the final outcome for the patient or the physician. An approach that this author suggests is that when an adverse event occurs, the physician follow the triple A mnemonic:

- **Acknowledge** the patients concerns with empathy, accepting responsibility for their care but not the cause.
- **Assign** a staff member who is well-informed of the situation to be the only other person to assist the patient with any concerns or questions, so as to be consistent in patient /provider communications and provide good patient care.
- **Avoid** premature conclusions and **a**ssess what actually happened and **a**ct according to your attorney's advice.

We now turn to the fourth step you should plan for, that is, what to do in the aftermath of a claim/ lawsuit? The good news is that physicians prevail the majority of the time a claim is made against them. Yet, the road to that outcome can be long, costly, and stressful. The Medscape survey revealed

that 53% of physicians spent more than 20 hours defending the claim and 33% more than 40 hours. In addition, 67% spent at least 1 or more hours in lawsuit-related meetings and 47% more than 10 hours. Eighty-one percent spent time in depositions.[4] The advice by the surveyed physicians for handling the deposition was: be factual, don't volunteer information, provide short answers, read all the records, don't guess, and document everything well beforehand to avoid problems. Be prepared for the long haul, as the length of a lawsuit was reported as < 1 year (21%), 1 to 2 years (39%), 3 to 5 years (30%), and more than 5 years (10%) The survey reported that 30% settled before trial, 14% were dismissed from the suit in early months, 12% received a defendant verdict, 9% were still ongoing, 36% were dismissed at some point, and only 2% had a plaintiff verdict or settled at trial. This is consistent with previous data reported as to the ultimate disposition of cases. Nevertheless, even if the physician prevails, the process is a long and painful one, with 33% of physicians believing it adversely impacted their careers and 43% saying the threat of a lawsuit is now constantly on their minds. Thus, it seems prudent to take steps to avoid claims or, at least, minimize its likelihood with the steps described above.[4]

29.3 Measures for Mitigating Consequences of an Adverse Event

Part of preparing for the aftermath of a claim is to make sure one's livelihood and family are well-protected. Just as life and disability insurance is very important for physicians, physicians should also understand and shop for the best policy. The Medscape survey reported that 17% of insurers required settlement and 41% encouraged settlement despite the fact that physicians prevail most of the time. The explanation is complex but usually includes a cost savings analysis. It is sometimes less costly for the insurance company to settle a case than to litigate it, even if the physician is adversely impacted. The physician needs to balance the coverage protection sought and resultant peace of mind with the costs. Coverage protection can vary according to state regulations. Some states such as Florida allow coverage as low as $250,000 per occurrence and $750,000 in aggregate per year, often referred to as

250/750 minimum requirement. Most states and hospitals require a $1,000,000/$3,000,000 minimum requirement.[15] Some argue that higher minimums invite lawsuits and that going bare (no insurance) is best, since attorneys are reluctant to pursue action that may not result in recoverable costs. Yes, attorneys can go after other assets, but that is limited by how a business is structured (incorporated, etc.) and the use of trusts or other arrangements that transfer ownership of assets to others. The use of such trusts or other mechanisms is not within the scope of this chapter. Suffice it to say, there is a price for everything in life and cons to going bare include: risk of losing hard-earned personal assets, control of assets by others (divorced spouse), legal and administrative costs of setting up and maintaining such arrangements, costs of defending lawsuits to prevent asset forfeiture, and cost of peace of mind, since suits can occur years after retirement when physicians are most vulnerable economically. Malpractice insurance should account for physicians at risk of a suit seeking high-economic damages including: (a) practicing in a specialty or geographic area where juries routinely award high damages, (b) owning high value assets, or (c) caring for high-income patients who pose a risk for higher economic damages should they be impaired. Once one decides to procure malpractice insurance, the best choice is "occurrence" coverage which covers any claims made for services provided during the purchased coverage. This coverage applies even if the policy expires (tail coverage). Insurance companies/employers do not like to provide "occurrence" coverage because it means keeping the books open to deal with future costs from former policy holders; instead, they will promote "claims made" coverage which means physicians are only covered for claims made and reported during the period you are actively purchasing coverage. Claims coverage is cheaper than occurrence but gradually increases as the risk of a lawsuit increases over time. A physician with claims insurance will need "tail coverage" from the same carrier to protect against claims made after a policy is surrendered. The cost of "tail" is usually very high and in the range of 200 to 400% of the full price of a mature, claims-made policy.[15] The other option is to purchase retroactive or "nose" coverage form your new insurer, which functions like tail coverage and is usually less expensive than "tail" coverage. Often, this is a third-party carrier that may limit coverage to 3 to 5 years preceding when the claims–made policy ends and may provide less financial coverage.

When considering a policy, other components such as exclusions, cyber-security limitations, defense costs coverage, and consent clauses are important to consider as well. Most exclusions are non-negotiable and include willful, illegal, or fraudulent acts but policies should be scrutinized for minimal exclusions. Defense costs/expenses should not be "inside" the coverage limits as they can significantly reduce the policy coverage. Always look for defense costs independent of the coverage or "outside" the coverage limits. Cyber-security coverage for privacy lapses that result in liability are best covered by a separate cyber-security policy. A "consent clause" requires the insurance company to obtain the policyholders approval before settling a case. This control by the policyholder can have implications since a settlement may be cheaper for the company but can have many adverse consequences for a physician, such as national practitioner data bank (NPDB) reporting, etc. Often, insurance companies will tie a "consent clause" to a "hammer clause" that says the policyholder will be personally responsible for any judgment due in excess of the settlement offer. It goes without saying the policy should be screened for such clauses and avoided. Finally, an insurance option that may exist for individuals employed by a state entity such as a state university is a "sovereign immunity" clause that may provide for restrictions on whether the employee physician can be sued or limits on the suit awards.[16] Often this is "occurrence" based and provides excellent protection for the physician, even to the point of minimizing reporting to the NPDB. However, the physician can still be subject to medical board regulatory actions if the claim meets certain criteria that require reporting to the medical board.

29.4 Consent and Arbitration

An arbitration clause is a statement in a contract that requires individuals to resolve their disputes outside of court with an arbitrator or panel of arbitrators. Arbitration may be voluntary or mandatory. Mandatory arbitration is being written into more employee contracts, which often requires an employee to waive their right to sue, participate in class action lawsuits, or submit appeals. Thus, the arbitrator's decision is binding. One of the issues with forced arbitration clauses are that these clauses generally bind the employee, but not the employer.[17] Furthermore, arbitration clauses are often written in a way that the employer retains the right for litigation.[17] Ultimately, arbitration is a private system without a judge, jury, or a right to appeal. Thus, laws that protect from any form of discrimination are unenforceable.[17] The Federal Arbitration Act is a national policy that enforces arbitration clauses.[18] Many states do provide exceptions to the general mandate enforcing arbitration. Thus, physicians should be aware of individual state laws regarding the Federal Arbitration Act prior to signing a contract.[18]

Conversely, arbitration clauses are also often utilized in patient intake contracts prior to treatment as a means to shield health care providers from undesired publicity and litigation. Many have questioned the legality of arbitration clauses in patient consent forms. Regarding this topic, arbitration clauses are subject to contract law. To prove that a valid contract exists, four elements must be met: (1) the parties possess the capacity to enter into a contract; (2) the parties mutually assented; (3) there must be a certain object for the contract; and (4) the contract must have lawful purpose.[18] If these criteria are met, the arbitration clause is considered valid and the Federal Arbitration Act then applies with some interstate variability.[18]

29.5 Conclusion

Most physicians (75% in low-risk specialties and 99% in high-risk specialties) can expect to be sued at least once during their career by age 65.[1] However, claims against physicians are falling, with dermatologists ranking very low (21 out of 28 specialties) in the incidence of reported claims versus other specialists with reported claims of only 1.1% against dermatologists.[2,3,4] Yet, dermatologists are falling behind other physicians, with a reduction in paid claims of only 2.5% compared to 17.9% for other specialties.[3] Some dermatology closed claims involving melanoma care have had astronomical awards in the millions, and a common cause for closed claims is dyspigmentation, which is a common occurrence in dermatology care.[3,5] Thus, dermatologists should acknowledge that a malpractice suit can occur, take steps to minimize adverse events, and have a system in place to handle adverse event occurs and a process in place to deal with the actual lawsuit and the aftermath of a lawsuit.

Appropriate and clear communication is a key ingredient to minimizing adverse events and subsequent legal claims.[7] Keeping in mind that "speed kills," physicians should use the informed consent and documentation process as an opportunity to slow down and build rapport and communication with the patient and other providers.[8] Checklists and protocols also can help prevent wrong site surgeries, help assure completeness of care, and are very useful for follow-up.[9] RCA is another tool by which root causes of faults or problems can be identified to assess what went wrong and how it can be prevented in the future.[10] It is important when conducting a RCA to be well versed in the state and local regulations and keep as much of the discussions oral rather than create a paper record that may be misconstrued.

When things do go wrong, apologizing to a patient is an ethical and personal decision each physician must make, but any apology should be well thought out and performed through a formal process rather than an impulsive act. Although there is data that apologizing may help in resolving adverse events, it is less clear is whether patients and physicians derive a significant benefit versus the benefit to health care institutions.[13,14] Regardless, physicians should approach adverse events in a methodical way and the **"AAA"** pneumonic for (1) **Acknowledging** a patients concerns, (2) **Assigning** a staff member to be readily available to handle patient concerns, and (3) **Avoiding** premature conclusions and actions until all the facts are sorted out, would seem a prudent way for physicians to proceed when facing an adverse event.

Assuming that, as per "Murphy's Law," things can and will go wrong, physicians need to be prepared for the aftermath of an adverse event. First and foremost is to have proper medical malpractice coverage, which usually means having occurrence-based insurance. When considering a policy, other components such as exclusions, cyber-security limitations, defense costs coverage, and consent clauses are important to consider as well.[15] Arbitration contracts or clauses are also either an option or sometimes mandatory. These can limit liability and expedite the long legal resolution process in some circumstances. One needs to be well versed with regulations regarding these for the physicians' state of practice. By taking these risk management steps, physicians can sometimes avoid or at least minimize the emotional and/or economic toll that an adverse event can entail.

References

[1] Grob G. OIG Final Report: Risk Management at Health Centers. Department of Health and Human Services. Available at: oig.hhs.gov/oei/reports/oei-01-03-00050.pdf

[2] Moshell AN, Parikh PD, Oetgen WJ. Characteristics of medical professional liability claims against dermatologists: data from 2704 closed claims in a voluntary registry. J Am Acad Dermatol 2012;66(1):78–85

[3] Kornmehl H, Singh S, Adler BL, Wolf AE, Bochner DA, Armstrong AW. Characteristics of medical liability claims against dermatologists from 1991 through 2015. JAMA Dermatol 2018;154(2):160–166

[4] Report MM. Medscape. Available at: www.medscape.com/slideshow/2017-malpractice-report-6009206#1. Accessed December 16, 2019

[5] Jena AB, Seabury S, Lakdawalla D, Chandra A. Malpractice risk according to physician specialty. N Engl J Med 2011;365(7):629–636

[6] "CRICO Home." CRICO. Available at: www.rmf.harvard.edu/. Accessed December 16, 2019

[7] Goldsmith LS. "An MD/Attorney Reveals: 5 Top Reasons Patients Sue Doctors - Medscape - Oct 23, 2018." Available at: www.medscape.com/viewarticle/902904. Accessed December 16, 2019

[8] McGahan JP. "Advice on Avoiding a Malpractice Lawsuit." MRI in Pregnancy: Gastrointestinal and Genitourinary Pathology. Available at: www.appliedradiology.com/articles/advice-on-avoiding-a-malpractice-lawsuit. Accessed December 16, 2019

[9] Gwande, NEJM article

[10] "Root Cause Analysis." Wikipedia, Wikimedia Foundation. Available at: https://en.wikipedia.org/wiki/Root_cause_analysis. Accessed December 16, 2019

[11] "Morbidity and Mortality Conference." Wikipedia, Wikimedia Foundation. Available at: https://en.wikipedia.org/wiki/Morbidity_and_mortality_conference. Accessed December 16, 2019

[12] "Loose Lips Sink Ships." Wikipedia, Wikimedia Foundation. Available at: https://en.wikipedia.org/wiki/Loose_lips_sink_ships]. Accessed December 16, 2019

[13] "Sorry Works!" Sorry Works. Available at: https://sorryworks.net/. Accessed December 16, 2019

[14] Patterson J. "Apology Laws Don't Help Doctors Avoid Malpractice Payouts." Vanderbilt University. Available at: https://news.vanderbilt.edu/2017/02/01/apology-laws-malpractice-payouts/. Accessed December 16, 2019

[15] Page L. "Buying Medical Malpractice Insurance." Medscape. Available at: https://www.medscape.com/viewarticle/889653. Accessed December 16, 2019

[16] "Sovereign Immunity—A Primer for the UF Health Care Provider." Self-Insurance Programs. Available at: http://flbog.sip.ufl.edu/risk-rx-article/sovereign-immunity-a-primer-for-the-uf-health-care-provider/. Accessed December 16, 2019

[17] "Arbitration." National Association of Consumer Advocates. Available at: https://www.consumeradvocates.org/for-consumers/arbitration. Accessed December 16, 2019

[18] Sachs S. The jury is out: mandating pre-treatment arbitration clauses in patinet intake contracts Journal of Dispute Resolution. Available at: https://scholarship.law.missouri.edu/cgi/viewcontent.cgi?article=1813&context=jdr–. Accessed December 16, 2019

30 The Ideal Schedule

Mona A. Gohara MD

Abstract

An abstract about scheduling cannot be too long, right? Who has the time? Let's keep it short and simple. We all approach our day differently. There is no "right" way, no ideal. That being said, the exchange of ideas, tips, tricks, and pearls generally lends itself to the potential for modifications—Modifications in the name of efficiency, happiness, productivity, and ease. The purpose of this chapter is to offer a wide variety of strategies pertaining to scheduling one's clinic day, vacations, family, and consulting time. The intention is not to initiate a revamping, but rather a consideration of how to change one or two factors which could make your life a little (or a lot) easier.

Keywords: schedule, sample day

Top 12 Things You Need to Know

1. If possible, schedule vacations in Q1 when patient volumes dip.
2. Try to have either early morning or evening hours to accommodate working patients.
3. Schedule follow-ups for midlevels, so that you can see initial office visits and spend time doing procedures.
4. Plan far ahead and try not to cancel/move patients within 60 days of appointments.
5. Have urgent add-on slots built into your clinic schedule, especially for (complex) medical dermatology practices where attending to patients in a timely manner is a necessity.
6. If you love to be busy, then plan on having plenty of well-trained staff from every touch point of the patient's visit. Spend extra on more staff to support you and your patients.
7. Reserve an early morning power hour—one problem per patient, no new patients. You will be amazed at how many people you can see. Morning is the best time because people who really want/need to see you will happily come at any time, on time, and the phones aren't busy, so your staff is free to help.
8. Allow 10-minute buffer slots.
9. Have a no-show charge policy (I think you have to if you are procedure heavy).
10. Have apology bags filled with goodies or little coffee gift cards prepared always for those who are upset by extended waits.
11. It is much easier to add than it is to take away. When starting out, it is preferable to conduct fewer sessions while you sort out what pace works for you and how you want to spend your time outside of clinic. You can always add more in the future once you are settled.
12. Monitor your schedule daily and anticipate scheduling issues in advance.

30.1 Introduction

As doctors, it is imperative to look out for the well-being of ourselves, our staff, and, most importantly, our patients. When basic human needs are not met, delayed or compromised, the work environment and feelings about the work environment suffer. With jammed schedules that force skipped meals, skimped sleep, or worse, shirked familial obligations, the physician burnout becomes a threat to productivity and can impact patient care. Overcommitment is a recipe for disaster. On the other hand, some have disdain for that feeling of being under committed or not being busy enough. That too may be a source of self-dissatisfaction. Either way, curmudgeonly vibes have zero benefit. So, how do those who appear balanced, professionally and personally, make it work? Is there an *ideal* schedule? We all know that the answer is unequivocally, no. I am content when I make time for my son's basketball games and my workouts. These activities make me happy and a better person to be around. Others may find that allotting time for clinical trials gets their engine revving. For each of us, there *are* ideal ways to allocate hours in a day. In my 15 years as a practicing dermatologist, I have indeed learned a few things about scheduling. First, I always start at 7 a.m., so that my patients who work can easily get an appointment. Some may choose evening hours for this exact purpose. Second, especially when your kids are young and not tied up in school or sports, consider taking vacations in Q1 when patient volume almost ubiquitously dips. Third, consider your approach to skin checks, and decide if capping the number you do each day works better. I personally do, at least, 4 an hour. Finally, schedule midlevels for quick follow-ups (warts, molluscum, and isotretinoin), so you can see more initial office visits, and do more procedural derm if that is part of your practice. These are just a few of my views. As there are many permutations of this panacea, I asked some of my esteemed colleagues how they make it work and how they run their offices, so that patient and self-satisfaction are maximized. But before I pass the proverbial mic, here is my scheduling pearl (SP):

> **Scheduling Pearl**
>
> Set one schedule intention each day. A schedule intention is something that you make sure you get done within a 24-hour period. Perhaps it involves taking a few minutes more with each patient or making sure to eat dinner with your family. I find that small victories are easier to obtain, extremely rewarding, and less overwhelming to think about.

30.2 The Schedule Pundits

30.2.1 Pundit: Dr. Ashley Wysong

Affiliation

Chair, University of Nebraska Medical Center, Department of Dermatology

Specialty

Mohs surgeon, cancer epidemiology

General Scheduling "Philosophy"

For Mohs surgery, the schedule is constantly being tweaked based on the number of rooms available, staffing, and complexity of cases. We assign a "star" complexity level to each surgical case to account for the length of processing in the Mohs lab as well as the length of reconstructions. My philosophy involves optimizing patient access while keeping a nice clinic flow with happy patients and staff.

A Sample Clinic Day

In a high-complexity surgical day, we typically attend to two patients at 7:00 am, two to four 7:30 am patients, and two 9:00 am patients for Mohs surgery. We perform suture removals, wound checks, and minor laser scar revision procedures in the afternoon, with no more than four to six patients scheduled at that time.

Making Time for Everything Else (Family, Administrative Duties, Consulting, etc.)

I live by the "work hard, play hard" mentality. I try to compartmentalize and be fully present at work and "turn it off" at home and on the weekends as much as possible. I also plan all of my vacation time at least a year in advance. I believe it is essential to schedule regular time away and it's fun to schedule trips and have something to look forward to! I've gotten better over time at saying no to requests that may not be in line with my larger career or personal/life goals. In addition, I try to block off "work time" on my calendar for specific administrative, research, teaching, or other tasks.

> **Scheduling Pearl**
>
> Plan far ahead and try not to cancel/move patients within 60 days of appointments.

30.2.2 Pundit: Dr. Jonathan Leventhal

Affiliation

Assistant Professor, Associate Program Director, Director of Oncodermatology, Department of Dermatology, Yale School of Medicine

Specialty

Medical dermatology, oncodermatology

General Scheduling "Philosophy"

In clinics focusing on (complex) medical dermatology and oncodermatology, it is important to have urgent add-on slots built into the schedule in order to be accessible to patients with acute rashes or dermatologic toxicities. With time, we developed a system by which referring clinicians can reach out to myself or my nursing team to communicate an urgent referral which can then be triaged and scheduled in a timely manner. Another important component that helps me run an efficient practice is spending a great deal of my administrative time reviewing charts for the week, with a focus on new consults and challenging medical derm cases. Patients appreciate this, and we can navigate through their complex histories with ease. Setting up smart phrases for my electronic medical record (EMR) and patient handouts save a lot of time as well and help reduce additional calls and questions.

A Sample Clinic Day

I attend to patients in three different settings, the faculty practice, our institution's cancer center, and a satellite practice. I generally see 5 to 7 patients every hour and practice six half-day sessions a week. Once a month, I run a procedure clinic for excisions in order to avoid using clinic slots in our busy tertiary care-centered practice.

Making Time for Everything Else (Family, Administrative Duties, Consulting, etc.)

Work-life balance is important. My philosophy is to set aside quality time to spend with my wife, friends, and family. This important time also allows for a mental break that reenergizes me to then devote uninterrupted time to finish notes and other administrative, teaching, or research endeavors.

> ### Scheduling Pearl
>
> Have urgent add-on slots built into your clinic schedule, especially for (complex) medical dermatology practices where seeing patients in a timely manner is a necessity.

30.2.3 Pundit: Dr. Ellen Marmur

Affiliation

President/Founder, Marmur Medical, & MMSkincare Associate Clinical Professor, Department of Dermatology and Department of Genomics/Genetic Science, The Mount Sinai Medical Center

Specialty

Mohs/procedural dermatology

General Scheduling "Philosophy"

I have Mohs mornings, skin check day, and cosmetic days. I try to keep like procedures together. These often become hybrid visits: when primarily a medical visit requests a cosmetic procedure and vice versa. Then, we sprinkle in add-ons or reschedules on top; however, the staff mindset is better when we have dedicated blocks.

A Sample Clinic Day

I see about 30 to 35 patients a day. Mondays and Wednesdays are primarily surgical and medical. Tuesdays, Thursdays, and Fridays are mainly cosmetic. Most visits include both types of concerns. I break at the same time daily for a multitasking lunch plus management update or consulting calls.

- **Monday:** 8 to 8:30 am follow-ups; 8:30 to 11 am six-ten Mohs until completed; 11 am to 1:30 pm add on follow-ups, plus finish Mohs reconstructions; 1:30 pm to 2 pm break for lunch and meetings; 1:30 pm to 5 pm skin checks often with cosmetics—hybrid visits
- **Tuesday:** 7:30 to 8 am management meeting; 8:15 am to 6 pm cosmetics often with medical concerns—hybrid visits
- **Wednesday:** 8 to 8:30 management meeting; 8:30 to 5:30 total skin checks and cosmetics—hybrids
- **Thursday:** 8:15 am to 6 pm cosmetics often with medical concerns—hybrid visits
- **Friday:** 8 am to 2 pm cosmetics; 2 to 5 pm research, meetings. Monthly full staff meetings 4-5 pm with refreshments like Rosé
- **Saturday:** One Saturday morning occasionally

Making Time for Everything Else (Family, Administrative Duties, Consulting, etc.)

- Family: Always be home for dinner three to five times a week. At work I wear an iPhone watch, so that they can always call me, and I tell my patients "sorry it is my child on the phone" and step out of the room. My kids are part of the office culture. They come visit with friends and help with mailings or simple tasks. I have my daughter's artwork in my office and family photos at my desk. Our office culture is that of an extended work family and I try to know their families too.

- **Administrative:** Learn to delegate and do not micromanage. Diversify your expectations. No one manager can be perfect, so split up the tasks with a little overlap. This way, if one person is underperforming (bad week), the second team member is able to help. Make sure you have dedicated meeting times, as you cannot manage a practice with "in between" conversations, texts, or emails. Meetings are essential. All-staff meetings once a month are a minimum. Breakout meetings with front desk, or back staff, only is helpful monthly too.
- **Consulting:** I feel that it is almost never worth it, unless you feel like it! Follow your heart. Media and consulting are lovely and fun but will not necessarily help to grow your practice. Be careful to keep your identity to what you prefer, pure dermatologist, media rockstar, or both, whatever feels most authentic. But do not do consulting or media just because others do it.

> **Scheduling Pearl**
>
> If you love to be busy, then plan on having plenty of well-trained staff from every touch point of the patient's visit. Spend extra on more staff to support you and your patients.

30.2.4 Pundit: Dr. Deirdre Hooper

Affiliation

Co-founder of Audubon Dermatology. Assistant Clinical Professor, Louisiana State University and Tulane, Department of Dermatology

Specialty

Medical and cosmetic dermatology

General Scheduling "Philosophy"

I have some basic rules that contribute to a more fluid flow. No new patients are booked in the first or last hours of the morning/afternoon. New cosmetic patients are asked at booking if they want to be injected that day or just consult.

We specifically ask patients, when booking, if they have cosmetic concerns apart from the medical reason they are booking and vice versa! I also always keep in mind that the patient who books the first appointment of a day generally has a focused concern; they usually come on time and don't bring a list. This is in contrast to patients who book late morning or mid-afternoon; most of the time they have nowhere else to be and they take longer.

A Sample Clinic Day

- Seven new patient slots a day scheduled mid-morning and mid-afternoon.
- 15 established slots a day.
- 15 cosmetic slots scattered through the day.
- Five work-in slots a day during late morning and afternoon or double booked first thing after lunch.
- All slots are of 10 minutes duration and the scattering of appointments allows me to take more time with injectable patients or complicated medical patients. For established patients, double book first and last couple of slots, which allows wiggle room if they come late.
- Power hour, 7 to 9 am, on one day a week; I can see 10 an hour during these slots.

Making Time for Everything Else (Family, Administrative Duties, Consulting, etc.)

Everything goes into the calendar—workouts, date night with hubby, kid time, and administrative duties.

> **Scheduling Pearl**
>
> Reserve an early morning power hour—one problem per patient and no new patients. I do this at 7 am every Wednesday and I love it. You will be amazed at how many people you can see. Morning is the best time because people who really want/need to see you will happily come at any time, on time, and the phones aren't busy, so your staff is free to help.

30.2.5 Pundit: Dr. Annie Chiu

Affiliation

MD, Private Practice Redondo Beach, CA

Specialty

Cosmetic dermatology

General Scheduling "Philosophy"

I may run behind, but I make sure every patient feels like all their questions have been answered. This is imperfect, and often patients are upset by waits, and I've probably lost a few patients due to my waits, but I do not feel right cutting off or limiting a patient's questions or complaints. I also rarely turn away "add on" procedures (cosmetic), as I feel sometimes patients don't know what they need when they schedule. And if you reschedule them, they may never undergo the procedure they need to achieve their best results.

A Sample Clinic Day

We aim for approximately 20 patients a day. 10-15 minute neuromodulator slots, 20-30 minute filler slots, and 20-30 minute laser slots. We schedule for numbing time. We also blocked 1-2 "buffer" 10-minute slots in the morning and one in the afternoon to help us run on time.

> **Scheduling Pearl**
>
> Allow 10-minute buffer slots. Have a no-show charge policy (I think you have to if you are procedure heavy). Have apology bags filled with goodies or little coffee gift cards prepared always for those who are upset by extended waits.

30.2.6 Pundit: Dr. Brittany Craiglow

Affiliation

Private practice and adjunct assistant professor, Yale School of Medicine, Department of Dermatology

Specialty

Pediatric and medical dermatology

General Scheduling "Philosophy"

My primary goal with my schedule is to be able to spend the time that each patient needs without having a waiting room full of people.

A Sample Clinic Day

On average, I see about five patients per hour. I book a double slot for all new patients with hair loss and try to see them at the end of the morning, as often many of these appointments run longer. I also leave time at the end of the day, so that I can add on urgent patients when needed.

Making Time for Everything Else (Family, Administrative Duties, Consulting, etc.)

For me the key has been moving to a part-time schedule. Seeing patients five sessions per week enables me to have more time to pursue academic interests, engage in some consulting work, and spend extra time with my family. Inevitably, I still often find myself working at night or on the weekends, but overall, I am happy with the balance that I've been able to achieve.

> **Scheduling Pearl**
>
> It is much easier to add than it is to take away. When starting out, it is preferable to do fewer sessions while you sort out what pace works for you and how you want to spend your time outside of clinic. You can always add more in the future once you are settled.

30.3.7 Pundit: Dr. Valerie Callendar

Affiliation

Private practice, Medical Director, Callender Dermatology & Cosmetic Center; Professor of Dermatology Howard University

Specialty

Aesthetic, medical, and surgical dermatology

General Scheduling "Philosophy"

Be organized, efficient, and prepared.

A Sample Clinic Day

Every day is different. I typically see 30 patients a day. If I am performing hair transplant surgery or aesthetic procedures, I will attend to less patients.

I see patients six days per week and sometimes on Sundays (VIP patients). My day begins at 8 am although I arrive at 7 am before anyone arrives.

- **Monday:** Medical patients 8 to 5 and cosmetic patients 5 to 6
- **Tuesday:** Surgeries 8 to 12:30 and medical patients 1:30 to 5
- **Wednesday:** Medical patients 8 to 9 and cosmetic patients 9 to 7
- **Thursday:** Surgeries 8 to 12:30 and cosmetics 2 to 5
- **Friday:** Medical 8 to 5
- **Saturday:** Cosmetic patients 9 to 2

Making Time for Everything Else (Family, Administrative Duties, Consulting etc.)

Three-fourths (75%) of the time my husband travels with me, especially in places we have not been before, and my son will join us if he can.

> **Scheduling Pearl**
>
> Monitor your schedule daily and anticipate scheduling issues in advance.

The key to a well-run clinic is an outstanding team that has your back. First and foremost, you must choose exceptional people for your staff, people who do excellent work, exemplify professionalism, and advocate for patients because it is simply who they are, and they could not do otherwise. Then, you must earn their loyalty and renew their energies by valuing these people, taking care of them, treating them extremely well, and making their work experience enjoyable and fun.

30.3 Closing Thoughts

30.3.1 Pundit: Arianne Shadi Kourosh

Affiliation

Director, Laser and Cosmetics, Brown University Medical Center

Director, Community Health, Department of Dermatology, Massachusetts General Hospital

Assistant Professor, Department of Dermatology, Harvard Medical School

In Her Words

The key to a well-run clinic is an outstanding team that has your back. First and foremost, you must choose exceptional people for your staff, people who do excellent work, exemplify professionalism, and advocate for patients because it is simply who they are, and they could not do otherwise. Then, you must earn their loyalty and renew their energies by valuing these people, taking care of them, treating them extremely well, and making their work experience enjoyable and fun.

30.3.2 Pundit: Dr. David Leffell

Affiliation

Chief, Section of Dermatologic Surgery & Cutaneous Oncology, Department of Dermatology, Yale School of Medicine

Respect for the Patient

Our patient satisfaction is at the 99th percentile nationally, and I think it is due to a common culture of caring about the patient and her or his needs and experience. Since our patients come from all over the region, I hear stories about those offices that run well and those that don't. I think the ones that operate well have strong physician leadership and administrative staff that follow the example set by the doctors in how they care for patients. The success of a practice depends on word of mouth recommendation and that grows out of how patients feel treated. That focus on patients and their needs has to be modeled at the top.

31 Delegating: Physician Extenders and Integration into a Practice

Kavita Mariwalla MD, FAAD

Abstract

An extender in dermatology can be a physician assistant or a nurse practitioner. In deciding whether a midlevel practitioner will be an asset to your practice, you have to assess if your practice actually has a need. In other words, what is your wait time? What is your personality? Do you have time for training and supervision? Will an extender actually be able to reduce your work burden? Would it be better for you in the long run to instead hire and partner with another physician? One of the common mistakes we make is that an extender should be hired instead of a physician. Most practices have a mix of both. To be successful in hiring a midlevel, thought should be paid on what to delegate to them or how to best integrate them into a functional practice environment.

Keywords: nurse practitioner, physician assistant, extender, midlevel, dermatology practice

Top 10 Things You Need to Know

1. Before hiring an extender make sure that you actually have adequate patient volume to make it a financially viable endeavor.
2. Assess your own personality and office flow to make sure you can accommodate a midlevel practitioner.
3. Decide whether you want to hire a physician assistant (PA) or a nurse practitioner (NP) based on how much supervision you are able to provide.
4. Assess how you want to schedule the extender — should they only attend to follow-up patients for example?
5. Be prepared to train your office staff to credential the extender on the phone, so that patients feel comfortable seeing them.
6. Use your extender as your extension not only in patient care but also in accomplishing administrative duties.
7. Clear lines of communication between employer and employee are key, especially when deciding to hire a midlevel to assist you in your office.
8. Pay scales vary, and I recommend a base salary with a production bonus.
9. Evaluate your reimbursements and overhead to assess how many patients you need your extender to see in order to make the partnership a profitable one.
10. The end goal is to deliver greater access to good patient care. Time is required for training but it should ultimately lead to an extender who can mimic your decision-making process and truly be an asset to you.

31.1 Introduction

This chapter is written from the perspective of a physician who will employ and supervise an extender. In the last few months, with a new Presidential Executive Order, extenders may no longer require physician supervision. As a result, the role a physician plays in employing a midlevel may change completely but as of the time of this publication it is too early to tell if this will create a shift in Dermatology.

As the practice of dermatology has transformed, so has the role of physician extenders. For one, many more extenders are used in daily practice than ever before. Second, the autonomy of extenders has changed and varies extensively from one state to another. So how do you make the decision to hire an extender or work with one in your current practice environment? The answer depends on who you are. Are you the employer or are you an employed physician? In this chapter, we explore the role of extenders and expectations of the relationship which can be mutually beneficial.

31.2 What Is an "Extender"?

In the field of dermatology, an extender can be a physician assistant (PA) or a nurse practitioner (NP). In most states, a NP can work independently; in other words, without the direct supervision of a physician. A PA, as the name implies, is a physician assistant; although in many states, a PA can actually own their own practice and hire a physician. According to a survey by the American Academy of Dermatology to assess the practice profile of dermatologists in the US, the employment of physician extenders, including NPs and PAs, increased from 28% in 2005 to 46% in 2014. PAs comprised the largest percentage of physician extenders.[1]

When we talk about an extender, the idea, quite simply, is to have a person in the office who can literally act as an extension of you. But what does that mean? When looking around at different practice models, there exist extremes of all situations. We all know of offices with outpost locations staffed primarily by extenders with distant physician supervision that is in line with state laws but may raise an eyebrow practically speaking. We have all seen extenders who bill themselves as board-certified experts in aesthetics on social media channels and who practice potentially outside the scope of what they were trained to do. There are also those practices which will not allow extenders to see Medicare patients and bill as "incident to" for all visits overseen by an extender (paid at 85% of MD rates) and ensure that a covering physician is a phone call away if the employing physician is on vacation. The best way to employ an extender is to first find out the applicable "rules" in your state. Must you physically be present in the building or can you be a phone call away? If you hire a NP, do you have less liability exposure?

Once you have figured out your state-specific rules, following are the questions to ask yourself when thinking about hiring an extender:
- What are your current wait times for a new patient and an established patient?
- Do you have the personality to trust another person to diagnose and treat your patients?
- Do you have time to spend training a new graduate from school or are you looking for someone with several years of experience?
- Are you available to directly supervise the extender and/or are you willing to take on the liability of that person practicing while you are not at the office concurrently?
- Is your office staff trained to be able to shuttle patients toward the extender?

Let's take a moment to explore the answers to these basic questions.

31.3 Question One: Wait Time

It is no secret that wait time is a problem in most dermatology practices. According to an article published in *Dermatology Times*, Merritt Hawkins conducted a survey of wait times for new patients seeking a skin check and observed that it increased to 32.3 days in 2017 compared to 28.8 days reported in 2014. Merritt Hawkins is a physician recruitment firm and found results according to ▶ Fig. 31.1. So if your wait time seems in line with these numbers, it may indeed be the right moment to expand access to your services. Conversely, if your wait time to see a new patient is under

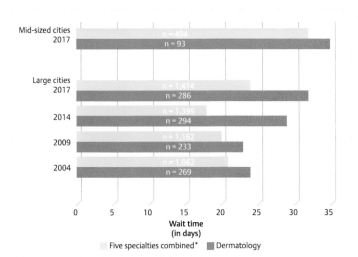

Fig. 31.1 Average wait times for new-patient appointments. *Cardiology, dermatology, family medicine, ob.gyn., and orthopedic surgery

Notes: Based on the results of a survey conducted from January 9, 2017 to February 13, 2017. Offices in midsized cities were included in the survey for the first time in 2017. Source: Merritt Hawkins.

21 days and an established patient less than 14 days, you likely do not need an extender.

When deciding to use an extender, different models have worked to decrease wait time. The first is to book low-acuity medical derm automatically with the extender. The second is to pass all follow-up visits to the extender and make sure all new patient visits are taken care of by an MD/DO. You will want to define if the extender can perform full skin checks and if you feel comfortable with them managing certain recurring visits such as psoriasis patients on biologics or patients on isotretinoin. Other options to consider are allowing your extender to run a spot check clinic one day a week or booking same day urgent visits with them. Another option is to have the extender run with you and perform all biopsies, conduct patient counseling, and complete your notes, call back and biopsy calls. In the author's opinion, the latter option is less efficient for the practice and underutilizes the training of the extender.

If you are an employed physician and find your individual wait time growing, asking for an extender whom you will supervise may be a winning combination for your panel and also the employer. However, if you are being asked to supervise an extender, I would ask to be compensated for this, as it is a risk you are now taking on and involves added work in terms of checking notes and being available to answer questions.

31.4 Question Two: Your Personality

Let's say you have built your practice from the ground up. For you, your practice is your baby and hiring another person to join you is a big step. It is time to really look inward and ask yourself: do you want to hire an extender or are you looking for another doctor? Yes, finding an extender will be infinitely easier than finding a board-certified dermatologist but that should not be part of the decision. What you should be evaluating is your inherent ability to trust an extender and his/her level of training. You have to know the pulse of your patient load. Does your office mainly attend to complex medical dermatology? Can you feel comfortable that an extender will offer the same level and quality of care that you do now? Will you allow the extender to offer identical services that you do? Are you looking for a partner to share in the overhead costs and administrative duties of the office? Keep in mind that board-certified dermatologists may

alleviate the worry of having to supervise someone else, but will seek partnership in a matter of 3 to 4 years. Which they may or may not be prepared to give. Do you feel that hiring a physician extender will actually grow your practice or do you have patients who will not be willing to be attended to by anyone other than an MD? Depending on your stage in your career, are you looking to pass your practice on to someone, or are you just trying to maximize your value prior to selling to a firm?

As part of your internal review of your personality, you should also make sure you are good at providing constructive feedback. Remember that you are the supervising physician and as such, you should be able to provide tips and not be timid about teaching and pointing out changes that need to be made in management plans.

Case One

One movement gaining traction in dermatology involves promoting the practice of dermatology by board-certified dermatologists only. As a board-certified dermatologist, I certainly support this movement, but it creates an inherent hypocrisy within the walls of my office. Having experienced the difficulty in finding a board-certified dermatologist to join me, I also know that my wait time is unacceptable and I cannot possibly work any harder than I already am. Therefore, in hiring an extender, I made sure the people I hired believe in the same role of the extender that I do. That being said, I am always in the office when they are and cosign every single one of their notes. Over the years, I find this works with my personality. However, I often find that patients do get confused as to the credentials of who is treating them. Many times patients will see me again after seeing one of my PAs and they will tell me that they saw one of the other doctors in the practice. I have found the following phrases to be helpful in these awkward situations. "Oh yes, you got to see my lovely PA. I've been following along with the notes which I reviewed each time you were in. Since you are doing so well, here is what I suggest.... or since your skin is being a bit more stubborn than we initially thought I am thinking we should try this." Patients are then assured that the care they were given was good, reviewed by me as the supervising physician, and they are in a practice where consistency of care is key. They are also clear as to who has treated them.

31.5 Interview Red Flags

Over the years, there are a few red flags I have come to rely on when interviewing an extender to see if they are the right fit for my practice. The first is how eager they are to learn aesthetics. My main goal is for my extenders to be available to help me on the medical derm side, so it is important that they are mainly interested in that. The second is their willingness to work evenings and potentially a weekend day. The third is how many patients they can handle in a day. I expect my extenders to see five patients an hour and be able to function with one MA in the room with them while one loads additional rooms. The extender must not only call their biopsy results but also work to check my patients' labs and make phone calls for my biopsies. While I am happy to do my own work, I have learned that if I am consistently the only one working late hours and weekends I can be resentful. For me, my goal is to hire an extender to make my life easier and not more complicated. If I am ultimately responsible for generating income to cover their overhead, I need to be sure they are also working to be profitable. I also offer a 3-year contract, fully aware that the first year anyone joins your practice is the most costly. This also mitigates to some degree the heartache of spending time training someone only to have them leave you after a year and join another practice.

31.6 Question Three: New Grad versus Experienced Extender

In my office, I employ two PAs and I have precepted NP students. My formula for personal comfort in bringing someone on has been as follows: For a new graduate, I recommend a one-year training period. During this time, the entirety of Bologna is covered in a structured way. For extenders with dermatology experience, I ask them to follow me in the rooms during all of my patient hours for a minimum of 3 months. I begin to book my follow-up patients with them once I am confident that what they say and do in the room will be exactly what I would otherwise do. I make it clear that I should be consulted for any complex medical cases. I personally then review all notes and cosign them, providing feedback on management and plans. Once a week I give a didactic on a common problem like melasma or high-risk medication management (of which isotretinoin

and spironolactone are considered on the list as examples) to ensure that we are all practicing in a consistent manner. At the conclusion of visits with some of my patients, I tell them to book follow-up with my PAs; if it is a quick follow-up, for biopsy results of a rash for example, I let them know that I am available to come into the room to answer questions at that time as well. Of note is the fact that a program called Dermwise is also available to help with training new graduates.

I also encourage my PAs to attend CME events and encourage their participation in the Society for Dermatology Physician Assistants. One cautionary tale is that sometimes PAs, who come from other practices, may not be used to the type of supervision you prefer. It can be challenging to undo bad habits; however, communication is key. Ultimately, the right fit between an extender and a physician is one in which each person understands their role in the patient care team. If those goals are aligned, the team composition is actually a seamless one.

If you decide to train your extender in aesthetic procedures, be aware that any training you provide is portable. In other words, the NP you train today could set up a practice, making house calls for toxin tomorrow. While we all like to believe our extender will stay with us permanently, that is often not the case. On the other hand, if you don't like performing cosmetic procedures, you may find it useful to hire a midlevel who possesses training in plastics or aesthetics to perform these on your behalf. Certain laser procedures are more economically performed by an extender rather than the physician (e.g., laser hair removal). Keep in mind that cosmetic patients are the most high-maintenance and any complications will be yours to own regardless of whether you performed the procedure.

31.7 Question Four: Supervision

The degree of supervision of an extender depends on the degree of the extender. For a NP, he/she can practice independently. Up until the latter part of 2019, for a PA, a supervising physician must exist "on the record." In some states, that means being a phone call away; in other states, it means being physically present for a percent of patients attended to or provide direct supervised care. It is best to check with your local state before assuming which role you can take. Also, be aware of rules provided by Centers for Medicare (CMS) for extender use in treating Medicare patients and billing them. In my practice, I cosign every note written by my PAs but this is a time-consuming endeavor. Via Executive Order in November 2019, much of this has changed but as of publication it is not clear what impact this will have in Dermatology.

In terms of liability, your extender's malpractice is typically tied to yours. In the majority of cases, where an extender is named in a malpractice suit, the supervising physician is also named.

Equally important to supervision is the marketing of the midlevel. Be clear and transparent with patients on your website as to who the midlevel is and his or her qualification. Make sure you have strict rules in place with your social media managers as to how to qualify them across the various platforms you engage in. Similarly, outline the ways in which your extender brands him/herself on social media and what they post, as it can be a reflection of your practice.

31.8 Question Five: Changing Your Office Flow

While bringing on an extender can be helpful, the equation only works if you can get the midlevel up and running to see their own panel of patients. One of the components of this success is training your staff from those who answer the phones to those who check in patients and book follow-up appointments. It may not be adequate for your staff to simply say that they are booking the patient with your extender to convert patients to them; instead, think of ways to promote the extender as a qualified person to treat skin. For example, a hold message that credentials all members of your provider team including the extenders, or an area on your website that discusses details including the training schools of the extenders. In our office, we have wallboards in all of the rooms where one of the rotating images includes headshots of everyone who treats patients and their schooling background.

In terms of revamping your schedule, consider whether you want to be the person who attends to all new patients and, then on follow-up, be clear with the patient that he or she will be seeing your extender. Be willing and able to pick up on cues from patients who may be hesitant to do this and offer to come into the room if they would like. In my personal experience, not providing patients with a choice to decline seeing the extender is a mistake. Another way to build up your extender's schedule is to block a segment of time each day for emergency visits or spot-check appointments. Similarly, consider asking your extender to call back all noncancerous biopsy results that require follow-up and have these patients book with them for follow-up.

31.9 Delegating to Your Extender

An extender will only be as valuable as the amount of time you initially spend with him/her, making it clear what your expectations are. Hiring an extender to function as an uber medical assistant is not only a financial mistake but will lead to an unproductive work environment as you move through the years. It is, however, important that you be willing to relinquish some control to give the extender administrative responsibilities. This will function as two roles. The first is to make it clear to the staff that the extender is part of the provider team. The second is that it alleviates some of the paperwork burden that most physicians carry themselves. For example, if you have a log of your biologic patients, make your extender in charge of staff who oversees this. Similarly, delegate checking labs that are sent to the office to your extender and aid in establishing a schedule for the nursing staff. The most successful models I have seen use an extender almost as a backstaff manager, allowing you to spend time with other administrative functions that you, in particular, are needed for (such as budgets, managing overhead, etc.). What you don't want is an extender who essentially works as an island; in other words, someone who comes in for their schedule and leaves immediately when finished. Expectations of your extender should include ways to alleviate your responsibilities, so that the extender is not just another person attending to patients and creating additional work for you to catch up on.

31.10 Pay

Initially, it is reasonable to pay a flat yearly salary. As extenders in derm have become more in demand, so have changes and expectations in pay scale. It is not uncommon for a midlevel practitioner to ask for a percentage of collections; be aware that this is illegal in some states. If you choose to pay a production bonus, there should be a formula other than straight collections. For example, consider patient satisfaction, timeliness for completing organizational tasks, and contribution to office efficiencies. Make the evaluation markers clear and review them on a regular basis when calculating any bonus. In most EMRs, a midlevel is a separate license cost. If you choose to prepay for a set amount of time for a license, there should be some clawback for this fixed cost if the midlevel leaves prior to that time. In addition, most extenders expect an allowance for CME, time for CME days, and paid vacation.

31.11 Conclusion

It is a tough decision to decide to hire a midlevel versus another physician. For some, finding a physician to join their practice has been unsuccessful or too costly. While midlevels can be a more economical option, I would caution you that it is not *that* much more economic and should not be the only reason you hire one because your time for training and supervision also has a value. There are some key introspective questions to ask yourself before deciding to bring a midlevel on which I think are helpful to honestly answer. Most midlevels, because of reduced patient load, are able to spend more time with patients; as a result, they can be an asset to your practice. In addition, they can help reduce administrative and paperwork tasks, which often fall with the physician. At the end of the day, keep in mind that a midlevel should be an extension of you, and to the extent that you have to invest time to make sure that this is the case, it can ultimately be a very productive and symbiotic relationship.

Reference

[1] Ehrlich A, Kostecki J, Olkaba H. Trends in dermatology practices and the implications for the workforce. J Am Acad Dermatol 2017;77(4):746–752

32 Managing Expectations of Staff

Laura Kruter MD

Abstract

Managing staff can be one of the most challenging aspects of running a medical practice, given the unfamiliarity of the role and lack of exposure to personnel management during medical training. This chapter aims to introduce the physician-practice owner to begin thinking like a manager. By working through introspection and self questioning, learning from real-life examples, and examining the provided resources, the reader will be equipped with new tools to put to use in daily practice management.

Keywords: management, staff, expectations, human resources, communication skills, self-evaluation, workplace satisfaction, burnout

---

Top 10 Things You Need to Know

1. Practice self-reflection consistently to help guide decision-making.
2. Consider structured sessions with a designated mentor or coach to help identify blind spots.
3. Be aware of your communication styles: strengths and weaknesses.
4. Examine how you come across to others by consulting with trusted friends or mentors.
5. Transparency is key in maintaining open channels of communication.
6. Listen to your staff and craft a thoughtful message before reacting.
7. Aim for consistency in treating staff members.
8. Maintaining an integrative, positive, and curious perspective can help managers unify staff.
9. Rather than focusing on managing expectations, focus on tailoring clear messages and supporting a workforce that reflects your culture.
10. Education and mindfulness are the best burnout prevention methods.

32.1 Introduction

We've all been there. Receiving unwanted news from our staff that a biopsy has been lost, a result miscommunicated, a log mishandled, or a negative patient review. We immediately begin to wonder if this isolated incident is the tip of an iceberg of gross systematic workflow errors or an assistant who had a bad day. The fallout of one incident is manageable, but often opens our eyes to how reliant we are on our staffs' competence, care, and goodwill. Inevitably, as everyone shifts uncomfortably, we assign blame, deflect or try our best to discuss calmly, and then begin to devise a plan or a system to avoid repeating the error. As we reflect on how to improve, the looming questions are what *should* we have done? What can we expect from our staff and colleagues and what can they reasonably expect of us? A more grounded question would be 'how can we shorten the gap between expectation and reality while leading a team and caring for patients?'

32.2 Section One Objectives

- *The importance of insight into your own strengths, weaknesses, and values*
- *Benefits of finding a mentor or formal executive/ professional coach*

Many management books or coaches will stress that the first step and *sine qua non* in managing well involves a deep dive inward to understand one's own strengths and weaknesses, values, and preferences. When we understand these, we can better visualize the work environment that reflects them and, over time, develop tools to manage staff more effectively. The goal of this chapter is to present some methodologies for effective and purposeful self-reflection, and then link these results to culture creation, practice, and maintenance.

The ability to self-reflect, not sporadically, but on a regular basis in a systematic manner is an invaluable tool that, when honed, can be readily accessed both daily and when challenges arise.

To start down this path, either hiring a professional executive coach or recruiting a trusted mentor is a great place to begin. Following are some questions one might discuss with one's coach initially:

- Which qualities most impressed you in relation to the managers and mentors you've worked with in the past (e.g., chief resident, attending, principal investigator, any other manger you worked with even outside of medicine)?
- Which qualities or behaviors did you tell yourself you'd never incorporate and why?
- What immediate emotions do you feel and what is your communication style when challenges or conflicts arise? Confrontational, calm, avoidant, or angry?
- Do you know how to delegate or find the need to take on everything yourself, or delegate but then micromanage?
- What qualities do you think you are modeling to your employees? How do you think they perceive you?
- What single investment in time or money would add the most value to the practice and you as a manager (e.g., staff, training, leadership development, or personal relationships)?
- Which aspect of the job do you most love? Which ones do you avoid or dislike concentrating your energy on (e.g., diagnostics, procedures, teaching staff, talking to patients, number crunching, or marketing)?
- What kind of ideal environment do you enjoy working in (e.g., calm, bustling, organized, or chaotic)? Have you been able to create this in your practice?
- How do you measure your success at work? How do you measure your staffs' success? (e.g., objective-performance measures, patient satisfaction, or financial performance)
- Do you enjoy helping your staff learn and grow, or would you rather just focus on patient care and delegate other work to your office/business manager(s)?
- What power dynamic are you most comfortable with? For example, must you be at the helm at all times or do you enjoy/are you able to let others lead?

These are just some examples of questions which would be invaluable to reflect on with a coach. The answers to each will likely not be simple—strengths and weaknesses will surface, as well as many more questions, if answered candidly. Choose weaknesses that might be improved and piece together how these get triggered—is there a time of the month, such as when expenses are due, or particular individuals or personalities who you find challenging? Write these down and develop a plan on how to better handle these situations and/or discuss them with your coach. Commit yourself to internal accountability. The way in which you would handle them may change with time, so revisit the plan often.

32.3 Section Two Objectives

32.3.1 How to Explore Other Perspectives to Improve Communication?

Once the practice philosophy and your preferences as a manager are clear, executing this vision becomes the next, and to some, most challenging step. In reality, most of us grossly overestimate how well others understand us. In our minds, as long as we've planned it out—intentions clear and our message perfectly crafted—there should be no confusion. However, what transpires (and we are all guilty of being on the other side) is that people interpret messages through a unique, individual filter, which is a blend of their particular world views, interpretation of language, assumptions, and emotional responses. A view that we, as the interlocutors, cannot always reliably predict or control. A real-world example is as follows: A new, ambitious, and go-getter medical assistant joins an established team and splinters the staff. His eager behavior and over-performance pleases one physician, who values performance above all, but antagonizes another physician who views this behavior as self-aggrandizing and disturbing to the normal flow. The confused, eager to please novice, without guidance, may end up isolated and unsure of how to adjust. An experienced, insightful manager may know to jump in quickly and help tweak the assistant's behavior and talk to the staff to ease the effect of a new competitor in the mix.

For most of us, subconscious biases and expectations shape how we perceive others and interpret their actions. As most of these perceptions are reflexive, overcoming them is an unrealistic goal, but increasing our awareness around this is valuable. Here are a few exercises to help flex those muscles, when you find yourself in a communication bind:

On perception of others:

- Is your first impression of a staff member based on bias and assumptions? Realize that, in the present, this person is part of *your* team, therefore make the most of it, open your mind to the idea that you may be wrong, and readjust your viewpoint to one of curiosity and desire to get to know someone rather than critique.

On perception of oneself:

- Are you surprised about how you're coming across, for example, thinking you are transmitting warmth or kindness but consistently met with a negative response? Ask a trusted friend to help identify signals that may be misinterpreted.

On communicating:

- Be explicit about what you're thinking, feeling, and intending. If saying things outright is challenging, practice by writing them down.
- Before communicating an important message, draft it in three to five different ways. Think of how you would tailor it to different audiences: perhaps composed of devoted disciples, fierce competitors, change-averse veterans, bubbly millennials, or experienced leaders. Then, think of your true audience and how you can approach each individual separately or mold your message to include nods to different personal dynamics?

Improving communication skills should be a deliberate process and, unless one is trained to do this from previous work experiences, this is an unlikely habit for a clinician to engage in naturally in a busy medical practice. Any effort to engage in this with both yourself and your staff will pay off greatly.

32.3.2 Real-World Scenario

Your experienced office manager of 4 years approaches you, requesting an unplanned raise. Timing is particularly poor financially, as you are about to go on maternity leave and also happen to be losing your other full-time provider without immediate perspective of a comparable stand-in. Once you shake off the surprise, scenarios of how to manage the untimely request without losing a crucial employee come into focus. Regardless

of whether it makes financial sense to offer the increase, key communication strategies are pertinent in dealing with any ask. Begin always by reflecting on the practice values and your image in the eye of the employee—the way the process is handled reflects your commitment and will be remembered and shared with the outside world. Consider competition, benchmark the salary with other practices, and review performance evaluations and budgetary expectations for the year. For some, improving work-life balance is as or more valuable than a raise—consider offering work-from-home options and educational opportunities and schedule changes to allow for more time off. A generous benefits package can offset a lower pay scale, framing a raise as an increase in total compensation rather than salary alone. Turning the tables and asking the employee "what would you consider in my situation" can also open the exchange and make the other feel heard.

Beware of obvious inconsistencies—if in the past, you've been quicker to acquiesce, prepare to candidly discuss your reasoning. Not doing so could potentially cause the employee feel personally undervalued. In 2018, 90% of job seekers stated they highly valued transparency in the workplace, and this should be no different in medical practices. Transparency does not necessarily mean opening books and nailing down a 5-year agenda, but implies clarity in negotiation and thoughtful explanation, where appropriate, behind choices made that impact staff members.

Walking the fine line between maintaining low overhead and managing a high-patient volume optimally can be a challenge, and at the core of this balance is maintaining a productive and stable workforce. Without a focus on this and employee morale, the risk of losing good staff to a higher paying or less busy practice is a constant issue. Offsetting this risk centers around making employees feel respected, recognized, understood, and impactful. Listening to and actively addressing feedback seems simple, but is uncommon enough to make a practice that does so effectively stand out. What conditions can be created to allow employees to find satisfaction in the work itself? Most practice staff have a lot on their plate and setting realistic expectations and revisiting goals openly shows staff that, though perhaps high, the standards to which they are held are not unreasonable. Meetings should not only be held to address concerns, disasters and how to fix them. They should also be an opportunity to highlight successes, praise staff, and focus on positive reinforcement. When you hit a target, genuinely involve your employees in sharing in your success, whether through monetary incentives, such as a one-time bonus, treatment/products, or public recognition, or one-on-one praise. If, despite best efforts, the outcome results in an employee parting ways, maintain professional standards with them until their last day. Former employees, just like former patients, continue to be calling cards for the practice and may always circle back to join the company in the future.

32.4 A Note on Managing Burnout

The crisis of burnout in medicine is a serious enough matter to deserve a chapter of its own. Top reasons for burnout in our current medical economy affects all specialties: attempting to maintain service and excellence amid an overbooked, chaotic environment; clashes in values and culture; accumulation of long hours, nonclinical work, and rigid schedules that don't allow for self-care or family time. Although pervasive, burnout manifests slowly, thus is often missed and explained away as something else. The first step is being attuned to signs in oneself and others: behavioral changes such as increased tardiness, frequent illness, signs of exhaustion, and personality shifts like acting withdrawn. Unfortunately, the notion that burnout is part of the job—taken for granted, not excused, and somehow compensated for with salary—is still commonplace. In reality, identifying, coping, and preventing this issue is valuable to the employee, their loved ones, their patients, and the practice itself. Ways to start protecting our teams against burnout include being thoughtful about flexibility in scheduling, task redistribution and role assignments, and increased focus on work-home balance and personal growth. Investing in resources is well worth a practice's time and money. See below to begin learning and set an example in your practice on how to take hold of burnout:

- wellmd.stanford.edu/healthy/stress.html: Diagnosing and coping guide for different classes of stress
- www.aafp.org/fpm/2013/0100/p25.pdf: An excellent guide with causes, questionnaires, and resources on physician burnout

A note on managing physician colleagues—the process of onboarding a new dermatologist colleague can be stressful, as it is difficult to predict how a functioning team will change in the presence of a new addition. Openness and inclusiveness will make the new member feel welcome, and frequent check-ins can ease the process on both ends. Among colleagues, much as with siblings, flares of competitiveness are normal; however, these tendencies can dominate and sour relationships unless quickly identified. Framing the practice as a collective can help integrate and shift perspective from a self-centered one to that of a team.

33 Pricing Cosmetic Procedures

Omer Ibrahim MD, Michael S. Kaminer MD, Jeffrey S. Dover MD, FRCPC

Abstract

The increasing transparency among people sharing their experiences with cosmetic surgery, along with the rise in prevalence of aesthetic procedures on the Internet and in social media, has led to an increase in demand for inexpensive and accessible minimally invasive cosmetic procedures. How do providers price cosmetic procedures to take advantage of this demand, while maintaining their reputation and skillset, and also differentiating themselves from other physicians? In this chapter, first we describe the differences between commodities and luxuries, and then we describe how cosmetic procedures are at risk of commoditization. Thereafter, we discuss how providers can measure their worth, time, and expertise, calculate profit margins for procedures offered, and effectively and competitively price match their luxury services within their area.

Keywords: pricing cosmetic procedures, commoditization, commodity, luxury, botulinum toxin, filler, laser

Top 10 Things You Need to Know

1. The prevalence and transparency of cosmetic surgery on the Internet and social media have led to a rising demand in inexpensive and accessible minimally invasive cosmetic procedures.
2. A "commodity" is a good or service whose wide availability typically leads to smaller profit margins and diminishes the importance of factors (such as brand name) other than price.
3. A "luxury" is a good or service for which demand increases more than proportionally as income rises. Luxury goods are products that are not necessary for daily life but tend to make life more pleasant for the consumer.
4. Commoditization of cosmetic procedures threatens to devalue and mass produce our specialized cosmetic procedures, debasing the position of the physician from artist and expert to injector and laser technician.
5. It is our duty to shift the conversation with the patient from "how cheap can I get this treatment?" to "how well can I look and feel after this treatment?"
6. Recognize your worth and make it known: do not go cheap on yourself.
7. Factors that condition pricing cosmetic procedures include consumable cost, time required to complete the procedure, overhead costs, and the number of treatments required to achieve a desirable result.
8. Price matching to fit your demographic area is important; however, keep in mind that competition is based on skill and results, not price matching of competitors and medspas.
9. Avoid discounting the luxuries you offer patients.
10. Pay attention to the following details: make sure that the visit, from the moment the patient enters your practice to the moment they leave and beyond, is a memorable experience that is worth the money they paid.

33.1 Introduction

The increasing transparency among people sharing their experiences with cosmetic surgery, along with the rise in prevalence of aesthetic procedures on the Internet and in social media, have led to an increase in demand for inexpensive and accessible minimally invasive cosmetic procedures. As a result, the clinician has been confronted with the following challenge: How do I price my cosmetic procedures to take advantage of this demand, while maintaining my reputation and skillset, and also differentiating myself from other physicians and from the community "medspa" down the block? How does a physician ensure that he or she is able to provide a luxury good, carefully wrapped in expertise, quality, and exclusivity, and yet still remain accessible and financially successful? In this chapter, we discuss the evolving changes in the aesthetic realm, the challenges faced by physicians providing cosmetic procedures, including the threat of commoditization, and suggestions on how physicians should value their expertise and price cosmetic procedures.

33.2 Commodity versus Luxury

According to the Merriam Webster dictionary, a "commodity" is "a good or service whose wide availability typically leads to smaller profit margins and diminishes the importance of factors (such as brand name) other than price."[1] In contrast, a luxury is a good or service for which demand increases more than proportionally as income rises.[2] Luxury goods are products that are not necessary for daily life but tend to make life more pleasant for the consumer. They are typically more costly than necessity goods and are often purchased by individuals who have a higher disposable income or wealth than the average. Luxury goods are uniquely in demand, and value the importance of brand, reputation, and quality. In general, individuals who pay higher prices for the objects feel that they are worth the cost.

Cosmetic surgeons and providers have the option of marketing and pricing their services as luxuries. In general, there are the following three groups of providers: (1) the low-price, high-volume, less frilled practice, (2) the middle of the road practice that provides great care and charges modest prices, and (3) about 10% or less of the practices that are high-end, charge high prices for luxury services, and have patients who are willing to pay more for these services in spite of the price, and sometimes, in fact, because of the price.[3,4] Therefore, providers of cosmetic procedures are faced with the challenge of whether to offer lower-priced commodities in exchange for more volume, or higher-priced luxuries in exchange for more revenue and less volume.

Before discussing how the struggle between commodity versus luxury affects cosmetic surgery, it is worthwhile discussing a famous conflict between commodity and luxury in the apparel and retail community, as this example not only highlights the contrast between these two types of goods, but also shows the potential benefits and risks that exist on both sides of the coin. Zara is a fashion retailer that was founded in Spain in 1975. From its infancy, the company set out to be known as a "fast fashion" company by way of quick production times, speedy deliveries, and,

most importantly, high-end appearing fashion but inexpensive and accessible to the masses. Repeatedly, Zara has been accused of "copycatting" the designs seen on the runways of major fashion brands.[5] Time and time again, the stores' shelves would be stocked just a few weeks later, many times ahead of other brands, with clothing that looked eerily similar to those of other retailers, but priced much more inexpensively.[5] Zara's goal of bypassing the luxury "stigma," and rapidly providing less extravagantly tailored, inexpensive, yet still somewhat chic clothing to the masses, was embraced wholeheartedly by consumers, leading to the expansion of the company internationally and its multi-billion dollar net worth today. Major luxury fashion brands, as well as smaller independent designers and boutiques, suffered financially from the commoditization of their designs and philosophies.[6]

In the cosmetic surgery world, a similar risk of commoditization threatens to devalue and mass-produce our specialized cosmetic procedures, debasing the position of the physician from artist and expert to injector and laser technician. Large and small practices alike and all physicians, even highly specialized, skilled, and experienced ones, stand to lose from this commoditization. The advent of social media, live streaming advertisements on televisions, tablets, and mobile phones, and multiple online forums and review-based sites, have led to record numbers of people being targeted by aesthetic companies, pharmaceutical representatives, and paid "beauty bloggers and influencers." Large corporations have launched national and international direct-to-consumer marketing campaigns, taking advantage of this unprecedented ability to reach the eyes and minds of millions of people. Terms such as "Botox," "Restylane," and "Juvederm" are quickly becoming household names. This wave of marketing has served as a double-edged sword. On one hand, greater awareness of cosmetic procedures can lead to greater acceptance and a larger potential patient base for the clinician. However, on the other hand, this direct marketing to the patient has led to the risk of these services being viewed as mere commodities and goods that require mindless dispensing without prior consultation, thought, expert opinion, and skill.

Lately, especially among the younger, millennial population, we have seen an increasing number of inquiries and phone calls in the form of "How much do you charge per unit of Botox?" "How much is one syringe of Restylane?" "How much do you charge for a Fraxel or an IPL treatment?" Often these callers are calling your practice as part of a price-shopping routine, and have already called other providers before you and will call more after you. In these scenarios, the provider's expertise has been overlooked, and patients are flooding into clinics with Instagram screenshots on their phones and magazine cutouts. They demand a product or service, without discussing their aesthetic concerns, a wide array of other potentially beneficial treatments, and risks, or even inquiring if the physician is properly trained to provide said service. More and more patients are asking "Do you have this product and how much does it cost?" rather than asking, "What would you recommend for this concern? What are all my options? Is this safe? Are you trained in performing this procedure?" It is our responsibility, and an opportunity, to shift this conversation and paradigm from commodity to a service with a hint of luxury, and how we price our cosmetic procedures not only solidifies our services as medical luxuries, but also ensures our future financial success and stability.

33.3 Recognize Your Worth and Make It Known

The first step in pricing cosmetic procedures and differentiating from others in a sea of commodities is to recognize your worth, skillset, and artistry. These qualities should factor into how to price procedures, how you interact with the aesthetic patient, and how you deliver quality services to optimize outcomes. No matter what the complexity of the chief complaint, the patient's concern can be as simple as a subtle lip augmentation or as complex as a full-face ablative resurfacing, your education, training, and expertise factor into the decision-making process and ultimate delivery of that service by assessing if the patient is a candidate, determining the patient's desires and goals, evaluating risk and benefit, deciding on the appropriate product or device, skillfully providing the treatment or service, and finally planning for potential future roadblocks and further treatments. Given the use of the clinician's extensive training to constantly optimize outcomes, maximize satisfaction, and mitigate risks, the aesthetic

treatment of a patient's concern is worth much more than just the price of the syringe or laser consumable.

Once you recognize your own worth and skillset, make that expertise known to your patients, at least some of who have been trained by the media, Internet, and popular opinion to see dollar signs and price tags. This can be exemplified by a personal anecdote (OI). One day, at the end of my visit a person, who was a friend of the patient on whom I had just conducted a laser resurfacing procedure, asked, "Restylane is X dollars, right? I want my lips done again, because I wasn't happy by the job done at the medspa. It's around X dollars here too, right?" Even though this was not an official consultation, and I would not be reimbursed for my time with the patient's friend, I decided to spend 3 extra minutes to shift the conversation. I respectfully overlooked the direct price-seeking question and asked, "What are you looking to achieve with your lips?" After seeking out his specific concern, I used this opportunity to educate the patient's friend and set myself apart from other providers he may have seen before me. We quickly discussed what hyaluronic acid fillers were, the subtle differences between each brand and kind, what can realistically be achieved with lip fillers, and what should be avoided. At the end of the impromptu 3-minute consultation, both the friend and the original laser patient were scheduled for lip augmentation the next week. A discussion of specific cost only took place the day of treatment. Both individuals left the examination room with confidence that their provider was honest, aware, and able to provide them with the most realistic and aesthetic outcomes safely and effectively. In fact, they paid more than they would have at the medspa, but left feeling cared for and satisfied, knowing that they paid for the syringe, an expert opinion, skill, and artistry. Remember the syringe is the commodity not the service. The patient is paying for the skill with which the material is used and placed to achieve a desired look.

Ensuring that patients know that you have much more to offer than just a product, like your time, training, expertise, and wisdom, is a constant endeavor that materializes not only in the examination rooms, but also on a broader horizon. Your ancillary staff, advertisements, websites, and social media pages should constantly and consistently highlight your accomplishments and sing your praises and your credentials: make your value known. Once you ensure that patients know that not all procedures are performed equally, then the prices of your services, taking into account your skill and expertise, will be warranted and accepted. This begins the process of elevating your high-quality expertise to luxury good status, thereby clearly differentiating it from a commodity.

33.4 Pricing Your Procedures

When pricing cosmetic procedures, several factors must be considered in addition to factors such as skill and training. First, the cost of the consumable or disposable for each procedure must be taken into account. When looking at two procedures that require the same amount of time and staff, the procedure with the higher consumable would logically be priced higher to cover the disposable and yield a net positive return for the practice.

Next, in order to quantify the actual return, or the practice gains from each procedure, one must also take into account overhead costs. For any procedure offered in a clinic, costs include consumables, capital expenses, service contracts, fixed costs such as rent, heat, and electrical bills, provider's time, and ancillary staff time. All these factors that keep a practice up and running are included in the overhead cost. Geographic location can also impact overhead cost in the following manner: keeping a practice running in or near a large expensive metropolitan city costs more than running a practice in a smaller, less affluent area. After taking into account the consumable and overhead costs, the profit margins can then be assessed for each procedure or category of procedures to ensure the practice is functioning smartly and cost-effectively. For example, let us assume a practice's overhead is 50%, and the cost of a certain syringe of filler is $200. The physician decides that the price of treatment with this syringe will be $600. Subtracting the consumable cost, the initial profit (before overhead deductions) is $400; many end their calculation there. They see the filler procedure is richly rewarded at a price of $600 and profit of $400. However, taking into account the overhead of 50%, the true profit from this procedure is $100 ($200 consumable, $300 overhead). Is this a fair return for that practice? To answer this question, it is helpful to compare costs to medical dermatology visits. In general, a medical dermatology visit can reimburse $100 to 150 per visit with a profit of $50 to 75 (50% overhead in this example).

Many a time, the general dermatology visits, especially in private practices, can be completed within 10 to 15 minutes, with quick follow-up visits taking even less time, and also posing less risk on the part of the clinician. In contrast, cosmetic appointments can require longer time given the nature of, at least, some cosmetic patients. In sum, the practice must answer the following question: For each procedure, what is the proper math to ensure that your practice is getting a fair profit margin? Once the math is calculated for each procedure or category of procedures, then the physician can decide if the service is even worth providing at the practice at all.

Another factor to consider when setting prices for cosmetic procedures is the time required to complete the procedure, and if the procedure is performed by the physician or nonphysician staff member. The physician's time costs more than the staff member's time, and, sometimes, the operative time of the procedure trumps the cost of the consumable and overhead. For example, if a certain laser procedure incurs minimal consumable and overhead cost, but requires a tedious hour of the physician's time, then the cost of the procedure should reflect that time. How much do you believe your hour is worth? What about the capital cost of the laser and the expensive yearly service contract?

In addition, the price of the procedure should reflect the number of treatments required to produce a positive result. If the procedure is intended to be part of a series of treatments, then the price should honestly and adequately reflect the fact that the patient will see an incremental improvement, and the price is meant to allow the patient to commit to a series of treatments.

33.5 How Expensive Should I Be? Price Matching and Discounting

Studies have shown that patients appreciate clinicians who are cost-conscious and make an effort to keep costs low for the patient.[7] Every provider should continually address the patient's cost limitations and offer treatments that fit within the patient's needs, goals, and budgets. However, cost-consciousness should not come at the expense of discounting procedures and undervaluing one's own skillset and expertise.

When deciding on a fair range of prices for your practice, some market research may be necessary to discern the approximate range of prices that are charged by physicians of equal caliber to you in your geographical area. Speaking with colleagues and friends, as well as local sales representatives, may help determine the range of prices that seem reasonable for your geographical location. When setting your prices in comparison to these ranges, keep in mind that competition is based on skill and results, not price matching with competitors and medspas. Setting prices so low to attract bargain hunters leads to an unstable and unreliable patient base. Setting prices that are extremely high can deter some patients. In general, prices should be adequately high to reflect the level of luxury you wish to exude, as people in general equate luxury and quality with price. Pricing your services as luxuries allows you to charge more, spend more time with each patient, and work less strenuously to make financial ends meet. In the early stages of your practice, charging more for a medical luxury initially means that you will be attending to fewer cosmetic patients. However, in dermatology, we have the option of filling gaps in our schedules with medical dermatology, as our cosmetic reputation gradually builds. Over time, assuming you are skilled and capable, the cosmetic schedule will fill up, and your higher prices will remain intact, which means your revenue will be much higher than earlier in your career. As such, setting higher prices from the start is an initial investment in your own schedule and reputation that will eventually allow you to bring in more, work less, and achieve a more favorable work–life balance. In the end, would you rather see twice as many patients for half the return, or half as many patients for twice the return?

33.6 Conclusion

Sometimes the delight and excitement in receiving a present is as much a result of the wrapping paper and bow on the box, as what is in the box itself. The entire package and presentation of a gift can enhance the experience of receiving that gift, making it that much more special. As such, don't forget the bow in offering cosmetic procedures. Pay attention to the details that heighten and perfect patients' experiences, so that when they pay for a rendered service, they are paying for the entire experience from the moment they walk through the door to the moment they leave the office. People pay for attention to detail, uniqueness and exclusivity. This is why small details like the Tiffany's signature blue box, Christian Louboutin's famous red soles, and Gucci's interlocked "G's" emblem are international symbols of luxury and uniqueness. These companies offer a sense of distinction that even a multibillion-dollar corporation like Zara could not offer the masses. Practices and offices that can invoke similar feelings of individualized care, indulgence, and exclusivity may retain patients and lead to higher patient satisfaction. Open, warm offices make patients feel safe and comforted. Warm, courteous, and communicative staff members make patients feel well cared for. Tidy waiting rooms, clean examination rooms, open hallways, and even colorful artwork on the walls have been shown to increase patient satisfaction and decrease patient anxiety.[7,8] Therefore, even the smallest details of the practice setup, its décor, and staff, can impact the prices of cosmetic procedures and patients' willingness to pay for these procedures.

References

[1] Merriam-Webster. Available at: https://www.merriam-webster.com. Published 2018. Accessed October 23, 2018

[2] Deloitte. Available at: https://www2.deloitte.com/content/dam/Deloitte/global/Documents/consumer-industrial-products/gx-cip-global-powers-luxury-2017.pdf. Published 2017. Accessed October 23, 2018

[3] Brewer J, Porter R, eds. Consumption and the World of Goods. New York, NY: Routledge; 1993

[4] Alsarraf R, Alsarraf NW, Larrabee WF Jr, Johnson CM Jr. Cosmetic surgery procedures as luxury goods: measuring price and demand in facial plastic surgery. Arch Facial Plast Surg 2002;4(2):105–110

[5] Business Insider. Available at: https://www.businessinsider.com/zara-forever-21-fast-fashion-full-of-copycats-2018-3. Published 2018. Accessed October 23, 2018

[6] CNN. Available at: https://money.cnn.com/2016/06/07/investing/ralph-lauren-jobs-layoffs/index.html. Published 2016. Accessed October 23, 2018

[7] Smith RJ, Lipoff JB. Evaluation of dermatology practice online reviews: lessons from qualitative analysis. JAMA Dermatol 2016;152(2):153–157

[8] Nanda U, Chanaud C, Nelson M, Zhu X, Bajema R, Jansen BH. Impact of visual art on patient behavior in the emergency department waiting room. J Emerg Med 2012;43(1):172–181

34 Integrating Cosmeceuticals into Daily Practice

Sarah Sawyer MD

Abstract

A skin care business can be a vital and rewarding part of a dermatology practice. Carefully strategized, this retail business can benefit physicians and patients alike. Some recommendations are to start small and grow, streamline the education of your staff, and delegate the discussions as you see fit. Avoid overloading inventory, becoming complacent at a certain level, and omitting staff buy-in when honing your skin care business.

Keywords: skin care, retail, aestheticians, loyalty programs, boutique

Top 10 Things You Need to Know

1. Commitment: Time, money, and focus are required for your practice. You can have a basic skin care business with minimal effort, but a GREAT skin care business requires commitment.
2. Project leader: An incentivized and motivated team leader is crucial. This person needs your vision and great training but should NOT be you.
3. Start simple: Initially, choose one line or a few favorite items from different lines that you can truly stand behind. Selling too many skews is confusing for staff and patients.
4. Goals and growth: Set a reasonable initial goal and expand that goal each month. Growth occurs best when staff is both aware of the goal and incentivized to achieve it.
5. Educate and indoctrinate staff: Provide products to staff with the caveat that the recipients understand their purposes and benefits. The staff are the product ambassadors and need to recognize the responsibility of receiving the product.
6. Devote space: A dedicated space, separate from examination rooms, should be established to discuss and sample your products. This space can initially be small and expand as your retail business grows.
7. Regimen cards: Print cards with your favorite regimens for specific conditions for quick reference.
8. Spread the word: Use social media platforms to educate your patients about your products and market your promotions. It may also be of help if your staff product ambassadors posted on an established schedule. Both you and your staff should share personal anecdotes and experiences about your favorite products.
9. Pair with procedures: Bundle products with particular procedures, such a lip antioxidant with perioral fillers, pigmentation products with peels for melasma, etc. This practice will add value and improve outcomes as well as introduce patients to your products.
10. Keep the excitement going: Incorporate products in blogs and newsletters. Consider a product of the month to keep the spotlight shining on your offerings.

34.1 Introduction

I am excited to share my personal experience with cosmeceuticals in my daily practice. Over the years, I have had both a modest skin care business and, now a more, lucrative skin care business. Although I have many fine mentors to thank for my success, I believe that trial and error, along with time and experience, have been my most valuable teachers.

I was fortunate to complete a cosmetic fellowship with outstanding dermatology proceduralists, including the late Richard Fitzpatrick, MD. For those of you who are not aware, Dr. Fitzpatrick founded Skin Medica. Under his mentorship, I witnessed a culture where the education of patients about skin care was a priority. I observed how cosmeceuticals could be successfully and responsibly incorporated into dermatology practice. Since this practice sold Skin Medica products almost exclusively, every staff member knew about the products in detail. Although I did not recognize it at that time, this focus and staff knowledge are the backbone of any successful skin care business. It was also at that time that I saw growth factors being incorporated into laser procedures, specifically laser resurfacing. This pairing of procedures and products is another concept that has helped me develop a good skin care business.

When I had the opportunity in 2016 to enjoy a large expansion of my office space, I opened a SkinCeuticals flagship store. My skin care boutique is a showcase for SkinCeuticals products. The focus on these products has allowed me to reach "the next level" in cosmeceutical sales. I have learned principles and many valuable tips that can certainly be used in the absence of any specific program or company. Our skin care business got much bigger, primarily because of the FOCUS.

Like many physicians, I was very concerned about the sale of products in my office. I am not a salesperson and I certainly did not want patients to feel pressured to purchase my products. If, however, we are recommending products that are benefiting our patients and improving their outcomes from procedures, this practice is a win-win. Although I agree with those who claim there are many excellent over-the-counter skin care products, having products in-house truly makes most patients happier because of the ease of acquisition and the ability to ask questions about the products. A physician taking ownership of a patient's skin care regimen makes them feel more confident about using it.

Regardless of how a physician feels about dispensing products, no dermatologist can argue against the point that we are experts in the field of skin and the many ingredients found in skin care products. I think, many a time, we take for granted what we know simply because we have known it for years and do not value it any longer. We are the most qualified people to coach a patient about a skin care program, just as we are most qualified to prescribe topical medicine.

The statistics on the business of skin care are shocking. Our patients are spending billions of dollars on skin care products that lack scientifically proven active ingredients, and most patients will travel to a department store or skin care store within a couple of days of visiting our offices if products are not introduced to them at the time of the visit. I am fascinated by how many patients choose skin care based on anything other than science. These same patients may insist that a board-certified core physician performs all their cosmetic procedures, but are perfectly happy using an expensive skin care brand that has no background science. I believe the reason for this discrepancy is focus, strategy, and time spent. The woman with no medical background behind the counter at a department store has time to spend with your patient and is focused solely on the sale of skin products alone.

For years I felt frustrated with myself and my medical assistants because we possessed no consistent strategy for carrying out a skin care discussion. By the time we finished a thorough consult regarding the available and relevant procedures, and answered questions, I was exhausted and running late. The clinic was moving much too quickly to incorporate the entire conversation in the examination room. It was totally unrealistic to rely on my very busy clinical team to conduct this, sometimes lengthy, discussion. A physician and his or her direct clinical assistants cannot leap the hurdle of time. Even though I had every desire to advise patients on skin care and the science behind my recommendations, I simply could not consistently have a conversation about it before I had to move onto the next patient. This one problem kept our skin care business stagnant for many years.

34.2 Our Skin Care Consultant and Project Leader

Although I was very reluctant to do so, the leap of faith I took to hire a skin care expert was a large part of the growth of our business. For years, I could not financially justify hiring an employee solely for this purpose, and certainly before the consultant was hired, our collections would not have supported an added employee. However, choosing the right person made the business grow to cover the extra payroll and added profit. The right person for this job should not only possess skin care and sales experience but also be willing to tackle other tasks in the office with any free time. Our skin care consult knows how to take before and after photographs, set up rooms, bring patients back to the clinic rooms, and much more.

We now have a system and strategy in place for me to vet my skin care brands and skin care expert within my consult, introduce the patient to the expert, and then let the discussion happen as I move to the next patient. I do like to mention a specific product or kit before leaving the room, so that the patient knows I am involved in the decision-making, but details are left to discuss once I have left the room. The important thing for patients to know during your time with them is that you are handing them over to a person who you trust to make recommendations on your behalf. Sometimes I will say "[skin care consultant], I would like for [patient's name] to use a morning and an evening antioxidant, then I'd love for you to find anything else that may fit her needs." The consultant walks the patient out of the examination room, spends time in the boutique if the patient desires, and answers any final questions the patient may have during the check-out process. Not only have our numbers improved, but I enjoy my day much more knowing that the skin care discussion, other than a few introductory comments, is off my plate and in the hands of a person I trust.

34.3 Choosing Products and Making Goals

There are many wonderful products available for dermatologists to dispense. I made my early decisions primarily based on my personal experience and knowledge. I think it is also vital to have good local support from representatives. When choosing skews, a representative who lives near your office, has helped others start skin care businesses, and has a good track record for attentiveness is a great resource. Goal setting can be difficult in the beginning. Attempt to go through a few "regular" months before setting a monthly sales goal, and keep the goal 5–10% above your average. Our best plan not only involves a monthly goal with a nice financial incentive (our staff splits 5% of sales based on hours worked) but also a "stretch goal" that offers a much better reward. Our "stretch goal," if met every month for a year, is rewarded with a weekend cruise for the staff.

34.4 Educating and Indoctrinating Staff

Taking time to train your staff is worth every moment when managed well. Start with a strategy and categorize the trainings, so that the information is truly absorbed. For instance, one session may be spent on sunscreens, then cleansers, and so on. Although your skin care consultant can plan these sessions, your involvement with the planning can make them most efficient. For the first few trainings, I felt stressed about the lost clinic time, but I now believe that the investment will reap benefits for years to come.

Make the products available to your staff, but link this perk to knowledge or sales goals. To start, we gave staff members each a few products to introduce them to the line, but this is not sustainable without limitations. SkinCeuticals has a trackable online didactic program with quizzes, so that we can reward those who make the effort. Also, products can be distributed as rewards for a great month of sales.

34.5 Devote Space

The issue of space is another limiting factor. Just as the skin care consultant was vital to solving the issues of time and focus, our boutique was critical to the issue of space. Skin care discussions should occur in an area that is not going to interrupt the flow of clinic. Also, a tester bar is necessary for patients to see and feel products before purchase. Our boutique is the size of a large examination room, but it certainly does not need to be this large. A simple corner or attractive display that has space around it is all that is necessary until your practice develops. Once sales increase, you can decide to devote more space if required. ▶ Fig. 34.1 is a photograph of our boutique.

34.6 Regimen Cards for Common Diagnoses

Develop several regimen cards for common conditions when you find yourself or your staff making a standard set of product recommendations. The diagnoses might include rosacea, hyperpigmentation, or acne. This can also be done if you have standard postprocedure recommendations. ▶ Fig. 34.2 is my regimen card for hyperpigmentation. This saves time and effort, and can prove to be a "last resort" if your normal system fails.

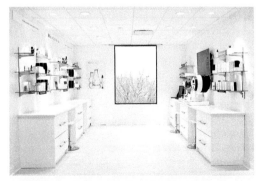

Fig. 34.1 A photograph of our skin care boutique.

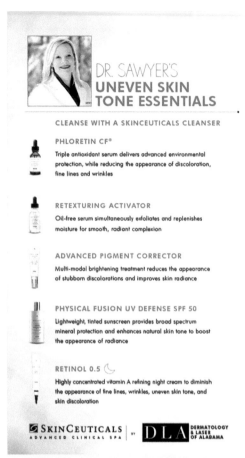

Fig. 34.2 A copy of my regimen card for hyperpigmentation.

34.7 Internet and Social Media

We have had several versions of online stores since our practice opened in 2006. While we have a local group that hosts our website, our store is hosted by DermPro. DermPro is an ecommerce service for aesthetic providers. They have a large menu of services, but our practice only uses online retail. They offer a membership program, gift cards, and content including videos and photographs of our products. They charge an initial fee and a monthly fee based on services used.

Social media is also a great place to showcase and promote your skin care range. We often include our favorite products in posts to exhibit a specific use or situation where a product is relevant to the experience. These posts can be based on seasonal activity and can be fun and educational. We like

to post about a staff member using a particular product for an issue specific to her, for example, an exfoliant for keratosis pilaris in the winter. When we promote a product or a bundling of procedure/product, we always post the same on social media and our website to raise awareness.

Despite our frustration, most skin care companies have online stores of their own with free shipping. However, some companies have developed strategies to drive patients to your practice or give you credit for the sale on the company website. Quizzing potential skin care representatives about their company practices on this topic may help you decide which companies will make better practice partners.

34.8 Aestheticians

Aestheticians are also employees who can elevate your skin care business. While we have had varied experiences with aestheticians through the years, our current aesthetic staff has become a large part of our skin care business. The opportunity exists, in your practice, for an aesthetician to guide your patients through a perfect skin care experience. An aesthetician provides a comfortable environment for your patients and also spends more time with them than anyone else in your practice. In the amount of time it takes to do a facial, superficial chemical peel, or dermaplaning, great education can take place about the skin care products sold by your office and why they are superior to others.

Before you refute this concept, let me tell you that I was the original naysayer of this level of service. First, I held a hard line that laser treatments are the only procedures that make major changes in skin quality. Second, I assumed that only young women would be interested in what I considered "entry level services." Finally, I assumed that an aesthetically concerned patient would either be a laser/filler/toxin patient or one who was interested in facials and dermaplaning. I couldn't have been more wrong in my assumptions. On many occasions, I have walked into a room and found one of my loyal laser patients glowing with the best skin they've had in years and more satisfied with our practice than ever. During the visit, they shared that they have added monthly facials to their existing maintenance plan of lasers and injectables.

Having a service performed by an aesthetician can be a luxurious act of self-care. The patients are not nervous or anxious as they might be before an injectable appointment. With this level of comfort, a patient is more apt to listen to the benefits of a great home skin care regimen. Many of my patients are very attached to our aestheticians. Our aestheticians are also my cheerleaders, and they encourage and educate our patients to try procedures or set up consults for beneficial procedures that they may have missed otherwise.

34.9 Loyalty Programs and Skin Care

For many years, we could not keep a full-time aesthetician busy. This, however, is no longer a problem after launching our first loyalty program, which is a VIP membership program with a monthly charge. Our VIP members receive one aesthetic service per month from a list of six services, 10% off on skin care, and 20 units of Botox. I have included our current flyer as ▶ Fig. 34.3. Although every practice is different, I believe I can offer some advice after beginning this program.

- MD services should not be offered as a monthly option. Typically, the MD schedules are the busiest.
- Make the services high value for the patient; however, ensuring that it does not create much of a financial loss to the practice. I did include Clear and Brilliant laser, which has a relatively high overhead cost, but my machine is many years old and was not as busy as I desired it to

Fig. 34.3 A copy of our current VIP program membership offerings.

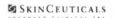 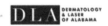

VIP

REWARDS
MEMBERSHIP

203.870.3303
201 OFFICE PARK DRIVE
SUITE 350
MOUNTAIN BROOK, AL 35223

Thank you for being a loyal patient at Dermatology & Laser of Alabama. We would love to have you in our **VIP Rewards Membership** program.

This monthly subscription gives members access to exclusive pricing on products, procedures & more.

The monthly membership fee ($169) will simply auto-draft from your account with 6 or 12 month membership options.

VIP Membership includes one service per month:

- Clear + Brilliant Laser procedure ($350 value - includes up to 3 treatments in the 12 month program or 1 treatment in the 6 month program)
- HydraFacial (30 minute - $200 value + $50 upgrade option for a 60 minute Luxe HydraFacial)
- Enhanced Facial or Chemical Peel with Dermaplaning ($225 value)
- Laser hair removal treatment for underarms ($200 value)
- Laser hair removal treatment for facial area(s) (up to $300 value)

As a VIP Member, you will also recieve 10% off all SkinCeuticals products, 10% off all MicroNeedling procedures & be the first to know about upcoming events, specials & promotions.

VIP Botox appointments are available to all members via our VIP direct scheduling concierge.

The 12 month membership includes 20 free units of Botox, a free 13th month of membership & the option to gift or transfer up to 2 services to family or friend accounts.

The 6 month membership allows 1 service transfer.

A $250 cancellation fee applies to both membership options.

Please, stop by or call 205.235.6994 for more information.

BIRMINGHAMSKIN.COM

217

be before I offered this program. I also limit this service to 3 per year.

- Avoid the urge to make the program too generous, so it does not need to be revised later once patients are accustomed to the perks.

This program got our first aesthetician very busy, and we have added two more part-time aestheticians in the space of one year. Our skin care sales have also increased because the aestheticians are spending an hour per month with each patient, discussing their skin and the products they should be using at home.

Our VIP program includes members of all ages and stages of life. It is a fantastic way for a new patient to "sample" our practice, but many of our VIP patients have been a part of my practice for years and have been going elsewhere for facials. The program is also beneficial for patients with specific problems such as acne and melasma, as well as those patients who are preparing for a special event. The automatic monthly income from our VIP program has surprised and delighted me. We have only one level of membership at this point, but other practices have up to three levels of membership.

34.10 Our Future Goals

While we have appreciated a few years of rapid growth, we have not reached our full potential. One practice I admire has their skin care expert available on a blog to write about products as well as field questions. In addition, I have always been interested in an auto replenishment service for interested patients. Finally, we have tried unsuccessfully to implement inventory management solutions. Although I have not employed either, two examples of inventory software are FlexScanMD, which can track by provider and barcodes, and Orchid Spa Software, which can also track patient points if your practice has a rewards program.[1]

34.11 Specific Financial Considerations and Benchmarks

When I began my practice, I did not know how to measure skin care sales other than by conducting comparisons with our past sales. Upon researching this many years ago, I came to know the general guideline that skin care should represent 8% of total practice revenue. I am now aware of benchmark data that is published every year regarding these numbers.[2] The following is a table of the range in skin care sales in dermatology offices:

Practice size	Revenue 25th %ile	Revenue 75th %ile	% of revenue
1–3 dermatologists	$120,000	$254,00	2.3–5.7%
> 3 dermatologists	$285,000	$926,000	2.0–8.9%

34.12 Common Pitfalls When Starting a Skin Care Business

- Avoid the urge to load up on inventory. For many years, I ordered 12 of everything when the representative approached me. This caused confusion and a lack of consensus among the staff.
- Do not place the skin care project leader responsibilities with someone who is already overloaded with other projects. Skin care tends to drop to the bottom of a list of priorities when this occurs.
- Don't forget staff buy-in when choosing a line or a product. If several of your key players are not excited about it, they won't sell it.
- Don't buy exclusively for discounts or free items such as travel-sized products.
- Don't stop the education process when sales improve. Have a plan in place for continuing education and for new employees to catch up.

Checklist for Introducing Cosmeceuticals

- ☐ Carefully choose a leader for your office skin care sales.
- ☐ Choose a space for your skin care display.
- ☐ Meet with company representatives to ask about the following:
  - Differentiating features of the company
  - Staff training
  - Staff product
  - Best selling products in your area
  - Geographic location of the representative
- ☐ Choose one or two skin care lines.
- ☐ Set aside time for the entire staff to train and bond over the skin care line. Start with four time slots of 2 hours each.
- ☐ Set goals for monthly skin care sales.
- ☐ At staff meetings, make skin care a priority in discussions. This is a good time to discuss sales from the previous month and any promotions available to patients in the following month.
- ☐ Recognize staff members who are putting forth great efforts.

34.13 Conclusion

One of the nice things about incorporating cosmeceuticals into your practice is that it does not require a large initial investment of money or time. I encourage all of you to participate at some level, and you will find that patients not only appreciate the convenience provided but also value the information disseminated about your products. As your practice evolves, your interest and satisfaction with it may increase, which can launch you to a new level. I truly believe that focusing on skin care is a good way of growing one's dermatology practice. Many savvy and successful dermatologists have made it an integral part of their practices, and made their skin care business a signature of the practice's personality. Good luck and best wishes!

References

[1] Gabi B. ASDS 2018 session entitled "Building Loyalty: Integrating Loyalty Programs into your Cosmetic Dermatology Practice"

[2] Allergan/BSM Consulting financial database, updated 2018

35 Building a Budget/Calculating Overhead

Matthew J. Elias DO, FAAD; Merrick D. Elias DO, FAAD

"The best way to stick to your budget is to start one."

– Anonymous

Abstract

Practices can succeed and fail if they do not track their revenue and expenses, create a budget, and learn how to benchmark that budget. In this chapter, we will teach you how to track what you are spending money on, how to categorize practice expenses into buckets, where your money is coming from, and then synthesize from the data a budget that you can stick to to create a thriving successful practice. In addition, you will learn how to benchmark your practice to other similar practices which would afford you the opportunity to discover areas where you can grow your practice and learn where deficiencies are in your practice. Budgeting is the basis for financial success and this chapter will provide you a foundation for success.

Keywords: budget, revenue, expenses, benchmarks, goal setting, negotiate

Top 10 Things You Need to Know

1. Create a budget and stick to it no matter what.
2. Make sure to dial in exactly where your revenue is coming from.
3. As a corollary, know where your expenses are going. Track both your revenue and expenses to the penny.
4. Benchmark your data.
5. While benchmarking is important, it should only be used as a guide as all practices function differently.
6. Benchmarking can show you very early on if something abnormal is happening to the fiscal health of your practice.
7. Creates timeline and goals and try to hit them, setting you up to hit the next goal; this can be done for both start-up practices and long-term highly functioning practices.
8. Research ways to earn cash back, points, travel rewards, rebates, etc. for all purchases and use them for each and every purchase. Don't forget for example to use eBates/Rakuten, etc. if you buy something on Amazon.com.
9. Create a "slush fund," so you can protect against unexpected expenses and stick to contributing to the "slush fund" no matter what.
10. Remember everything is negotiable and use this approach when dealing with all vendors. They need your business, not the other way around, so if the deal isn't to your liking, walk away, and its likely they will return to try to earn your business. This can be applied to all vendors, not just devices and large purchases but medical equipment like sutures to Internet services like websites, blogging, etc.

35.1 Introduction

The financial health and success of your practice can all be traced back to your budget. Unfortunately, many practices never create a budget and many others create one but never utilize it when making financial decisions. If you understand budgeting and follow your carefully planned out budget, you can keep your finances on track and prevent many issues that can cause failure of a practice such as poor staffing decisions, embezzlement, overhead issues, etc.

Physicians by nature of their focus on the sciences in school are typically highly lacking in finance and business. This is further compounded by the fact that we are not taught business in medical school or residency, so it is imperative you take the time to understand exactly how the finances of a medical practice work and this starts by learning how to create and maintain a budget.

If your practice is up and running, you may have the advantage of knowing where your revenue is coming from but be at the disadvantage of following your budget once it is set. If you are a practice start-up, you will be at a disadvantage in being aware of your revenue streams, making it more difficult to plan your budget; however, it will likely be easier for you to implement your budget once it's created and sticking strictly to it, thereby preventing any untoward practice events.

35.2 Methods for Identifying Revenue

To begin building your budget, it is imperative you identify your revenue sources and payer mix. If you are a start-up, you will be best served by using a conservative estimate that grows slowly over the first few years. There may be many ways for you to guesstimate future revenue in a start-up by obtaining information from practice consults or financial institutions that may be lending you money to start your practice.

To find your revenue, start by identifying what codes you are billing for and how much revenue was generated for each code by the payer. For example, a new patient skin check with a 99203 code may generate $100 from Medicare but $120 from a private insurer. By knowing what codes are reimbursing and which insurers are reimbursing, you will be able to create a matrix that will identify where you are most profitable, allowing you to try to grow your practice by growing the more profitable visits/procedures and better payers. By the same token, you can utilize this information to review your contracts, renegotiate with payors, and even potentially drop lower performing visits and insurers.

35.3 Methods for Calculating Expenses

Now, that you have a handle on where revenue is coming from, it becomes imperative to learn what expenses to track and how to track them appropriately. What to track and why will vary from one practice to another as will the detail level that the physician owner will need. If you are more of a high-level manager, it is best for you to produce reports that flow with your style for you to review but be down to the detail level for others like your office manager, CPA, or attorney to track, whereas if you are detail-oriented, it may be best to get down to line items for your

review and have the same level of detail as your office manager, CPA, or attorney will need/want. The most important concept to remember is to be detailed as possible and to not just use the limited categories of IRS tax forms; even if you won't review that much detail yourself, it is necessary to have the data to properly budget your practice.

Sample categories to be tracked can be many and varied, including physician dermatologists and midlevel wages and benefits such as medical/dental/vision insurance, retirement plans, CME, identity theft protection such as Lifelock or Identityforce, and supplemental insurance such as Aflac. Employee categories can be similar and should be accounted for as well. General categories may include EMR and PM or RCM costs, rent and utilities, repairs and maintenance, capital equipment purchases or leases, professional organization dues such as the AAD or ASDS, all forms of insurance including professional liability insurance (MedMal), other forms of business insurance such as business overhead and business interruption insurance, EPLI insurance, etc. Legal and accounting fees, marketing, janitorial services, charitable donations, meals, supplies, taxes, licenses, uniforms and laundry, travel for conferences. Discretionary categories may include owners' automobiles, life insurance policies of the practice owners, student loans, etc. All of these categories can be further broken down to individually track down the physician or staff member level. For example, Dermatologist X utilizes 3x as many supplies as Dermatologist Y but generates 5x the revenue. Data points like this can be exceedingly important budget-wise and show why it is essential to be as detailed as possible.

It may be necessary to have category overlap such as organization dues since some organization membership dues like the AAD may be a general category expense, while others like REAL may be a discretionary physician expense. It is best not to combine categories like a broad category of "supplies," rather administrative supplies such as printer ink, pens and letterhead should be kept separate from clinical supplies like gauze, band-aids, etc. Remember the more categories to a point, the better as you can break out the data points in a multitude of ways, leading to following your budget and pinpointing problems like embezzlement, theft of office supplies, incorrect staff ratios, etc. in a much easier way.

However, it is important to remember that as detailed as the categories can be, do not get too detailed where you can't make a decision. Using our supplies example again, there is no reason to break down supplies into band-aids versus gauze versus dermablades, as it won't help you make decisions, whereas if the category is clinical supplies and gauze goes up by 10% (it is always best to look at both the percentage and total dollar value of a category, as 10% of one item may not be much while 10% of another may be a lot of money) but dermablades and band-aids go down by 5%, it may balance out and keep your clinical supplies neutral. If you get too detailed down to the actual product level, you will go crazy chasing each item, whereas in this case, even though individual item prices changed, it was cost neutral to your budget. Also, remember different staff members will be involved in the expenses and others may be involved in the budget creation, so it is important for staff to be aware of what belongs in which bucket.

Once each individual practices, unique categories are created and categorical expenses are tracked, they should be subtotaled by category. By subtotaling expenses by category, you can accommodate unique situations like practice furniture and casement renovation, or disaster situations like hurricanes and floods, and isolate the anomaly in the budget, so as not to affect future budgets by creating a new separate apart from the rest of the budget category for these one-off or emergent expenses. Once all the subtotals are created, they should be added to learn the total outflow or expenses of your practice.

35.4 Methods for Creating a Budget

Now, that you understand the inflow of money or revenue in your practice and have learned how to breakdown the outflow or expenses, it is time to learn how to build a budget. The easiest way to create a budget is to use benchmarks which are readily available from third party national organizations like Medical Group Management Association (MGMA) on a national level and may be attainable on a local or regional level. These benchmarks can be used to reflect each expense category as a percentage of practice revenue.

"The 2018 MGMA DataDive All Surveys package arms you with the full array of data to identify the areas that you can improve your practice operations, manage your practice costs, and even attract and retain quality physicians and staff." MGMA DataDive includes provider compensation, management and staff compensation, cost and revenue, practice operations, and better performers.

MGMA DataDive Provider Compensation allows you to "slice compensation and production data for over 140 physician specialties and 60 nonphysician provider specialties based upon your organization's profile (practice size, region, and MSA), generate visualizations depicting compensation relative to production, and analyze trend data..." It also provides you the complete picture of compensation, "including total pay, bonus/incentives, retirement and more productivity—work relative value units (RVUs), total RVUs, professional collections and charges, and benefit metrics—hours worked per week/year, and weeks of vacation."

MGMA Data Dive Management and Staff Compensation Data allows you to understand staff compensation and benefits and the relationship between benefits and total compensation across varying regions, practice size, and specialties like dermatology.

MGMA Data Dive Cost and Revenue is probably the single most important data benchmark tool available to a practice, as it seeks to set and maintain a budget. "MGMA's DataDive Cost and Revenue online platform lets you uncover answers about how your organization's financial and staffing metrics compare to others in the industry. Achieve superhero status with data as your super power: Right-size your staffing levels for peak performance, examine how your cost structures compare to the best-in-class, determine how payer mix impacts revenue, and learn how people, process and technology affect collections and accounts receivable."

MGMA Data Dive Practice Operations may not be necessary as comparative data for developing a budget, but it is interesting nonetheless to a business owner Dermatologist in that "this platform provides operation benchmarks to common questions like: What should my average patient wait time be? Should my practice open on Saturdays? Is my staff turnover rate too high?

Do we have more no-shows than other practices? Should I outsource to a call center or hire more staff?

Finally, the last MGMA DataDive is the Better Performers data set for which they have "identified the gold standard of medical practice performance, so you can be the star. By scouring data submitted by practices across the country," they've "assembled the metrics and practices of high-performing groups."

Once you have your benchmark data like that provided by the MGMA data above, you can tease out all the categories that you have identified in your expense report for dermatology in your region and the type of practice you have, that is, sole provider versus group. Now, that you have both your data for each category and the benchmark data, you will begin to see where budget should lie and can easily begin to craft a budget for your practice. For example, if you are a solo general dermatologist in New Orleans, LA, and you have three medical assistants with a combined salary + benefits of $100,000/year, but the MGMA dataset for cost and revenue says you should have an annual MA salary + benefits of $125,000, then you are either understaffed or performing better than the benchmarks. Either way, it will allow you to set your budget appropriately for your practice, as you will know if your practice is humming along and performing exceedingly well; at the $100,000/year level, you can set your budget at $100,000/year, allowing you some leeway elsewhere, or if you and your staffed are overstressed you will know you should increase your budget to $125,000/year to accommodate for another employee to make your practice run smoothly. It is vital that you review the benchmark data at least every year, so your practice stays up-to-date with the current reality of practicing dermatology in your location.

In certain situations, you may need to adjust your benchmarks as they apply to your budget. For example, if your wait time for a new patient to see you is months, you may not require much money to go toward marketing; on the other hand, if you introduce a new cosmetic service to your practice, you may require a larger expenditure toward marketing. If benchmark data says 4% of your annual revenue should go toward marketing and you are booked out, you may adjust that down to 1% in your budget, while if you are introducing that new cosmetic service, you may

increase your budget to 6%. In certain situations, the adjustment will remain year over year, while in other cases, it will need to be reevaluated on a yearly, budgetary basis.

The benchmark data should be used as a basis for the budget of your dermatology practice, but it should not by any means be the end all be all for your practice, as every practice functions differently and your budget should be a function of your actual practice. It is good to compare your budget to the benchmarks and make adjustments as needed. These comparisons should be done on a regular basis typically annually as should the comparison between your budget and your practice's actual financial data which should be done more frequently, either quarterly or monthly. When comparing your practice data to your budget, you should be able to quickly pick up on inconsistencies and learn why they are happening. For example, are you overstaffed compared to the revenue you are generating, are you understaffed, or is your staff working too much overtime? If you collect $250,000 in June and your budget is set for $250,000/month, and your staff compensation + benefits is budgeted for 20% of $250,000 or $50,000, but in actuality it is $62,500 in June, something is wrong. If you compare these percentages to another variable item like clinical supplies (gauze, band-aids, dermablades, etc.) and find that that percentage is stable, budgeted for 5%, and is still 5% of $250,000 in June or $12,500, then you are likely seeing the same amount of patients as you were in previously months, what you budgeted for, and your staff is working too much overtime. On the other hand, if clinical supplies go up to 10%, this likely means you are seeing more patients and your staff is thus working harder, but you experience a collections issue, as you and your staff worked harder but collected the same amount. Comparing all of these datasets can lead to unbelievable knowledge about your practice, allowing you to make informed decisions as you grow and move your practice forward.

When opening a practice, there are many things to think about. Creating a realistic timeline early on is imperative. This will coincide with your budget and help you when calculating overhead and revenue. Once you have established your practice location, there are many things to consider relative to your budget. Memberships in local, state, and regional medical societies will be a recurring expense. Deciding to join the local chamber of commerce or other local groups can add expenses early on. Expenses like rent, utilities and various business-related taxes often increase slightly every year and must be accounted for. When signing or extending a lease, try to get as much rent abatement or tenant improvement allowances to help defray early costs. You will have plenty of variable ongoing costs such attorney and accounting fees. While it is difficult to calculate how much you may spend on this in a given year, it is better to estimate high and come in under budget. All it takes is one bad employee to make those attorneys' fees soar. The various insurances, which were discussed earlier in this chapter, can also increase yearly. Remember that a yearly budget is fluid and some line items may increase or decrease during the year. If you have cable and Internet and the company raises its rates, you may be over budget. A good office manager (or yourself) can try to call and negotiate with these types of companies when that happens.

Annual dues do not just include memberships to organizations like the AAD, but may include state medical licenses, DEA, CLIA, NICA, and a host of others. Hospital dues and CME fall into a similar category. It's important to account for these, particularly when starting a practice. Annual inspections, recertifications and repair on medical equipment such as autoclaves along with your fire extinguisher are further considerations. Should you decide to purchase a device that has consumables or requires a service contract after the first year, you need to remember to add this to your budget when you do an annual review. Sometimes you may purchase equipment or a device midyear that you were not planning on. It is imperative to adjust your budget at that time to account for this new expense. You may realize that you were under budget on advertising and can take it from there or you may decide to increase advertising to help promote the new device. If that happens, you need to adjust the budget further. Remember there are multiple ways to market your practice, via social media, that do not cost anything but time. An initial website can be created by yourself or a family member, but as your practice grows, you may wish to have it done professionally. This is another recurring cost that you must pay attention to when creating a budget.

As we continue to think about expenses germane to a medical practice, we must budget for maintenance services inclusive of janitorial, laundry and, depending on your lease or if you own your office, snow and common area maintenance (CAM). Nota bene: CAM is usually calculated and included in your monthly rent if leasing. Other utilities such as gas/electricity, water, telephone, Internet, and television may be negotiated into your lease (partially or fully), but it not need to be accounted for as well. Some of these charges can vary monthly.

Other ways to help cash flow and keep yourself under budget include using cash back credit cards, warehouse and online shopping (especially for consumable paper goods and office supplies), and purchasing recurring used items when they are on sale or have incentives attached to them. Moreover, you can offset some expenses such as travel to conferences if you get miles/points on your credit card. There are many websites to review the best deals on credit cards. If a capital equipment purchase allows you to use a credit card, you may find the CME course you need to take is covered, provided you pay off the credit card charges immediately and don't incur interest. What seem like small things can add up and help keep you at or under budget come year end. If you are going to use credit cards or have any loans, make certain to pay off any interest as soon as you can. If you find that you will be carrying a balance, particularly early on in your practice, make certain to account for that in your budget. Participating in a group purchasing organization (GPO) may have a similar positive effect on your company's bottom line. Remember, any place you save money can be reinvested back into your practice.

There is a great deal of information to process when creating and adjusting your budget. Creating a "slush fund" or surplus fund may help you stay within your budget. Having a certain amount of cash or a percentage of revenue in this fund will protect you against unknown expenses that occur every year. A piece of furniture or equipment may break and you need to repair or replace it. Whatever comes your way, within reason, you have accounted for it. Should you not need the money in this fund, it is best to roll it over to the following year, as you will eventually need it.

Furthermore, you must account for salaries and staff recruitment. Once you settle on how many staff members and what you are willing to pay them, you must figure out your own salary structure. Will you take a small base salary and then take bonuses and distributions? Can you afford to take a higher salary? What are the income tax benefits and laws where you practice? There are expected salary considerations such as annual raises or holiday bonuses. You should even build some staff overtime into your budget. If you have salaried employees, they should be the ones to stay late, so that you can avoid paying overtime. Unexpected salary concerns include when a good employee asks you for a raise midyear, you hire additional personnel, or you replace an existing employee with a higher salaried one. It may be cheaper to give the raise to a good employee than the expense to recruit, hire, and train someone new. A hidden cost savings is that patients often like seeing a familiar face in the office. You don't want the reputation of always having new employees. Having to pay unemployment benefits or negotiating with a terminated employee can increase your budget as well. Make sure to document everything in the employee's personal file to limit this expense.

Ultimately, it is paramount to remember that everything is negotiable. Review the biggest line items regularly and compare prices from different vendors. The amount you save may just pay for that well-deserved vacation you will need.

36 Evaluating Pharmacies and Patient Coupons

Peter A. Lio MD

Abstract

While there are many steps that are required to get a medication to a patient, one of the final steps involves paying for it at the pharmacy. Historically, prescriptions were available for most insured patients, but this has changed rapidly in the past several years. Specialty pharmacies and patient coupons and rebates have become commonplace, for better and for worse. While there are short-term advantages to utilizing these resources, they may pose long-term harm to the health care system, placing practitioners in a very difficult position.

Keywords: pharmacies, specialty pharmacy, coupons, rebates, prior authorization, drug pricing, pharmacy benefit manager

Top 10 Things You Need to Know

1. Drug pricing is much more complex than it may seem.
2. The actual cost of a medication to the patient and the system is often obscure.
3. If a patient cannot obtain your prescription, your "treatment" will be considered a failure.
4. Some companies have designated specialty pharmacies to help lower prices.
5. Remarkably, both branded and generic drugs have specialty pharmacy programs.
6. The working of business models of specialty pharmacies remains somewhat unclear and their total cost to the health care system may be significantly higher.
7. Coupons and rebates may have similar pitfalls in that while they allow for price reduction, they are also likely to influence prescribing behaviors, sometimes in favor of more expensive drugs.
8. While they may make certain medications available to some patients, they add even more layers of complexity and bureaucracy to a system that is already faltering under the weight of such overhead.
9. Doing the "right thing" is not entirely obvious when it comes down to the individual patient, making this area hotly debated.
10. With greater transparency, there is hope that prices will come down and accessibility will be improved.

36.1 Introduction

Any discussion of the cost of prescription medications in the United States is fraught with powerful opinions. Many of these opinions make an emotional appeal such as "How could this company charge so much for this drug?!" While there is no doubt that medications are too expensive in general, and most would agree our health care system is probably not sustainable in its current form, a deeper exploration of this question is needed in order to properly assess it.

Everyone has felt the sting of a patient who says "That doctor only spent five minutes with me, how could the bill be that high!?" Or one who remarks: "That dermatologist froze **one** spot and it took all of about 10 seconds, I cannot believe the fee!" Clearly, in such cases, the value of the service is worth more than the simple cost of goods or time it takes to convey the seemingly bland conclusion "That mole looks benign." A cashier at the grocery store could give the exact same advice, but clearly it wouldn't have the same value as when rendered by a board-certified dermatologist with years of training and experience, and who is responsible (and liable) for the correctness of the diagnosis. With this example, it becomes clear that evaluating "worth" is perhaps not quite as simple as stating "This probably costs them $0.05 to make!" Having said that, we shall go no further than to say that while medications are too expensive, they will probably never be as cheap as we (and our patients) would like them to be. This reality has necessitated a number of workarounds to bridge the gap of high medication prices, including specialty pharmacies and rebates or coupons for patients. In this chapter, we will discuss these methods from several perspectives, including the most pragmatic one: a busy clinician trying to get patients better.

36.1.1 Adherence and Access

As a clinician, one of the most challenging issues is adherence: getting the patient to use the prescribed medication is crucial to treatment success. However, adherence is fundamentally impossible without access: if the patient is unable to obtain the drug in the first place, the work carried out during the course of the visit would be useless. While there are many steps that are required to get medication to a patient, one of the final steps involves paying for it at the pharmacy.

Historically, prescriptions could be obtained by most patients. In fact, as recently as 30 years ago, the majority of prescriptions filled at retail pharmacies were paid directly out of the pockets of patients.[1] Gradually, health plans began to offer medication coverage to compete for new members, initially at a relatively low cost. Many can still remember a time when even branded drugs were usually covered without issue. Indeed, although this might be considered lacking taste now, Dr. Walter B. Shelley once quipped "A generic drug is about as good as a generic doctor."[2] Such sentiment, needless to say, has shifted significantly since that time.

Complexity, price, and prescription spending began to increase dramatically during the 1990s. Experientially, early rejections for branded prescriptions could be easily remedied with a prior authorization (PA)-paperwork submitted to the insurance company to justify the prescription. Over the years, this process has become increasingly difficult and time consuming, acting as a powerful deterrent to the point where many clinicians exclusively use generics the only exception being when no viable generic exists for a drug. For a time, there was a state of equipose, but more recently, the situation has seemingly worsened yet again. Two factors in particular have pushed things into untenable territory. First, the stratospheric rise in the cost of generics has made many of them completely unaffordable without insurance help— a gigantic change from the typical $4 triamcinolone cash-pay price of 5–10 years ago. Second, necessary help from insurance has progressively waned over time.[3] This toxic combination has left patients in a bind and holding an unpayable bill. It has also left clinicians relatively impotent and unable to execute treatment plans.

While it seems obvious that systemic improvements are necessary to get to the root of these cost issues, they unfortunately do not help the patient with atopic dermatitis next Tuesday, and the dizzying complexities of the system (see ▶ Fig. 36.1) place such discussions far beyond the scope of this chapter. Instead, we will focus on some of the short-term solutions, although some may be more harmful than helpful, and examine specialty pharmacies and rebates or coupons.

36.2 Specialty Pharmacies

In the current mire of drug pricing complexity, one solution that has become increasingly popular has been the concept of a "specialty pharmacy." As there are many middlemen involved with getting a drug to a patient from a prescription, it is clear that with each step, there is a cost and profit. It does not take a sophisticated analysis to include that any item, even a relatively inexpensive one at the start, can balloon in price as sequential markups occur with each intermediate handler.

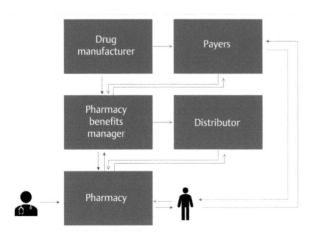

Fig. 36.1 Some of the relationships diagrammed to illustrate the labyrinthine complexity of getting a prescription from a prescriber to a patient in the United States.

Referring to ▶ Fig. 36.1 again, we can see that the manufacturer may set a price, but then either a distributor or pharmacy benefits manager (PBM) can alter that price, as can the final pharmacy, each potentially increasing the original price of the drug. By cutting out some of the intermediaries, it seems reasonable that having a designated pharmacy allows for a company to, at the very least, better track the price on its way to the consumer, and ideally pass on the efficiency savings by offering a lower price. Sometimes, this price is so low that a "cash pay" price is favorable, such that a medication can be affordable to a patient even without insurance. Increasingly, insurance plans have begun to strongly encourage—if not mandate—the use of special mail-order pharmacies. While there can be great cost savings for the patient this way, it is unclear if even these company-sanctioned pharmacies offer real savings to the insurer itself.[4] However, these are generally different than those working directly with drug manufacturers, adding further complexity for both patients and clinicians.

Arguably, this type of arrangement could be ideal with its benefits, but there are indeed several negative aspects to this setup as well. First, from a patient perspective, it can be off-putting to have to use a strange new pharmacy, sometimes one that is intimately connected with a drug company. There are potential privacy concerns that could occur with this closeness; more superficially, a lack of convenience and familiarity with one's neighborhood drugstore. In addition, such a relationship could theoretically deter competition between pharmacies, allowing for paradoxically higher prices despite the intention. Further, because different companies require different pharmacies, it is not uncommon to have to send different prescriptions to different places for the same patient, making for a complicated discussion that can be confusing for all. Perhaps most importantly, there are ample opportunities for graft and abuse in such closed systems, as we have unfortunately learned in spectacular detail with a well-known example from the recent past.[5]

For better or for worse, many companies have taken the route of selecting a pharmacy, or pharmacies, that will hopefully guarantee a price for most patients. Interestingly, this has not been limited to branded products, as there has even been an entry into a specialty pharmacy for select generic products that claim zero cost for most patients.[6]

How can this work? Does this not sound too good to be true? Ultimately, it is difficult to fully know the business models of these approaches, as there may exist differences from product to product and company to company. However, the unifying concept seems to be similar to the concept of Robin Hood: by charging a high cost of drug for those who are actually covered, they can subsidize some number of noncovered or poorly-covered prescriptions. Sadly, the relatively inexpensive actual cost of most of these medications allows for massive price inflation to be able to do so, even when only a relatively small percent is covered.[7] While this certainly makes for a compelling promise to patients, it is likely not sustainable in the longer term, increasing overall health care costs, especially for the "good" insurance companies that actually try to cover such medications.

36.3 Coupons and Rebates

Company coupons and rebates to the patient certainly have initial appeal, as they allow for a significant price reduction to the patient while serving the function of a tangible reminder of this for both patient and pharmacist. Like samples, having a coupon or rebate card may make one more likely to recommend a specific product, and such financial incentives have a measurable effect on patient behavior, making them more likely to obtain and use the prescription, at least in some settings.[8]

On the flipside, such incentivizing almost certainly encourages the selection of more expensive drugs at a cost to the entire system.[5] Expenditures for specialty drugs have been increasing at more than 10% annually, and one large study of more than a quarter million prescriptions found that, in most cases, coupons reduced monthly cost sharing to less than $250, a point at which patients were far less likely to abandon the medications.[9]

As a concrete example of this, at least at the time of writing, both tacrolimus and pimecrolimus have gone generic, which should be a wonderful thing for patients who need non-steroidal treatments for atopic dermatitis. However, the price for 30 g of tacrolimus 0.1% ointment is over $200, while the price for 30 g of pimecrolimus is over $300, as listed on a popular website that features drug pricing.[10] On the other hand, while crisaborole (branded only, there is no generic available yet) is listed at over $700 retail, a current program from the manufacturer promises $10 for those with insurance that covers the drug, $70 for those with insurance that doesn't cover it, and $100 for those who pay cash.[11]

Perhaps more than any made-up example, this somewhat ridiculous (but all-too-real) clinical scenario sums up the difficulty in answering the question "which is cheaper?" If you, as a patient, needed a Food and Drugs Administration (FDA)-approved nonsteroidal treatment for your atopic dermatitis and had a high deductible like so many Americans, from a cost perspective, the $10 would certainly be more palatable than $300, and even the $100 cash pay would be far better than the double or triple of the cash pay generic price. And, for this example, I forgot to mention that the crisaborole is for 60 g, which is double the amount, making this example even more extreme!

Now, this is of course only focusing on costs, and similar examples could be illustrated for acne products, rosacea products, and products in every other area of medicine. It is important to mention that the *value* may be different than the simple cost of a medication, and while it is beyond the scope of this chapter, it is worth pointing out that there are initiatives that seek to calculate value for both patients and prescribers, such as the Institute for Clinical and Economic Review (ICER).[12] Becoming familiar with such reports can help guide treatment selection and avoid costlier choices that may actually be less effective for patients, and is an integral part of a general cost stewardship for health care.

As one might expect, there is no easy answer related to coupons, and beyond discussions pertaining to cost, important ethical questions have been raised, including whether giving away such coupons helps pharmaceutical companies influence one as a prescriber.[13]

36.4 Conclusion

Perhaps it is a cliché to say that medicine in general, and dermatology in particular, is in the midst of a time of enormous change. With pressure from all sides, never before has the relationship between patient and physician been more imperiled. Adding to this is the increasingly high-cost of medications, against the improbable backdrop of worsening insurance coverage, making many prescription therapies functionally unobtainable for a growing number of patients.

We await more sweeping changes that will hopefully lower medication pricing, increasing accessibility, and yet continue to allow profit for companies who ostensibly push the field of medicine forward with new therapies to fulfill unmet needs. In the meantime, however, we are forced to find practical solutions to tide us over and solve the day-to-day problems faced in a busy clinical practice. It is with some trepidation then that we turn to both specialty pharmacies and coupons/rebates to help meet the needs of our patients in those situations for which the alternatives are simply not feasible.

References

[1] American Patients First. Available at: https://www.hhs.gov/sites/default/files/AmericanPatientsFirst.pdf. Accessed October 22, 2019

[2] Shelley WB, Shelley ED. Advanced Dermatologic Therapy II. 2nd ed. Philadelphia, PA: WB Saunders; 2001

[3] Rosenberg ME, Rosenberg SP. Changes in retail prices of prescription dermatologic drugs from 2009 to 2015. JAMA Dermatol 2016;152(2):158–163

[4] Johnsrud M, Lawson KA, Shepherd MD. Comparison of mail-order with community pharmacy in plan sponsor cost and member cost in two large pharmacy benefit plans. J Manag Care Pharm 2007;13(2):122–134

[5] McLean B. The Valeant Meltdown and Wall Street's Major Drug Problem. The Hive. Available at: https://www.vanityfair.com/news/2016/06/the-valeant-meltdown-and-wall-streets-major-drug-problem. Published June 5, 2016. Accessed February 13, 2019

[6] Dobkin HE, Zirwas M. Price discrepancies among mobile medication applications for common dermatologic prescriptions: Observational cost analysis. J Am Acad Dermatol 2017;77(6):1181–1182

[7] Price Discrepancies Among Mobile Medication Applications for Common Dermatologic Prescriptions. PracticeUpdate. Available at: https://www.practiceupdate.com/content/price-discrepancies-among-mobile-medication-applications-for-common-dermatologic-prescriptions/61165. Accessed March 10, 2019

[8] El-Sadr WM, Donnell D, Beauchamp G, et al; HPTN 065 Study Team. Financial incentives for linkage to care and viral suppression among HIV-positive patients: a randomized clinical trial (HPTN 065). JAMA Intern Med 2017;177(8):1083–1092

[9] Starner CI, Alexander GC, Bowen K, Qiu Y, Wickersham PJ, Gleason PP. Specialty drug coupons lower out-of-pocket costs and may improve

adherence at the risk of increasing premiums. Health Aff (Millwood) 2014;33(10):1761–1769

[10] Prescription Prices. Coupons & Pharmacy Information - GoodRx. Available at: https://www.goodrx.com/. Accessed March 10, 2019

[11] Learn How to Save on EUCRISA (crisaborole) ointment 2%. Eucrisa. Available at: https://www.eucrisa.com/eucrisa-4-you. Published March 22, 2017. Accessed March 10, 2019

[12] Home - ICER. ICER. Available at: https://icer-review.org/. Accessed March 10, 2019

[13] Zilbermint M, Schiavone L. To give or not to give: the challenge of pharmaceutical coupons. J Clin Ethics 2018;29(4):319–322

37 Deciding What Services to Provide

Elizabeth K. Hale MD

Abstract

With a broad range of modern dermatologic procedures at our disposal and new technologies continually evolving, dermatologists have to choose carefully and selectively which services to offer. Considerations like patient demand and physician expertise are important, but so are such practical concerns such as office space, equipment, time management, insurance, and workflow. More abstract factors like your brand, your philosophy on patient relationships, and your goals for media exposure also come into play. This chapter introduces the many aspects you should consider when choosing what services your practice will offer. It walks you through the issues that will influence your choices, as well as the consequences of your decisions, enabling you to take a comprehensive, clear-eyed view of how your services will shape your practice.

Keywords: services, conditions, equipment, treatments, procedures, lasers, cosmetic, medical, surgical, and skincare

Top 10 Things You Need to Know

1. Is the service I am considering offering covered by the insurances I accept? Am I willing to accept less net revenue to get insurance-covered patients into my practice? Can I convert those patients into full-paying clients for elective procedures?
2. How much of my time is required with each patient to properly administer the service? Diagnosing and prescribing topical medication for a rash takes substantially less time than laser hair removal. How will administering this service fit into my practice's workflow and schedule?
3. Can the service be provided by an MD only, or can a physician extender administer it? If it is the latter, am I comfortable delegating? How will this service impact my staff training, wait times for an appointment, liability, quality of care, and patient experience?
4. What equipment do I need to have in order to offer this service? Does my budget limit me in terms of purchasing a multiuse device or can I afford a higher-end, specific laser that is more effective but can only be applied to this service?
5. How much space will the equipment and administration of the service require? Do I have the necessary space, and can I commit the space for the time needed to offer this service to patients?
6. What benefit do I provide over other competing practices offering the same service? Better word-of-mouth? More expertise or experience? State-of-the-art technology? Lower pricing? Less wait time for an appointment?
7. Is this a service that will have longevity within my practice? Am I confident I will see a return on the investments I will need to make with regard to equipment, training, and marketing this service?
8. Is my staff well-informed enough about this service to properly introduce it to patients and answer basic questions about it? Can they confidently explain and "sell" this procedure?
9. How does offering this service reflect on my brand or fit into my practice's market positioning? Is it consistent with what my current patients expect from my practice, and will it draw in new patients who are a good fit for my practice?
10. Is my brand more about being a reliable, efficient service provider or a lifelong provider of holistic dermatology solutions for my patients? Am I interested in investing the time and energy required to cultivate close relationships with my patients, and am I willing to accept the consequences in terms of my schedule and patients' ease of access to me?

37.1 Introduction

In episode seven of the ninth season of *Seinfeld*, Jerry dates a dermatologist. He finds her musings on saving patients' lives grandiose, assuming her practice likely consists of popping pimples and telling patients to "put some aloe on it." That is, until a former patient approaches the doctor to thank her for saving his life from skin cancer. But Jerry is not alone in his ignorance of what exactly it is that we as dermatologists actually do for patients. The popular understanding of what comprises dermatologic services is vague at best. The confusion is exacerbated by the increased use of physician assistants and other physician extenders to meet the patient demand for skincare services, and the prevalence of nonmedical practices offering many of the cosmetic services dermatologists provide, in a non-clinical setting.

What services you choose to provide as a dermatologist will inevitably reflect your interests, talents, and priorities as a practitioner, and will also be a major determinant of how patients view your brand. But there are numerous more practical factors that come into play when deciding which conditions you will treat and which procedures you will offer. ▶ Table 37.1 will help you wrap your head around the possibilities. As you imagine your practice offering each service, take a holistic, clear view of how your choices will influence your day-to-day operations.

37.2 General Service Categories

Whether you're practicing in a high-tech medical building in a large city or serving the population of a rural fishing village, your options for which services to offer will fall into the following three basic categories:

- **Medical:** Medical dermatology covers the common skin rashes and chronic diseases that every patient will likely suffer from at one time or another. It is the largest service category, responsible for 56% of the dermatology industry's revenue.[1] This category encompasses dermatoses such as acne, psoriasis, eczema, warts, and common environmental rashes such as poison ivy. Medical dermatology has

Table 37.1 Common dermatologic services[a]

Category	Service	Description
Acne treatment	Visible light treatment	Blue, red, and blue + red light therapy for acne
	Topical or oral prescriptions (Isotretinoin)	Prescription treatment for acne
	Photodynamic therapy (Levulan Kerastick, Metvixia, Ameluz, red light, blue light, Vbeam Perfecta)	Laser-activated photosensitizer treatment for acne
	Photopneumatic therapy	Intense-pulsed light (IPL) and vacuum therapy for blackheads, whiteheads, and some inflammatory acne
	Infrared light treatment	Infrared light to treat pimples
	IPL	IPL therapy for acne
	Laser treatment (Smoothbeam, Isolaz, etc.)	Laser treatment for acne
Acne scars	Microneedling (EndyMed Intensif)	Skin smoothing and reducing appearance of rolling acne scars
	Infini	Microfused radiofrequency microneedling treatment for acne scars
	Fraxel (Re:pair, Re:store), Clear + Brilliant, or Clear + Brilliant Permea	Nonablative and ablative fractional laser resurfacing to reduce appearance of acne scars
	PicoSure	Picosecond laser treatment for acne scars
	Pixel laser, Active FX, or Deep FX	CO_2 fractional skin resurfacing for acne scars
	eMatrix	Sublative rejuvenation to address acne scars
	Chemical peels	Superficial peels to reduce acne scars
	Vbeam Perfecta	Pulsed dye laser for erythematous acne scars

(Continued)

Table 37.1 (*Continued*) Common dermatologic services[a]

Category	Service	Description
Antiaging	Botulinum toxin injections (Botox, Dysport, or Xeomin	Injectables to treat dynamic wrinkles
	Chemical peels	Superficial peels to address photoaging
	Dermal fillers (Restylane, Restylane-L, Restylane Lyft, Defyne, Refyne, Juvéderm Voluma, Juvéderm Vollure, Juvéderm Volbella Juvéderm Ultra and Ultra Plus, Sculptra, Radiesse, Belotero, or Versa)	Injectables for volume enhancement and wrinkle reduction
	Erbium:YAG	Ablative laser resurfacing for skin rejuvenation
	Nd:YAG	Q-switched laser for wrinkles and laxity
	Photofacial	IPL treatment to reduce signs of skin aging and sun damage
	ThermiTightor ThermiSmooth	Controlled radiofrequency treatment for wrinkle reduction and skin tightening
	Fraxel, Pixel, or Dermal Optical Thermolysis	Ablative fractional laser resurfacing for skin rejuvenation
	Fraxel re:store, Clear and Brilliant Permea, Laser Genesis, or Affirm	Nonablative fractional laser resurfacing for skin rejuvenation
	Platelet-rich plasma (PRP)	Autologous plasma injection for skin rejuvenation
	Ultherapy	Ultrasound energy to lift and tighten skin
	NovaThreads or Silhouette Instalift	Thread lifts for subcutaneous lifting
	Exilis Elite	Radiofrequency and ultrasound therapy for skin tightening
	Microneedling (EndyMed Intensif)	Facial tightening, wrinkle reduction, and nonsurgical lifting
	PicoWay, PicoSure, or PICO Genesis enlighten	Picosecond laser treatment for rejuvenation
	eMatrix	Sublative rejuvenation
	Alma ClearLift	Nonablative lasering for skin rejuvenation
	Infini	Microfused radiofrequency microneedling treatment for skin laxity
	Protégé Elite, Profound, or Thermage	Radiofrequency treatment for skin tightening
	HydraFacial	Multistep facial treatment to improve skin tone and texture
	CO_2RE, AcuPulse, UltraPulse, or Pixel	CO_2 fractional ablative laser resurfacing for skin rejuvenation
Body contouring	CoolSculpting	Cryolipolysis treatment for fat tissue reduction
	Kybella	Injectable enzymatic reduction of fat on submental area
	Liposonix	High-intensity focused ultrasound technology to target and destroy fat cells
	Thermage	Radiofrequency therapy for contouring and tightening
	SculpSure	Laser lipolysis for chin contouring, fat reduction in abdomen and flanks, back, inner thighs, and outer thighs

(*Continued*)

Table 37.1 (*Continued*) Common dermatologic services[a]

Category	Service	Description
	Endymed Intensif RF Microneedle	Microneedle treatment for body toning, tightening loose skin
	BTL Vanquish ME	Selective radiofrequency fat reduction
	UltraShape Power	Ultrasound treatment for fat in the abdomen, hips, and thighs
	Velashape III	Vacuum, infrared light and bi-polar radio frequency technology for body contouring and cellulite appearance reduction
	truSculpt	Radiofrequency treatment for fat removal and skin tightening
	Cellfina or Velashape	Minimally invasive cellulite treatment
	ThermiSmooth Body	Controlled radiofrequency treatment for cellulite reduction
Hair removal	GentleMax Pro, GentleLase Pro, GentleYag-Pro, or Vectus	Nd:YAG, alexandrite, or diode laser for removal of unwanted hair
	IPL	IPL therapy for removal of unwanted hair
	Electrolysis	Electric current therapy for removal of unwanted hair
Hair restoration	PRP	Autologous plasma injection for hair regeneration
	NeoGraft	Follicular unit extraction (FUE) hair transplantation
	Finasteride (Propecia), corticosteroids	Prescription medication for hair regrowth
	Capillus	Low-level laser light therapy to stimulate hair regrowth
Veins	Sclerotherapy	Injectables to eliminate varicose veins and spider veins
	Endovenous laser therapy (EVLT)	Laser treatment for spider veins and small varicose veins
	Radiofrequency ablation (RFA)	Radiofrequency treatment for large varicose veins
	Excel V KTP	KTP laser for spider veins
	Vbeam Perfecta OR GentleMax Pro	Pulsed dye laser for leg veins, and facial and spider veins
	IPL	IPL therapy for spider veins
Pediatric	Acne acquired and congenital nevi (moles) atopic dermatitis (Eczema) diaper rash hemangiomas of infancy keratosis pilaris molluscum contagiosum psoriasis ringworm scars vascular malformations/birthmark (port wine stains, spider angiomas, or pyogenic granulomas) vitiligo warts	Various

(Continued)

Table 37.1 (*Continued*) Common dermatologic services[a]

Category	Service	Description
Skin cancer or actinic keratosis	Mohs micrographic surgery	Surgical removal of cancer using microscopic control
	Cryosurgery	Freezing using liquid nitrogen
	Excision	Surgical tumor removal
	Curettage and desiccation	Tumor removal and electric current
	Radiation therapy	Treatment using high-energy rays or particles to kill cancer cells
	Photodynamic therapy (Levulan Kerastick, Metvixia, Ameluz, red light, blue light, or IPL)	Laser-activated photosensitizer treatment for actinic keratoses and some skin cancers
	5-fluorouracil (Carac, Efudex, or Fluoroplex), chemical peel, Diclofenac (Solaraze), Imiquimod (Aldara or Zyclara), Ingenol mebutate (Picato)	Topical treatment for actinic keratoses
	excel V, Vbeam Perfecta, Fraxel Re:pair, or Fraxel Re:store Dual	Laser surgery for actinic keratoses
	Melafind	Imaging system for melanoma detection
Mole/wart/skin tag/pigmented lesion /tattoo removal	Cryosurgery	Liquid nitrogen and compressed carbon dioxide (CryoCorrect) freezing technique for benign skin lesions
	Electrodesiccation, hyfrecation, or currettage	Electrosurgery for removal of skin lesions
	PicoWay, PicoSure, or PICO Genesis enlighten	Picosecond laser treatment for benign pigmented lesion and tattoo removal
	Q-switched nanosecond laser	Q-switched laser for dark spot and tattoo removal
	Fraxel Re:store Dual or LaseMD	Fractional skin resurfacing treatment for sun spots, tattoos, birthmarks, nevi, and melasma
	Alex TriVantage or Nd:YAG	Q-switched laser for tattoos, pigmented lesions, or melasma
	IPL	Light therapy for pigmented lesions
	Fraxel	Nonablative fractional laser resurfacing for tattoo removal
	CO_2 laser	Ablative CO_2 laser treatment for sun spots and uneven coloration
	Pixel laser	Fractional skin resurfacing for pigmentation
	Skin surgery	Surgical removal of moles, cysts, lipomas, and benign lesions
Vascular Lesions/Redness	Vbeam Perfecta or GentleMax Pro	Pulsed dye laser for vascular lesions
	Cynergy	Pulsed dye and Nd:YAG combination laser for port wine stains, hemangiomas, and telangiectases
	Photofacial	IPL treatment for rosacea and vascular imperfections
	excel V	Dual-wavelength laser for vascular lesions
	IPL	IPL treatment for rosacea and facial redness

(*Continued*)

Table 37.1 (*Continued*) Common dermatologic services[a]

Category	Service	Description
Feminine Rejuvenation	FemTouch, V-Lase, or FemiLift	Laser treatment for vaginal rejuvenation
	ThermiVa	Radiofrequency treatment for vaginal rejuvenation
Hyperhidrosis	Botulinum toxin	Injectable to control excessive sweating
	Iontophoresis	Electric current treatment for excessive sweating of hands and feet
	MiraDry	Noninvasive treatment for elimination of sweat and odor glands

[a]This table is not entirely comprehensive

no shortage of cases (see ▶ Table 37.2 for some numbers related to the most common conditions) and includes all-important total body skin examinations (TBSEs) that every patient should be advised to appear for regularly. But patient contact can be fairly limited to solving a specific, temporary problem. While medical dermatology services offer steady recurring cash flow with procedures usually covered by insurance, physicians often treat each case as a discrete problem to be solved, possibly forgoing a deeper connection with the patient.

- **Surgical:** Dermatologic surgery, also known as procedural dermatology, includes treatments as diverse as skin cancer surgery and Mohs micrographic surgery, liposuction, hair restoration, chemical peels, and in some cases, blepharoplasty and facelifts. It encompasses a broad spectrum of services that range from medically necessary to cosmetic. Every dermatologist practices some basic dermatologic surgery (cryosurgery, excisional surgery, etc.), but those who pursue fellowships in Mohs surgery can focus more on this practice and serve as a referral center for other dermatologists.

- **Cosmetic:** Cosmetic dermatology accounts for 21% of dermatological revenues,[1] but its share is growing as disposable income, population age, and our culture's focus on maintaining a youthful appearance continue to rise. Services within this category include the use of botulinum toxin and other injectable fillers, lasers, peels, and microneedling to improve the skin's appearance and laxity; treatment of spider and varicose veins; and lasers and other technology for body contouring and removing tattoos, age spots, and skin discolorations.

Table 37.2 Prevalence of common skin conditions in the United States

Type of skin condition	Approx. number of prevalence (in million)
Hair loss	80
Acne	50
Atopic dermatitis	28
Rosacea	17
Psoriasis	8
Skin cancer (annual)	2

Source: Data based on American Academy of Dermatology. https://www.aad.org/media/stats-numbers

Your services will likely span all of the above categories, and patients seeking a treatment that falls into one service area will often transition to services available in others. Someone coming to your office for neuromodulator injections can become a candidate for rejuvenative laser surgery; a patient requiring surgery for melanoma may have sun damage that can be addressed by lasers and injectables.

The bread-and-butter offerings of every dermatology practice are skin checks, skincare, and injectables. Skin cancer surgery is by far the most commonly performed procedure by dermatologic surgeons (see ▶ Table 37.3). But cosmetic lasers, neuromodulators and soft-tissue fillers are catching up quickly. As far as nonsurgical cosmetic procedures go, injection of botulinum toxin is by far the most popular. ▶ Table 37.4 depicts the top five nonsurgical cosmetic procedures of 2017, which will give you a sense of the extent to which Botox, Dysport, and Xeomin dwarf all other services. While many cosmetic procedures were

Table 37.3 Total number of procedures performed by ASDS members in 2018

Type of procedure	Approx. number of procedures (in million)
Skin cancer treatments	3.5
Laser/light/energy-based procedures	3.5
Injectable neuromodulators	2.1
Injectable soft-tissue fillers	1.6
Body sculpting	0.6
Chemical peels	0.5
Microneedling	0.3
Vein treatments	0.1

Source: Data based on American Society for Dermatologic Surgery. www.asds.net/portals/0/PDF/procedures-survey-results-infographic-2018.pdf

Table 37.4 Top 5 nonsurgical cosmetic procedures performed in 2017

Type of procedure	Approx. number of procedures (in million)
Botulinum toxin (botox, Jeuveau, Dysport, and Xeomin)	1.8
Hyaluronic acid (Juvederm Ultra, Ultra Plus, Voluma, Restylane Lyft, Restylane Refyne, Restylane Defyne, and Belotero)	0.8
Nonsurgical fat reduction (CoolSculpting, Sculpsure, Emsculpt, VASER Shape, Liposonix)	0.17
Hair removal (laser or intense pulsed light)	0.14
Chemical peel	0.13

Source: Data based on American Society for Aesthetic Plastic Surgery. www.surgery.org/sites/default/files/ASAPS-Stats2018.pdf

once limited to particularly high-end, urban, beauty-obsessed clientele, they are now so common and popular that most dermatologic practices offer them, regardless of location.

At my practice, CompleteSkinMD in Manhattan, our mission is to address patients' skin health as well as their cosmetic objectives. Our patient relationships are generally close and long-standing, and we cater to the medical, surgical, and aesthetic needs of our clientele synergistically: a patient coming in for a lesion biopsy may come across a pamphlet for Fraxel and ask about what it can do, or a regular Botox patient will realize the importance of a full-body skin check. Our service offerings reflect our approach, and are always changing to adapt to patient needs, industry developments, and technological innovations; yours will too.

37.3 Your Brand

Your practice's services must, of course, be about your patients and what they want and need. But they're also about you: your passion, your training, your style as a physician, and how you want your office to run.

One of the main reasons I chose dermatology as my specialty is because dermatology patients are motivated patients. They have a condition or malady that they can see, that bothers them, and that they want help with. They're usually seeking out

treatment themselves, looking for solutions, and willing to do their part to get better. That makes for a rewarding physician and patient experience. I can really help my patients because they really want my help. I can make a measurable difference in their lives, whether it is diagnosing and curing them of skin cancer, or helping them look better and feel more confident in their appearance.

Within dermatology, I chose to follow my passion, which is sun protection. The sun is dermatology's most prolific driver of patients, causing 86% of melanomas,[2] 90% of nonmelanoma skin cancers,[2] and 80% of signs of skin aging.[3] There is no shortage of conditions, both medical and cosmetic, caused by the sun, and my interest in this area has helped shape what treatments I provide. From Mohs micrographic surgery for skin cancer and cryosurgery for actinic keratoses to chemical peels and lasers for sun spots, the procedures available in my office reflect my dedication to addressing skin issues caused by the sun. Your particular area of interest should and will drive your decisions about what services to offer.

Your brand as a dermatologist determines how you will be known in the field, and embracing your true passion provides an organic credibility in your chosen area of specialty. Know your areas of expertise as well as your limits. My focus on sun protection also means I don't keep up with the newest immunologic therapies in, say, severe psoriasis, and so I defer to experts in that area for patients who need it.

My commitment to providing services related to sun protection, skin cancer prevention, antiaging and rejuvenative therapies, and my close work with the Skin Cancer Foundation, have led to media opportunities and exposure that lead many of my colleagues to assume I employ a publicist (I don't). Instances of being interviewed by a magazine for a beauty article about SPF myths, or appearing on a morning television show to give tips for keeping skin safe at the beach, reinforce my brand and promote my services. But I stay in my lane: if I'm asked to give an opinion on something like female hair pattern hair loss, I will pass. That's not my area of expertise, and not necessarily part of who I am as a service provider.

My interest in sun protection is not the only aspect of my "brand" as a dermatologist. I choose to get to know my patients well, which means spending more time with each of them at every visit. I treat them holistically, addressing medical and cosmetic issues rather than focusing on a more limited area of treatment. I perform all treatments myself, rather than having a physician extender handle things such as injectables and lasers.

The upside of these choices is that my clientele is very loyal, and willing to pay more for my services, knowing that they will receive the highest level of care. The downside to my approach is that my schedule is packed, and patients have to wait longer to schedule an appointment with me.

I am fortunate to have patients willing to wait longer and pay more to see me, but other approaches are just as valid. Increasingly, dermatologists rely on nonphysician clinicians (NPCs), also known as physician extenders, in their offices to provide services that don't require a medical license– even doctors who may grouse about nonmedical clinics undercutting business by offering low-cost injectables and lasers. NPCs help maximize the time you can spend on cases that can only be handled by a physician, speed daily workflow, and allow your patients to book an appointment more quickly and obtain treatment more affordably.

Are you willing to spend a valuable chunk of your workday removing hair from someone's back, knowing how much time hair removal takes? Only you can answer that question. Consider the extent to which you are willing to devote your time to treatments that can be performed by a nonphysician, and your comfort level with entrusting these procedures to NPCs in your office. Understand your state's scope-of-practice laws as they apply to nonphysician clinicians (they vary widely), and be aware of how medical liability insurance companies you work with treat services that are provided by an NPC rather than a physician. Above all, think about the effect these decisions will have, both positive and negative, on your patients' experience and ultimately your practice's brand and reputation.

37.4 Equipment

Imagine you are opening a restaurant. The type of food you can serve will be heavily influenced by your kitchen equipment. You'll need a broiler if you're going to offer steaks, and a wood-fired oven for artisanal pizza. You may believe sous vide is the future, and decide to invest $2,000 in an immersion circulator. Or forgo a deep fryer because your menu is all about raw food.

Dermatology services are very much the same way. Nearly every service we provide requires some kind of equipment, be it a syringe of filler or a very expensive fractional resurfacing laser. In order to think about your practice's services, you must first think about your practice's equipment.

There are dozens of lasers that do amazing things and that will prove to be an asset to your business; however, they are expensive. They require space (sometimes with ventilation and/or specific electrical outlets), maintenance, and training. They run the risk of breaking down, becoming obsolete, or being misused by inexperienced practitioners. You will want to strategize carefully about what equipment you bring into your practice and how it will fit into your slate of services. If you have the opportunity to work in an academic or large group-practice setting, that's a great way to gain exposure to a range of equipment, and get a sense of what works best for you.

The intimidating cost of equipment is likely to be your first concern. It's most cost-effective to buy a machine outright, but leasing is available, as are short-term trials to try before you buy. Keep in mind that the cost of maintaining lasers goes beyond the initial outlay of capital. Often, you'll get a limited service contract with your purchase, but once that expires, you have to make choices. You can end up spending $10,000 a year for a laser service contract that never breaks down. If you opt not to have a contract, when your laser breaks, the cost al la carte can be prohibitive. Some laser companies won't send out their technicians to help service your equipment, and you'll have to find your own.

Apart from the hardiness and durability of the laser itself, there are consumables to consider. Things like tips for Fraxel or Thermage can add up and affect your profit margin on services. Be aware of ongoing future costs, and ensure considering technical servicing and consumables in your purchase negotiations.

It's also a good idea to maintain good relationships with laser companies; your association with them is going to last the life of your device, which will hopefully be a decade or more. There are some laser reps I work with whom I can text pretty much any time and receive immediate tech support. Others leave my practice administrators on hold for hours when we need help. If you have a problem, or it's time to upgrade, reps can work with you to keep your equipment current with more favorable terms and arrangements.

My practice has 12 lasers, and some of my colleagues in larger group practices in New York have 30 or more. Single-function machines are the best at their jobs, but are priced accordingly. When starting out, many physicians begin by investing in a less-expensive technology, or a multi-use platform device. An intense-pulsed light (IPL) machine is polychromatic, and can treat vascular lesions, acne, wrinkles, brown spots, unwanted hair, and other conditions. In comparison, a pulsed dye laser (PDL), for example, is more powerful, but usually produces only one wavelength and will address only vascular lesions. Be mindful that if many of your services are heavily reliant on a single machine, you're going to have a major problem if that piece of equipment breaks down.

My advice is to invest in tried-and-true lasers that will allow you to offer popular treatments for conditions you can reliably expect to treat. If I had to pick only two lasers to have in my practice, I'd definitely go with a pulsed dye vascular laser and a fractionated resurfacing laser. Pulsed dye lasers utilize selective photothermolysis to treat cutaneous vascular conditions such as rosacea, port-wine stain birthmarks, hemangioma, leg spider veins, erythematous acne scars, surgical scars, stretch marks, and warts. Fractional resurfacing creates microthermal treatment zones which stimulate the production of collagen, addressing sun damage, brown spots, enlarged pores, skin texture and tone, wrinkles and fine lines, and acne and surgical

scars. I use Vbeam and Fraxel daily in my practice, so the positive impact on my profit margin makes the cost of the machines worthwhile.

Beyond these two workhorses, there are plenty of other machines to consider. If you are interested in offering tattoo removal, you'll want a Q-switched laser or a picosecond laser. To tighten skin and improve crepey texture, you may wish to offer radiofrequency therapy like Thermage, ultrasound therapy like Ulthera, or platelet-rich plasma therapy, which will require a centrifuge (in some case, the centrifuge can be yours at no cost, but you'll be on the hook for kits for each treatment). Hair removal is in extremely high demand, and can be addressed with long-pulsed alexandrite and diode or Nd:YAG lasers, depending on the patient's skin and hair type. Body contouring is increasingly popular among patients, as liposuction is declining, and there are many technologies that you can choose from in order to provide it, for example, CoolSculpting, SculpSure, Zerona, truSculpt, and more recently Emsculpt.

The options can be overwhelming. To help you get started, ▶ Table 37.5 lists popular equipment to consider, and the services each will allow you to offer to your patients.

Table 37.5 Primary types of lasers and other technology

Category	Examples
Vascular (pulsed dye laser)	Vbeam or excel V
Pigmented lesion/Tattoo removal	Q-switched (Ruby, Alexandrite, or Alex TriVantage), Pico (PicoWay, PicoSure, or PICO Genesis enlighten)
Hair removal	GentleMax Pro light sheer diode
Nonablative fractionated resurfacing	Fraxel
Ablative fractionated resurfacing	AcuPulse
Acne Laser	Smoothbeam or Isolaz
Radiofrequency/ultrasound skin tightening	Thermage or Ultherapy
Fat removal/body sculpting	SculpSure, CoolSculpting, or Emsculpt
Microneedling ± radiofrequency	Infini, Vivace, EndyMed Intensif, or Fractora
Endovenous laser ablation (EVLA)	CoolTouch

37.5 Training and Experience

Of course, services don't depend on equipment alone. Your training and experience are important factors in determining what procedures you can offer. I advise physicians to focus on specific services and do them really well, rather than try to be a dermatological jack-of-all-trades. There is an adage attributed to psychologist Abraham Maslow who states, "I suppose it is tempting, if the only tool you have is a hammer, to treat everything as if it were a nail." Don't fall into that trap. Use your unique capabilities, skills, and experience in a focused way. Do what you do best, and be willing to let some patients and cases go to other providers with complementary expertise.

Although you've completed your formal medical education, you'll find there's still a lot to learn. After medical school, I completed a fellowship in skin cancer and laser surgery, but today's fellowships increasingly include procedures such as hair transplantation, body contouring, and injectables. Another way to gain valuable experience with particular procedures is by way of professional and academic appointments. After leaving full-time academics, my first job as a private practice physician was with a large group practice that possessed equipment and offered procedures I could not possibly have accessed on my own. Working for an established practice that offers services you wish to provide is a great way to build your expertise. You can even moonlight for a practice while you build your own, until you have the necessary experience, training, and capital to provide the services yourself.

Now that I have my own practice with my sister, I still need to stay up-to-date on the latest procedures, so that my service offerings stay current and competitive. As a Clinical Associate Professor of Dermatology at the New York University Langone Medical Center, I have the opportunity to work closely with dermatology residents who keep me on my toes. I highly recommend seeking an academic appointment, so that not only can you give back to future generations of dermatologists, but also benefit from the students' modern perspective, and possibly gain exposure and access to new developments in the industry.

Conferences and workshops are a must for dermatologists, and an important way to get familiar with procedures you will want to offer in your office. For lasers, a great source of information about and exposure to new devices is gained from the annual conference of the American Society for Laser Medicine and Surgery (ASLMS). For dermatologic surgeons, there's the annual meeting of the American Society for Dermatologic Surgery (ASDS), which covers skin cancer surgery, Mohs surgery, practice management, and cosmetic dermatology. There is also the annual meeting of The American College of Mohs Surgery (ACMS).

37.6 Customer Demand

At the end of the day, the services you will want to offer are those that your patients want. The best way to find out what procedures your patients are interested in is to ask them. If your practice is not yet open, check the websites of other dermatologists in your area to see which services they offer. You may even want to call their offices and ask how long the wait time is for an appointment for a particular service, which may give you a better indication of how in-demand it is.

Once your office is open, patients will call asking whether you offer, say, botulinum toxin, lasers, platelet-rich plasma (PRP), or treatment of cellulite. Make sure your receptionist takes note of these requests if they're for something you do not offer. When you notice you're having to turn away a critical mass of patients, it's time to give that service careful consideration. Think about whether it's something you want to do, can do well, and to which you can allocate the necessary resources of money, time, space, and training.

If you have a website with a search function, poke around the analytics to see what search terms visitors are entering, or what pages they came to your site from for additional insight into their interests. When a new beauty treatment gets written up in *Harper's Bazaar* or is mentioned by Kendall Jenner on Instagram, you can expect patients will start asking about it. The media is where patients learn about what's new in dermatology, so make sure you keep up with popular magazines, websites, and blogs.

Keep in mind that you don't have to be a strong proponent of every service you provide. Business is business, and you want to make your patients happy. Occasionally, this might mean employing a first-iteration technology that you think still needs fine-tuning, or performing a service whose results are not as dramatic as you might wish. In those cases, be honest with your patients. Tell them you provide the service because it is helpful in some cases, and it's the best approach you have for the patient's complaint, but share your reservations. Being straightforward about your confidence in any procedure is crucial to maintaining your credibility and setting reasonable patient expectations.

A woman in her 60s came into my office seeking facial tightening. She exhibited significant jowls and laxity of her lower face and neck. "I would love to get a face lift," she admitted; however, she was afraid to go under the knife: a good friend of hers had suffered serious complications from plastic surgery recently, leaving my patient terrified of undergoing general anesthesia and risking adverse side-effects from surgery. She was hoping for a nonsurgical treatment to address her complaint. I was straightforward and clear. "We have a device called Thermage," I explained. "It offers radiofrequency skin tightening, so it's not surgical. I think it is the best nonsurgical technology out there. But it offers only modest benefits. On the other hand, there is very little risk to the procedure, no down time, and costs about one-tenth of what lower face lift and neck surgery will cost." I showed the patient some before-and-after photos, and she agreed the results weren't quite as dramatic as she'd hoped to achieve. I indicated that we lose facial volume as we age, so that in addition to Thermage, fillers could help address the laxity in her jowls. I made sure she understood that because of her age, she may have to repeat the procedure every year or so to maintain her results. After giving it some thought, my patient opted for the Thermage and filler combination treatment. She understood the results would not equate with what she'd achieve through surgery. But given her aversion to anesthesia and her concerns about complications, the nonsurgical approach made the most sense to her. She understood her options, had realistic expectations, was satisfied with her results, and continues to come back for regular treatments.

Services are not the only thing your office can offer that patients will want. Think about what products you may want to sell in your office. This is a service in itself: in addition to offering your patients convenience, you are ensuring that they will choose products appropriate for their skin, that complement the services you have performed, and that will be efficacious. The opportunity for patients to buy skin-care products directly at your office is helpful for them and profitable for you, so don't overlook this aspect of your practice.

37.7 Insurance Considerations and Profit Margin

Insurance is rarely fun to think about, but it's an important consideration when choosing what services to provide. On the one hand, offering procedures covered by insurance can be a useful strategy for getting patients in the door. On the other hand, these services will add far less to your bottom line than elective procedures.

At my practice, we offer photodynamic therapy (PDT), but many other dermatologists do not, simply because it would bring in patients for a service that isn't financially sustainable. Each treatment requires a stick of Levulan costing around $300, an hour of in-office wait time for the patient before the procedure can be performed, and a nurse to apply the light. What I recoup from insurance for PDT is simply not enough to cover the costs of consumables, space, and staff. We continue to offer it because we believe in its efficacy and since we don't take a lot of insurance, our losses are minimized by full-paying patients. But many dermatologists who are more reliant on insurance have understandably stopped offering PDT. Others look at such procedures as loss leaders. Offering services covered by insurance can help you establish a patient base, and you can have a reasonable expectation that many of these patients will stick with your practice for elective procedures as well.

Just because something is covered by insurance today doesn't mean it always will be. Sadly, dermatology is often at the top of the chopping block when reimbursements are cut. However, patients are often willing to pay for noncovered procedures to maintain a more youthful appearance and feel good about themselves. These days, as the population ages, stays in the workforce longer, and maintains image-centric social media accounts, many patients view dermatology as essential for both their personal and professional well-being. While many of our services may be considered luxuries, they are ones that patients are reluctant to cut out even when they're otherwise looking to reduce their spending.

In addition to insurance reimbursements, you need to think about your costs for every service you provide. Real estate, staffing, equipment maintenance, and consumables are all considerations that will affect how much profit you can earn from offering a particular service. Botulinum toxin provides an illustrative example. When patients come in seeking neurotoxin injections, they'll usually ask for "Botox" by default, perhaps not even realizing that it is a commercial brand name with competitors that offer virtually identical results. Two alternatives are Dysport and Xeomin, the cost of which are significantly less than Botox.

In the past, when a patient asked for Botox, I would always use Botox, even though it was more costly for my practice than other alternatives. More recently, however, clinical evidence has indicated that Dysport may actually have an earlier onset and longer duration than Botox. Armed with this information, I began explaining the potential advantages to my patients requesting Botox, and offering the option of Dysport. Within a couple of months, I'd converted about half of my patients to Dysport, giving them added treatment benefits, and saving my practice thousands of dollars every month.

37.8 Adding New Services

While I hope this chapter will help you choose which dermatological services to provide, your job is by no means done once you have that list. We are fortunate to work in a dynamic field with constant innovations that help us improve patient care and outcomes. Services are invented, developed, improved, and replaced frequently. You will need to keep abreast of the latest developments in the industry, so you can assess the new services you may want to offer.

How do you stay current? Stay engaged in the dermatologic community by taking courses, attending professional association meetings, and reading academic journals. Membership in organizations like the Skin Cancer Foundation is a great way to keep up-to-date and establish contacts with leading practitioners in dermatology. Such associations can also help you get media exposure. If a local morning news show in your area is doing a story on skin cancer, professional dermatology organizations will recommend local

members for interviews. One of my earliest media appearances occurred when Laura Bush had a squamous cell carcinoma removed from her leg in 2006, and the Skin Cancer Foundation arranged for me to speak about the skin cancer to Katie Couric on CBS News.

Product and laser reps are another convenient way to learn about new skincare products and technologies. Sure, they're trying to sell you something, but often what they're trying to sell you will inspire your future service offerings. Once you've decided to offer a new service, let reps meet with your staff to educate them about the new product or procedure. Make sure every customer-facing member of your team, from front-desk receptionist to nurses, understands the new product or service well enough to provide a brief explanation to patients who may ask about it over the phone, in the waiting room, or in the examination room before you arrive. Your staff is the front line of your practice and an extension of your brand, so it's crucial that they be able to speak knowledgably about every service your office provides.

Once you and your staff are ready to introduce a new service, it's time to let your patients know about it. Adding the service to your website and procedures list is not enough—you'll want to do a little targeted marketing. Consider an email blast to let your mailing list know that you now offer SculpSure or that you're welcoming a new picosecond laser into the armamentarium. Educate patients about new services through evening workshops (offering some wine and cheese and a discount on the service you're highlighting is always a nice touch). Prominently place brochures describing the service and its benefits in your reception area and treatment rooms for patients to peruse while they're waiting.

Be cautious of trends that may not last. It's best to make sure a procedure is safe, popular, and here to stay before investing in it. Of course, nothing lasts forever. For example, microdermabrasion, long a procedure of choice for patients seeking rejuvenated skin, has been declining in popularity, passing the torch to more individualizable, effective, and longer-lasting procedures. Some of the services you provide will inevitably go out of fashion, or fade into obsolescence when something better, cheaper, or with fewer side effects comes along. Accept it when it happens and embrace the future.

37.9 Conclusion

Deciding what services to provide ultimately comes down to supply and demand: what services can or must you offer to bring in enough patients and revenue to make your practice viable? Within that broad parameter, you can think about what you love to do, how you relate to patients, how you want your practice to be viewed as a brand, and what resources you can or want to invest now and in the future.

I highly recommend starting slow, and avoid investing heavily in equipment, staff, space, and marketing for services you aren't sure will be useful drivers for your business. In my practice, we operate by the adage that the customer is always right. In the case of services, let your patients be your guide, and always build your slate of services with their objectives in mind.

References

[1] IBISWorld. Available at: https://www.ibisworld.com. Published 2018. Accessed November 13, 2018

[2] The Skin Cancer Foundation. Available at: https://www.skincancer.org/prevention/sun-protection. Accessed November 13, 2018

[3] Flament F, Bazin R, Laquieze S, Rubert V, Simonpietri E, Piot B. Effect of the sun on visible clinical signs of aging in Caucasian skin. Clin Cosmet Investig Dermatol 2013;6: 221–232

38 Evaluating a Laser for Purchase and Calculating a Return on Investment for a Device

E. Victor Ross MD

Abstract

The purchase of an energy device is a big investment for any practice. The astute practitioner should examine all the nuances of the transaction. Most importantly, the buyer should match the technology to common skin conditions that present to the practice. In this brief chapter, we discuss some of the trials and tribulations associated with an energy-based device purchase.

Keywords: return on investment, purchase, laser, energy, device

Top 10 Things You Need to Know

1. Make sure the device application menu matches the common concerns among your patients.
2. Test drive any device before purchase to assess efficacy and ergonomic features.
3. Review the history and reputation of the vendor.
4. Discuss potential purchase with a trusted colleague, preferably one not in your immediate geographical area.
5. Always negotiate for better terms as far as lease, purchase, or service agreements are concerned.
6. Determine if a device is delegable with respect to your particular style, as well as in accordance with your local state laws.
7. If the device applications are to be largely delegated, ensure that the operator (nurse, PA, NP, etc) has an opportunity to provide feedback regarding ease of use prior to purchase.
8. Move the device around your office to ensure easy transport from one room to another.
9. Ensure electrical compliance with your physical plant.
10. Ensure that air conditioning is sufficient to maintain a comfortable room temperature during prolonged device use.

38.1 Introduction

A literature search of "lasers AND business AND skin" returns few titles, and even fewer which refer to the business of cosmetic laser dermatology.[1] In any practice, the first question should be "why should my practice purchase, lease, or rent a laser/energy device?" Lasers and other equipment are expensive, and practices must determine the cosmetic needs among their patient base.

When practicing in the 1980s, a dermatologist could treat a large range of conditions by simply purchasing an electrosurgery device, sclerotherapy equipment, and chemical peeling agents. Some of these same conditions are now treated by more expensive devices. However, for practices that concentrate on cosmetics, older prelaser technologies are normally insufficient to provide the full range of services in today's highly active cosmetic arena. Some conditions, for example vascular lesions and excessive hair, cannot be treated in a reproducible and rapid fashion, without a laser or other light-based technology.

The large array of technology available in modern dermatology is daunting, ranging from visible light technologies for red and brown dyschromias to cannula-based subdermal heating apparatus. In our practice, about 50% of our "effort" is directed toward reducing red and brown dyschromias. Accordingly, a good starter investment for most practice demographics includes a visible light technology such as a pulsed dye laser, 532 nm laser, or an intense pulsed light (IPL).

Laser hair reduction (LHR), although still the most common cosmetic procedure, has been commoditized, and ever lower prices have reduced profit margins. However, there is still a place for LHR with strategic marketing; also, once other potentially more lucrative procedures have been offered, many patients will also request LHR. It, in fact, might be considered a "gateway" procedure for other procedures that offer a higher return on investment (ROI). Not having a capable device could drive that patient to another practice. Other potential types of equipment include radio frequency (RF) needle devices, deeper heating devices, body contouring equipment, and ablative and nonablative lasers (both fractional and non-fractional).

It is best to have at least one device for each of the most common applications. I liken it to a baseball position division of labor—having a catcher, pitcher, etc. Different devices play different roles, but to be comprehensive, the practice should have a well-suited player at each position. However, depending on the size of your practice, decisions might be required regarding optimizing offerings that allow for a high ROI, and ultimately ROI drives all of these procedures.

One reasonable source for a panoramic view of the various available technologies and their pricing is the Aesthetic Buyers Guide, published quarterly to show "what's on the market." Any practice should look at local pricing for particular procedures and how that relates to the number or procedures per week or month within the context of "clinic costs" for the procedure. Ideally, any laser should be used often, or the deprecation will outpace the ROI.

Like an airliner, more use means more profits. A laser sitting in the corner depreciates (▶ Fig. 38.1) and takes up space. There are some technologies that require so-called "consumables" both virtual and real. By "virtual" we suggest that the part does not truly wear out but rather "times" out, meaning that after so many iterations, a new tip or cannula must be placed on the base unit, or some time-based feature must be reset to continue (like putting in a coin for more time on the old pay phones). In other cases, the consumable part might become contaminated by contact with the skin, such that a new handpiece tip is required simply for sterility.

Purchase price. The purchase price of a laser is sometimes a bit unclear (see ▶ Fig. 38.2). Often there is a base price, but with options (akin to buying a car) as well as extended service warranty options. There is typically room for negotiating, particularly when considering two or three brands of similar equipment. Today, the reliability of laser equipment is at an all-time high. Components are sturdy and reliable, electronics are more stable, and many systems offer real-time diagnostics online or through a USB port. Software upgrades likewise might be available through a USB port. The first step in assessing a potential purchase involves appraising the laser with respect to wavelength, spot size, power, speed, ergonomic compatibility, and mobility, all within the context of specific cosmetic applications. Then a quick review online from reputable manufacturers should provide for 3 to 4 "players" in that category. What constitutes a reputable manufacturer? The term not only includes laser specifications, but also service availability, quality of workmanship, reliability, and support after the sale. As much of the equipment can be similar in specifications, the eventual purchase might come down to price, relationship with the local sales staff, and service availability. The price usually includes base equipment plus potentially extra hand pieces and service options. For example, for IPL, a range of handpieces can be selected, from those that target red and brown dyschromias and HR-dedicated hand pieces to full-fledged lasers that are powered by the IPL base. In some cases, one must rely on advice from colleagues, peer-reviewed papers, and the word of the company representative.

Another consideration is the range of procedures that are offered in the practice. For example, if one is an expert chemical peeler, the need for an ablative laser is reduced. Or if one routinely performs sclerotherapy, a 1,064 nm for leg veins might prove to have a poor ROI, unless, for example, the use is extended to other lesions, such as small facial

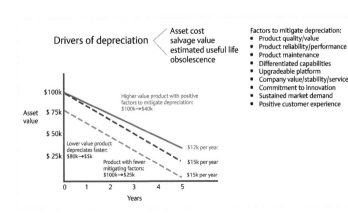

Fig. 38.1 Graph showing drivers of depreciation.

veins, venous lakes, exophytic vascular malformations, and/or LHR.

If one performs liposuction, then perhaps noninvasive body contouring is not as necessary as one that does not perform minimally invasive liposuction. On the other hand, a noninvasive body contouring option could extend the range of options for patients who are not interested in something as invasive as liposuction. Many practices want to offer a whole buffet of services to their patients, but unless one is sharing the

devices among many MDs, PAs, or NPs, the number of uses of the laser would not justify the initial cost and upkeep.

Used equipment: The question of used equipment often comes up at meetings. The web is full of tantalizing offers for deeply discounted equipment. Sometimes devices are advertised as refurbished or come with a warranty. Lasers, like luxury automobiles, are sophisticated creatures with multiple moving and nonmoving parts; like automobiles, various parts "give out" at different

PRODUCT DESCRIPTION	QTY	Unit Price (in USD)	Total Price (in USD)
ICON™ INTENSE PULSED LIGHT (IPL) SYSTEM Optimized Pulsed Light (OPL) System. Complete with on-site installation & clinical in-service, and one (1) year equipment warranty. System includes: 1 each Icon Base Module, Heat Exchanger Module, Chiller Module and Cart 1 each Starter Kit, Power Cord and Boom 1 Freight	1	$250,000	$250,000
SKINTEL® Melanin Reader	1	included	included
IPL HANDPIECE OPTIONS:			
Max Rs™ IPL Handpiece - Red Super	1	included	included
Max G™ IPL Handpiece - Green with treatment adapter	1	included	included
Max Ys™ IPL Handpiece - Yellow Super with treatment adapter	1	included	included
Max Y™ IPL Handpiece - Yellow	1	included	included
LASER & SPECIALTY HANDPIECE OPTIONS:			
1540 Fractional Laser Handpiece, Non-Ablative with XF™ & XD™ microlenses	1	included	included
1540 Fractional 15mm microlens (Optional)	0		
2940 Fractional Laser Handpice, ablative with Groove & Blue Optic	1	included	included
Purple 2mm Optic (Optional)	0		
Green Optic (Optional)	0		
Marketing Package: Printed and electronic marketing material support including: product brochures, print-ready files, web and media files, before and after photos.	1	included	included
Hospital Discount			($94,500)
Icon™ sysytem sold with multiple IPL's and at least one Laser or Specialty Hand pieces will include 2 consecutive days of clinical in-service			
Quoted Price Valid for 30 days from above date. Price do not include sales, duty or excise taxes, including medical device taxes which are the responsibility of the Customer to pay and will be billed separately.			$155,500

ACCEPTANCE OF AGREEMENT

By signing below, the Customer (i) is reprenting to _____ that it has the requisite corporate authority to execute and deliver this Customer Purchase Agreement ("Agreement") and has the required licensing from the applicable state medical review board to operate the Product purchased by this Agreement, and (ii) is entering into a binding agreement for the purchase of the Product and/or services described above and accepts all of the terms and conditions as stated in this document (including the following page(s)). This Agreement is subject to _____ terms and conditions of sale contained or referred to herein and the Customer expressly disclaims any additional and/or different terms and conditions or any terms and conditions on the Customer's purchase order. Federal law restricts the sale of the products to a licensed practitioner.

Customer Signature (Authorized Representative)   _Date_   _Area Sales Manager Signature_   _Date_

a   Delivery Date: _____

Fig. 38.2 (a) A sample purchase contract.

[illegible]

Terms

Prices are FCA, Westford, MA Incoterms 2000 in U.S. dollars

Payment Terms: 15% non-refundable deposit required with purchase order.
Balance due net 30 days with prior credit approval. (VISA/Mastercharge/American Express accepted.)
Payment is not contingent upon installation and/or acceptance.
1.5% interest due monthly on overdue balances.

All Sales are final. [illegible] Grants no right of return.

Due to continuing improvements, prices and specifications are subject to change without notice.

[illegible] reserves and the Customer grants to us, a security interest in all Products sold and all proceeds to secure the full payment.

Warranty Information

Return Goods Authorization Service

Product, damaged or otherwise, will not be accepted by return shipments without prior approval from [illegible] Customer Service Department. Authorization for return is at the sole discretion of [illegible]. All returned Product must be accompanied by a RETURN MATERIALS AUTHORIZATION number issued by [illegible]

Icon™ Optimized Pulsed Light (OPL) System Warranty

[illegible] Inc., warrants to the original purchaser of any new laser system except for laser consumable/accessories, that the equipment is free from defects in materials and workmanship, under normal use and service, for a period of twelve (12) months from the date of shipment. Laser consumables and accessories are warranted for a period of thirty (30) days from the date of shipment. Replacement parts other than the items stated above that are purchased outside of this warranty period are warranted for a period of thirty (30) days from the date of shipment.

ICON™ IPL Handpiece Warranty

[illegible] Inc., warrants that the handpiece is free from defect for a period of two (2) years or 100,000 pulses, whichever comes first. All other parts of the device are covered for the remainder of the original warranty. When the IPL handpieces have exceeded 100,000 pulses, they are considered consumed items to be replaced. Customer must contact [illegible] to purchase a replacement.

1064+ Handpiece Warranty

[illegible] Inc., warrants that the handpiece is free from defect for a period of one (1) year or 50,000 pulses, whichever comes first.

1540 Handpiece Warranty

[illegible] Inc., warrants that the handpiece is free from defect for a period of one (1) year from the date of shipment or 100,000 pulses, whichever comes first.

2940 Handpiece Warranty

[illegible] Inc., warrants that the handpiece is free from defect for a period of one (1) year from date of shipment.

Optics, Microlens and Adapter Warranty

[illegible] Inc., warrants that the microlens and adapter are free from defect for the same period as the handpiece on which the accessory is applied.

Chiller, Heat Exchanger & Skintel™ Warranty

[illegible] Inc., warrants that the chiller, heat exchanger and Skintel is free from defect for the same period as the base unit on which the component is applied.

[illegible] is an Equal Opportunity Employer.

THE OBLIGATIONS OF [illegible] UNDER THIS WARRANTY ARE LIMITED, IN ITS EXCLUSIVE OPTION, TO REPAIR OR REPLACE PARTS AND MATERIALS WHICH PROVE TO BE DEFECTIVE.

These Warranties are null and void a) where the Product is unpacked, installed, serviced, and/or repaired by person(s) other than an authorized [illegible] service representative; b) where service is required due to the Customer's failure to operate or maintain the Product in an manner consistent with the specifications and guidelines set forth in the Product's operator manual; and/or c) where service is required due to attempted or actual dismantling, disassembling, alteration, and/or modification of the Product by person(s) other than an authorized [illegible] service representative.

Additional services, including, but not limited to telephone support, repair, maintenance, and refurbishment of equipment, may be purchased.

THE FOREGOING WARRANTIES ARE THE SOLE AND EXCLUSIVE WARRANTY OBLIGATIONS OF [illegible], AND THE REMEDY PROVIDED ABOVE IS IN LIEU OF ANY AND ALL OTHER REMEDIES. THERE ARE NO OTHER AGREEMENTS, GUARANTEES, OR WARRANTES, ORAL, WRITTEN, EXPRESSED, IMPLIED, OR STATUTORY, INCLUDING, WITHOUT LIMITATION, WARRANTY OF MERCHANTABILITY OR FITNESS FOR A PARTICULAR PURPOSE. [illegible] SHALL NOT BE LIABLE FOR LOST PROFITS OR ANY INDIRECT, INCIDENTAL, SPECIAL, PUNITIVE OR CONSEQUENTIAL DAMAGES DUE TO ANY CAUSE WHATSOEVER EVEN IF ADVISED AS TO THE POSSIBILITY OF SUCH DAMAGES. THE CUSTOMER AGREES THAT [illegible] LIABILITY IS SO LIMITED.

This Agreement shall be governed by and construed under the substantive laws of the Commonwealth of Massachusetts. The Customer agrees to submit all disputes arising out of, or relating to, this Agreement to a court in Boston, Massachusetts.

AUTHORIZED USE

Use of the Product is permitted only for individuals who are: (i) authorized to treat patients, as defined by the applicable state medical review board in the jurisdiction in which the Product is operated; or, (ii) under the supervision of such licensed physicians.

The Customer is responsible to ensure that all operators have the requisite skill required to use the Products as defined by the applicable state medical review board in the jurisdiction in which the Product is operated. Customer will, at all times, ensure that it and its employees and agents are and remain in full compliance with all federal, state, and local laws and statutes, including without limitation state medical agencies and certification boards, relating to this Agreement or the Product or their use.

The Customer acknowledges that proper operation of the Product requires use of supplies specifically engineered to meet [illegible] compatibility, quality and performance standards. Accordingly, the Customer Agrees to use only supplies provided by or expressly authorized by [illegible] and never to buy supplies from any other supplier for use with the Product. Customer use of supplies not provided or expressly authorized by [illegible] will void all warranties and extended warranties on the Product.

Upon completion of training. Customer shall become an authorized provider of [illegible] products and authorized in connection therewith to use the [illegible] trademarks solely in its promotion and delivery of services utilizing [illegible] products, and in accordance with any trademark guidelines pubished by [illegible], which may be updated from time to time. Specifically, [illegible] trademark guidelines strictly prohibits Customers from purchase and/or use of internet domain(s) adn business name(s) consisting of or incorporating any of the [illegible] trademarks. Customer agrees not to purchase and/or use internet domain(s) or business name(s) consisting of or incorporating any of the [illegible] trademarks. Customer acknowledges [illegible] exclusive ownership of the [illegible] trademarks and that its use thereof inures solely to [illegible] benefit. Customer shall not attempt to obtain registration of any [illegible] trademark, and shall not debrand, rebrand or private label any [illegible] product or service.

TERMINATION OF USE

Customer acknowledges that its use of the Product (including the Software) is subject to compliance with the usage and other requirements described in this Agreement (including, without limitation, the "Authorized Use" provisions above). Customer's authorization to operate the Product and license to the software will terminate automatically in the event Customer fails to comply with such requirements. In such event, in addition to any other remedies available to [illegible] under applicable law. Customer expressly agrees that [illegible] will have the right to cease selling Products to the Customer, including but not limited to SculpSure Drives, supplies and consumables.

b

Fig. 38.2 (b) A sample purchase contract.

rates. There are many variables that play a role in laser reliability. One is the architecture of the device itself. For example, most RF devices will enjoy a higher rate of reliability than their laser counterparts based on intrinsically simpler designs that put less stress on components. Let's look at a typical solid state laser. The laser head is the most important part of the device, comprising the laser rod, lamps, mirrors, and reflectors, etc. all coupled to a cooling supply that maintains the head at a peak operating temperature. The lamps are "ignited" by a power supply comprising a cascade of capacitors and resistors. For high powered lasers, there is normally a water pump as well, and the beam is delivered normally through a fiber or articulated arm. All of these parts are immobilized by fixing them to an optical bench that is covered by a plastic skin, and the whole assembly moves along on wheels. For all to go well, the various components must all work in harmony and are only as strong as their weakest link. Often mirrors, fibers, lamps, and lenses are routinely near their damage thresholds such that with every laser pulse a virtual symphony of "stressful" events is occurring over less than a second.

Still, a used laser, like a used car, can be a good deal, where the laser is relatively new and not overused. Laser systems depreciate quickly. Some components fail due to use, like lamps, whereas other components can simply wear out from time (and disuse), such as a gasket drying out and allowing fluid to leak out of a cooling supply circuit.

In developing a plan for used equipment, one should assume that, as part of the purchase, a vendor might supply some warranty. Once that warranty expires, one would might rely on a third-party vendor to supply service. Our experience with third-party vendors has been variable. Sometimes, the specific service engineer has industry contacts that allow him/her to obtain difficult to find parts, and some experienced engineers "know" how to cobble a bunch of parts from a warehouse to keep a device running. In other cases, we have had third-party vendors who have taken a small problem and created a big problem, only to walk away without any resolution. We also had an experience with an engineer who was unable to recalibrate our older pulse dye laser to specs despite installing new lamps, a new dye kit, and other parts for the laser head. When an engineer arrived from the manufacturer, he quickly noted that the dye kit serial number showed a dye that was approximately 10 years old. In these cases,

we have had to bring in the original manufacturer engineers with significant expense. Accordingly, we tend to use the service engineers from the original manufactures for those pieces of equipment that are still adequately new, so that the original manufacturer offers bona fide service contracts and/or service agreements.

The test: before any purchase, a prospective buyer should test the laser in the office. Although canvassing exhibit halls and websites can be helpful, the actual "test drive" is imperative, as much for ergonomics and practical issues as for results. The footprint should be compatible with the clinic floorplan; portability could be a key factor in decision-making. Electrical compatibility and air conditioning limitations should also be considered. Most lasers will require at least a 20 ampere maximum current, and either a 120 or 220 V plug.

In our own clinic, we often begrudgingly move heavy equipment from one room to another, where the door shams act like speed bumps to create wear and tear on these delicate "optical benches" on wheels. We have removed these strips at the base of our doorways to make these inter-room odysseys more palatable. A good example of the "issue of portability" is the difference between two of our vascular lasers. One has a smaller footprint, runs on 120 V, has all four wheels that rotate, and has very few protruding parts. The other laser is heavier, has a larger footprint, possesses back wheels that do not turn, and has a delicate fiber that extends forward into the workspace. We routinely move the former laser from one room to another with minimal effort, whereas the latter we almost never transport across "room" lines.

The real test of a device involves arranging for a set of patients to be treated as part of an overall evaluation. This exercise can be frustrating, as the prospective buyer is simultaneously evaluating ease of use, immediate efficacy, pain issues, all with limited experience with that particular new technology. Also, some results, such as noninvasive body contouring or fat reduction, might require weeks or months to assess the final results.

ROI: In one article, the authors in a facial plastics practice examine the acquisition of a fractionated CO_2 laser as a model.[2] The emphasis was on ROI under a 5-year lease compared with a 3-year lease. They found that, for example, if we consider lasers (often costing from \$50,000 to more than \$150,000), the practice should devise a simplified form of return on investment:

38.2 ROI formula

The ratio should always be optimized. For example, a practice charges $500.00 for a pulse dye laser procedure for the entire face. The number of procedures being performed might vary, but if one were to perform approximately 20 procedures per week with that particular laser, then one would have $10,000 of revenue from that particular device for that week. There are two cost categories that can be identified: the fixed costs, including device acquisition of maintenance, and the variable costs. The fixed costs do not vary based on the number of procedures, and in general would include lease payments or any additional service agreement costs. Variable costs include those that are directly related to the number of procedures performed, including all labor costs and the price of consumables. The total cost per year for operating the laser is the sum of all fixed and variable costs. Depreciation and amortization are used in most accounting analyses. We include a rough depreciation laser chart that characterizes some of the contributors to the rate of depreciation (▶ Fig. 38.1).

The return on investment was estimated for a 5-year rate on a 5-year lease, and a 3-year rate on a 3-year lease.[2] With a 3-year lease, the ROI was significantly lower than the 5-year results. The reason the 5-year produced a better ROI is because more revenue was generated on a yearly basis (vs. monthly payments), while cost did not

$$\frac{\sum Total\ revenue - \sum Total\ cost}{\sum Total\ cost}$$

increase year-over-year. Over the life of the asset, the total fixed cost with a purchase is less than that with the lease. For example, if a physician were to purchase a 50,000 laser with cash, then the practice would pay $50,000 and roughly $4000, a year for the service contract. This scenario results in a total 5-year fixed cost of $70,000. However, if the physician were to lease the laser over 5 years with warranty, the total fixed cost would be higher. By leasing, the physician pays an additional fixed cost due to the debt service (roughly $8,000 more). In all the cases, the 5-year ROI had a higher rate than the 3-year ROI, with the amount of debt servicing for most lasers with leasing ranging from 7.9 to 14% of the total fixed cost.[3] Also, the provider should contact her insurance carrier to ensure that adding lasers would not increase the cost of malpractice coverage.

There are some potential benefits to leasing (▶ Fig. 38.3). One is that, typically, you can customize a lease plan that would fit the practice's budgetary needs. Payments might be lower than conventional financing if the device were to be purchased. Also, as device technology changes fast,

Fax

Email

Cost	$73,900.00

Dollar Buy-Out Finance Lease Agreement			
TERM Months / Rate	1st w/ Acceptance	90 Days Deferred	**6 Months Deferred!** Practice Builder Financing 6 Months at $99.00!
36/5.49%	$2,221.12	$2,270.87	
48/5.49%	$1,711.15	$1,753.23	6 Months at $99.00 $99.00 Followed by
			48 Months $1,801.21
60/5.49%	$1,405.61	$1,443.50	OR
			60 Months $1.485.58

1. All payments/fees exclude applicable taxes.
2. Your proposed lease financing is subject to credit / documentation review and approval by Heartland Business Credit.
3. A one time documentation fee of $150.00 is charged with contract acceptance.
4. You may pay-off your Heartland Agreement early without penalty.

End of Lease Terms/Definitions:

The $1 Buy-Out Finance Lease is a finance lease agreement. The lease payments should/can be treated as a capital depreciation expense (depreciable asset). This financing program protects your cash reserves, helps manage your cash flow, and simplifies budgeting with fixed monthly finance payments.

Fig. 38.3 A sample lease terms.

leasing provides the ability to manage some of the technology risks associated with owning.

All key components of the transaction should be agreed upon in writing before the purchase of the device (▶ Fig. 38.2). Training is important for the staff and the provider. Most companies will have an obligatory training session for the staff and physician, which is included as part of the purchase. However, this feature is normally not included with used laser purchases. Some companies require a precertification process for used lasers before they are willing to service the device with their own technicians.

A better understanding of the equipment will allow the provider to extend use over a broader range of applications, and in some cases, "teach an old dog new tricks." For example, a long pulsed alexandrite laser that is optimized for hair removal can often times be used for some vascular lesions and pigmented lesions, so long as the provider has a good understanding of basic laser tissue reactions.

38.3 Repairs

Inevitably, some of this very expensive equipment will require service: either preventative maintenance, which might include replacement of lamps and other internal gear, or replacement of hand-pieces and cleaning of the various components inside the casing. One critical aspect of the contract should be the time between calling in the concern and action taken by the manufacturer. Normally, if the device is on a service contract, it receives priority over the pay-as-you-go service, even if offered by the same manufacturer (▶ Fig. 38.4). Optimally, the company should respond within 48 hours to repair or replace a component and get the device running as soon as possible. In case of a more comprehensive breakdown, the company should provide a stand-in unit until the repair is completed. This condition should be in writing in the laser purchase contract. One should read the provisions of the service contract carefully. We have included a typical first page of a service contract; however,

---

COMPREHENSIVE SERVICE PLAN TERM

The term of this Comprehensive Service Plan Agreement is for 12 months (the 'Term') commencing on 4/9 18 (the 'Start Date') and expiring on 4/8/19, subject to the terms and conditions below and/or attached herto. The Term and any service periods set forth hereir are not tolled or extended for any period during which Equipment is being repaired by Cynosure, Inc. ['Cynosure'] or if the Equipment is replaced by Cynosure during a service period.

☐ **1 Year Coverage / $10,950 USD***
Luminary Pricing - $8,760*
- Service Coverage of Elite +™ base unit provided
- Non-disposable parts and labor included
- 20% discount off consumables and accessories
- Unlimited technical support

Cynosure, Inc. Representative:

EQUIPMENT COVERED		EQUIPMENT COVERED	
DESCRIPTION		DESCRIPTION	
	Elite+	ELM+0129-R	

COMMENTS

Above offer expires 4/27/2018
applicable taxes are not included in above price
20% Luminary Discount Applied

GENERAL TERMS AND CONDITIONS

By signing below, the Customer is entering into a binding agreement for the purchase of service coverage described above and accepts the quotation terms and conditions as stated on pages 1 and 2 of this document. This agreement is subject to Cynosure Inc.'s terms and conditions of sale contained or referred to herein or attached hereto; the parties expressly disclaim any additional and/or different terms and conditions.

SIGNATURES

Printed Name		Printed Name	
Signature	Date	Signature	Date
Title		Title	
Customer		Cynosure, Inc	

Fig. 38.4 A sample service agreement.

the second third and fourth pages (not included) list many "small print" items that should be read carefully before signing the agreement. For example, moving the equipment from one location to another might invalidate the warranty with some manufacturers. Also, one should be careful to make sure the warranty covers accessories such as handpieces and fibers. At times, these components can be warrantied at additional costs; however, some companies include those as part of the warranty package depending on the level of warranty (often with names such as "bronze, silver, or gold").

The salesperson's knowledge may vary from one manufacturer to another and from one salesperson to another. At worst, they should know some basic details and possess some comparative data on hand with respect to their device and competitive technologies. However, the onus is on the buyer to make sure they have done a good study of the various equipment to make the best choices. The buyer should check the company's website for details such as specifications, scientific and white papers, and testimonials.

Some newer devices allow for onboard diagnostics without the presence of an engineer, but even in these cases, the engineer often takes advantage of some Internet-based data to convey to the home base to optimize repairs. For some newer equipment, the trend has been for several years in the laser industry to return smaller pieces of equipment to the manufacturing facility and have it serviced there, with a replacement item sent during the interim. These provisions should be included in the purchase agreement. Service by third-party vendors is often the only option for devices that are older and no longer supported by the manufacturer. Sometimes the owner will receive a letter in the mail noting that a particular piece of equipment is no longer serviced by the manufacturer, and with that normally comes in enticing offered to buy the newer equipment.

In the US, there are several manufacturers that have been stable for over 20 years (although ownership might have changed over that time). Some companies, although they are strong in markets outside the US, enter into the American market ill-prepared for the long haul and then have to pull-up stakes, leaving the practice with an orphaned product. It is best to look at the long-term track record in the American market or, at least, try to determine from the manufacturer their commitment to the American market, and

if there are provisions for service if they were to abandon the US market. There has been great consolidation in the laser industry in the US over the last 10 years. Often times, companies will have a distributorship here in the US, but sometimes those relationships only last for a short period of time, which can make service challenging. Also, sometimes buying from distributors becomes challenging because the representative will have a large array of devices and possibly other "sidelines." It follows that their knowledge of one particular device is often incomplete.

Laser systems are available either as stand-alone or platform systems. Stand-alone systems tend to be of single wavelength with one hand piece (HP) designed for specific purposes such as a long pulse alexandrite 755 nm laser for LHR. Platform systems possess the ability to attach multiple HPs and address a large range of indications. The HPs could be a hair removal HP or an IPL HP for treating vascular lesions or even a near infrared HP offering skin tightening treatments, etc. At any given time, one or two HPs can be attached to the system and can be changed as desired. The software of the system recognizes the HP attached, and the settings can thus be changed as required. Each of these two areas has its advantages and disadvantages and these are enumerated in ▶ Table 38.1.

One issue with multipurpose systems is that if one component of the system breaks down, the entire platform is often disabled. With multiple single indication systems, although versatility might be compromised versus a platform system, if one system is down, the remainder of the systems are operational. Also, with platform systems, only one patient can be treated at a time, so that, for example, if one were pantomiming LHR in one room with a platform system, another patient could not be treated for blood vessels on the nose in the other room.

Another item as part of the business proposition is that barriers, blinds, as well as goggles for safety will have to be purchased. Also, provisions for a laser safety officer, typically a nurse or the main provider in the clinic, should be established and standard operating protocols should be framed for the various lasers.

Lessons learned: In a recent article, out of Modern Aesthetics in January February 2019,[4] Dr. Peter Capizzi relates some of the lessons that he has learned. The article, like the ROI one from 2010,

Table 38.1 Comparison of stand-alone versus platform systems (https://aestheticsjournal.com/feature/aesthetic-lasers-should-you-buy-new-or-used)

Stand-alone lasers	Pros	Cons
	Tend to be robust work horse systems	Take up more space
	Dedicated machine for selective work	More expensive to own multiple systems
	Ability to treat multiple patients simultaneously if more than one stand-alone systems available in clinic	More number of service visits if systems are of different make
		Higher maintenance costs
Platform system	**Pros**	**Cons**
	Cheaper to own with ability to treat different indications	In case of breakdown of platform, all HP may not work
	Takes up less office space	Only one patient/indication can be treated at a time
	Less number of service visits needed	HP needs to be used carefully as each HP tends to be expensive
	Probably lower maintenance costs	Not as robust and perhaps less effective when compared to stand-alone systems
	Easier to transport amongst different centres	

focuses on ROI. Dr. Capizzi noted the most important thing about taking in a particular technique or product is (1) does it work? (2) how does it fit into the practice? and (3) how can I make it easy for my staff to deliver and implement it? He cautions that implementation is usually more difficult than the actual purchase.

I would agree that many procedures, which are stated to only take 15 or 20 minutes, might only take that long if the entirety of the procedure, except for the very heart of the procedure, is performed by allied health personnel. Sometimes, the challenge involves assessing an emerging technology which is enticing but has had inadequate time to show proven and consistent results. Particularly in the area of noninvasive skin tightening, we have noted that, even though sometimes results are quite impressive, that as a group these procedures tend to be quite expensive and not always predictably effective. Sometimes, you bring a product into your practice simply not to lose that potential part of your business to a local competitor. The other consideration is a domino effect, where the patient has a procedure with the relatively new device that spins off into procedures with an older and more established equipment.

A physician colleague noted that approximately 20 years ago he purchased a laser under the assumption he would use it to treat leg veins, as that was the initial marketing emphasis by the laser community. Although his leg vein practice increased because of the marking associated with the machine, most of the patients were still treated with traditional sclerotherapy. So, sometimes a machine becomes an expensive marketing tool.

Also, one needs to make sure that you are performing procedures for conditions that are common and are consistent with the demographics of your region. If you are treating primarily darker skin patients, the requirement for a vascular laser, particular for treating facial veins, might be low.

Ensure the company provides marketing materials and there exists a contract for the duration of the materials they will supply; another concern is competition in the local area. If you are introducing a new technology to your practice, but there are several like-devices in the same geographic area, then a prospective patient might only come to your practice based on either the reputation of the practice, patient loyalty based on other procedures performed in your practice, or if you are offering a lower price.

The purchaser should make sure that he has full command of the specifications of the device. For example, some companies will list a maximum fluence that is quite high, but the upper range might be only within the context of a very small spot size and/or long pulse duration. Again, this is another compelling reason for performing test treatments with the particular device; only then will the practitioner observe the nuances and day-to-day practical issues that might be associated with a new technology. For example, a large spot size is preferable for LHR. The practitioner should examine the area covered per unit time within the context of the price to look and see if that device will generate more income or other opportunities. A round spot size of 10 to 24 mm is available in conventional LHR systems. Some newer hair removal systems have even larger spot sizes (up to 23 × 38 mm) and up to 4 cm^2/s.

One should examine the beam profile in real life and with a very low fluence on burn paper to establish uniformity of the energy across the entire spot. A top-hat beam profile is particularly preferable for Q-switched lasers, thus preventing uneven energy distribution over a given area and "hot-spots." With respect to scanners, the prospective operator should examine the attachment for ergonomics, speed, and ease of use. For example, the scanners should be attached and detached from the arm relatively quickly. Scan density, pattern of scan, pulse width, fluence, etc for fractional lasers should all be assessed. Devices should optimally have variable on time and off times (repeat mode rates). The hand piece of an IPL should optimally have in-built cooling; however, some state-of-the-art systems rely on an optimized spectral output to reduce the need for active cooling of the sapphire or quartz crystal.

Many devices lasers require some form of cooling for protection of the epidermis immediately before, during, and immediately after a laser procedure. Many devices have in-built cooling either in the form of cryogen spray, contact parallel cooling or simultaneous air cooling. It is important to ensure that cooling is working properly to prevent any accidental epidermal injury. Some of the cooling devices work independently and must be turned on, particularly the air cooling devices. Most modern contact cooling and cryogen spray devices are integrated into the whole system.

There typically are two laser manuals: one that goes into detail about the operation of the device and the other emphasizing treatment guidelines for specific parameters and certain applications and skin types. Many modern devices have these suggested settings built into a graphical user interface driven menu. Alternatively, the safe settings are suggested settings that can be taped to the side of the device for rapid access. At least one company offers an in-built melanin ureter to assist in choosing optimal parameters with visible light and near infrared technologies. In these cases, the melanin reader interprets the local skin color and provides, through Bluetooth connection, recommended settings based on the real-time melanin assessment, all within the context of the fluence, wavelength, application, and spot size associated with that particular hand piece.

All lasers are shipped with their specific eye protecting glasses with the recommended optical density (OD) to block out the harmful rays from entering the operator's eyes. Often times, only two sets of glasses are provided.

The representative should know that you are looking at other systems. Sometimes a company will offer package deals, where 2 or 3 lasers might be purchased at a considerable discount versus purchasing one device at a time. Some of these package deals can be quite compelling.

The buyer should obtain quotes from different companies for similar systems. All medical lasers depreciate as soon as they are sold. Also the buyer, MD should investigate that the cost of goods and other issues go into the manufacturer's suggested retail price (MSRP) for the laser; another factor is demand. Companies can charge more for devices in high-demand regardless of the cost of goods.

Installation should be performed by the company representative. During the time of installation, the installation report should list the serial number, make/model number, installation date, warranty period, and instructions regarding the electricity provision for the system.

A checklist for signing a contract is shown in the text box (▶ Box 38.1). The exact format will vary according to the system, company, cost and payment terms, and conditions.[1]

To summarize, some important points to consider while purchasing a laser system are shown in text box (▶ Box 38.2).[1]

38.4 Conclusion

The purchase of devices for a clinic is a major investment, both physically and emotionally, for the entire practice and staff. Once all the aforementioned considerations are made, a logical decision can be made regarding equipment acquisition.

References

[1] Aurangabadkar SJ, Mysore V, Ahmed ES. Buying a laser—tips and pearls. J Cutan Aesthet Surg 2014;7(2):124–130

[2] Jutkowitz E, Carniol PJ, Carniol AR. Financial analysis of technology acquisition using fractionated lasers as a model. Facial Plast Surg 2010;26(4):289–295

[3] Krieger LM, Shaw WW. Aesthetic surgery economics: lessons from corporate boardrooms to plastic surgery practices. Plast Reconstr Surg 2000;105(3):1205–1210, discussion 1211–1212

[4] ROI: getting it right. Modern Aesthetics Supplement, 2019:3–18

39 Evaluating Costs of Fillers and Toxins: Brand Loyalty versus Offering Everything

Ellen Marmur MD

Abstract

The high cost of fillers and toxins makes them a critical part of the business of cosmetic dermatology. This chapter helps to explain how to judge what products to purchase and when to buy them. Learning the business needs of your practice takes years as your practice evolves, thus your methods of evaluating the costs of fillers and toxins will mature. Taking inventory regularly, analyzing your peak points of sales, and anticipating the kinetics of your return on investment will all help you understand your annual profit and loss reports. You will learn how to start an inventory system. You will also receive insight into the pros and cons of participating in brand loyalty programs. Forming valuable professional relationships with company representatives may allow you to articulate what exactly you need for your patients and for your professional training while also availing you to advice about healthy ways to market your practice successfully. Whether you are in a solo or group practice, this chapter emphasizes the value of keeping a keen focus on your business needs over the pressure of bulk purchasing to achieve tier status or other sales forces.

Keywords: fillers, toxins, inventory, brand loyalty, tier programs, marketing

Top 10 Things You Need to Know

1. Learn everything there is to know about every new Food and Drugs Administration (FDA)-approved filler and neuromodulator from the best board-certified dermatologists.
2. Offer your patients only the products you trust the most.
3. Buy what you need only when you need it. Do not stockpile or try to game the rebate system.
4. Value your work—do not undercharge or overcharge. Just make certain you invest your time in training and expertise.
5. Do not succumb to the pressures of single brand loyalty. Maintain your integrity as a serious doctor and offer your patients what is best for them, not what is best for your relationship with a company. This is what makes you superior to business to business types of cosmetic offices, such as some spas or new franchises that are based on the bottom line.
6. Have frequent and honest conversations with your sales representatives and their managers about your goals and needs, and ask them what they can do to help you. They can offer advice on operations and also provide you with professional support.
7. Have frequent and transparent conversations with your trusted colleagues and ask how they run their practices, from operations and HR to work–life balance and marketing.
8. Participate frequently in professional meetings to hone your skills and update your knowledge.
9. Create a network for your office manager with other trusted office managers of a range of practice types, so they are a collective resource; of course, with permission from your colleagues.
10. Offer your patients access to the loyalty programs offered by each company. Every patient loves a little discount or rebate, even the wealthiest!

39.1 Introduction

Evaluating costs of fillers and neuromodulators can be extremely confusing, but with a little research you can simplify your business plan. Deciding which fillers to offer can be simply based on preferences or can be more complex based on pricing, rebates, support, and brand relationships. When building a cosmetic practice, it may be too costly to offer a full range of FDA-approved injectables. Busy cosmetic practices are able to track data of their use of different fillers and toxins to guide their ordering. Regardless of size, no practice should succumb to sales pressures to purchase large inventories in order to maintain preferred tiers in loyalty programs. Simply put, buy what you need when you need it in amounts that are not a burden to your overhead.

As your filler and toxin practice grows, establishing authentic relationships with each company through sale representatives and their managers is valuable. Ask them what their company's prospective new products are launching in the next 12 months. Ask them what they can do for you to grow your practice: organize training sessions in order to improve your techniques, meet with their medical science liaison to discuss the latest in techniques and research, establish collaborations with other local practices or medical centers, share their tips and pearls in practice management and marketing, or finally ask for an invitation to be a trainer or speaker for their company. These relationships not only convey your interest but also allow you to conduct very direct communication about the best business methods for your practice with respect to purchasing and managing this expensive inventory. Try to make time for the sales representatives and ask to meet their management and other leadership personnel. Your understanding of the company's products, it's rebate or tier system, and comparing that to the benefits of the new group purchasing organizations are important when assessing your practice's return on investment.

When evaluating the cost of a filler or toxin, also include brand safety in its value to your practice. Product safety is priceless. This includes the extent of research, efficacy, percent and types of adverse reactions, and the ability to reach a clinical support team at a moment's notice. Offering everything that is FDA approved may be tempting, but only offering the most trusted and effective brands is worthwhile.

Once you feel comfortable with more than one product, offering a variety of the most effective and trusted brands provides more financial control. If a practice stays brand specific, what leverage do they possess to negotiate the best price available? Yes, most practices negotiate the cost of products. The tier-structured pricing available from most vendors does offer additional discounts for quantity of product ordered, but that model does not allow you to take advantage of special promotions that all brands offer at different times during the year. If you have three trusted brands, you can take advantage of multiple brand promotions, and very often you can get one brand to match another's offer, therefore keeping your pricing as low and competitive as possible.

39.2 Tracking Inventory, Pricing, and Promotions

One key to the financial health of the cosmetic filler and toxin business in any practice is tracking inventory. It sounds much easier than it is and every practice struggles with it. To get started, one easy tip involves requesting your monthly or quarterly ordering information from your sales representatives tracked on simple spreadsheets. Have your front desk and office manager perform a daily, weekly, monthly, quarterly, and annual reconciliation of your invoices, inventory, and sales reports. If your practice management software does not have an inventory tracking system, you can begin tracking inventory on a spreadsheet or purchase an inventory tracking system that can integrate with your practice management system. There are many comprehensive inventory tracking systems readily available. Keeping track of daily inventory provides the following information at a glance:

- **Accountability**: All inventory received translates into revenue (nothing goes missing).
- **Trends**: Review daily usage for trends by brand, price, and category.
- **Intelligent purchasing**: Decisions made based on data and not blind loyalty to brand.
- **Reduction in overhead**: Inventory control eliminates expiration date waste and guarantees all necessary products are available.

This inventory tracking sheet shows brand, units/box, price/box (converted to price per syringe where applicable), daily inventory by date, and cost of inventory on the shelf (see ▶ Fig. 39.1).

This annual inventory tracking sheet shows brand, products, units/box, cost/box (translated to cost per syringe where applicable), and units used per month and per location (see ▶ Fig. 39.2).

Your annual inventory tracking sheet should also track brands, products, units/box, cost/box (translated to cost per syringe where applicable), and units used per month and per location.

Your brand partners should be able to produce this information monthly, quarterly, and annually. By tracking your own inventory, you can match your brand/partner information to your practice management charges and inventory tracking for the purposes of accountability. Trends in use by brand/product and location are easily assessed which translates into intelligent purchasing. "Why would I want to order more of Brand X if the

A	B	C	D	E	F	G	H	I	J	K	L	M	N	O	P
	UNITS	PRICE		11/19		Total	Price of		11/20		Total	Price of		11/21	
	Per box	Per box		Location 1	Location 2	Units	Inventory		87th street	Park ave	Units	Inventory		87th street	Park ave
GALDERMA															
Restylane - L	1	$300.00		25	10	35	$10,500.00		26	8	34	$10,200.00			
Restylane - Defyne	1	$300.00		25	10	35	$10,500.00		27	7	34	$10,200.00			
Restylane - Refyne	1	$300.00		25	10	35	$10,500.00		22	9	31	$9,300.00			
Restylane - Lyft	1	$300.00		25	10	35	$10,500.00		28	5	33	$9,900.00			
Restylane - Silk	1	$300.00		25	10	35	$10,500.00		24	8	32	$9,600.00			
Sculptra	2	$300.00		25	10	70	$10,500.00		24	9	66	$9,900.00			
Dysport	1	$300.00		30	20	50	$15,000.00		25	15	40	$12,200.00			
ALLERGAN															
Botox 100 cosmetic	1	$300.00		30	20	50	$15,000.00		25	15	40	$12,000.00			
Juvederm - Ultra XC	2	$300.00		25	10	70	$10,500.00		23	9	64	$9,600.00			
Juvederm - Ultra plus XC	2	$300.00		25	10	70	$10,500.00		20	5	50	$7,500.00			
Voluma XC	2	$300.00		25	10	70	$10,500.00		21	8	58	$8,700.00			
Volbella XC	2	$300.00		25	10	70	$10,500.00		24	7	62	$9,300.00			
Vollure XC	2	$300.00		25	10	70	$10,500.00		20	6	52	$7,800.00			
Kybella	2	$300.00		5	5	20	$3,000.00		4	5	18	$2,700.00			
MERZ															
Belotero	1	$300.00		25	25	50	$15,000.00		23	21	44	$13,200.00			
Xeomin	1	$300.00		30	20	50	$15,000.00		25	15	40	$12,000.00			
Radiesse volume advantage	2	$300.00		25	25	100	$15,000.00		21	23	88	$13,200.00			
ADDED NEW INVENTORY															
TOTAL COST OF INVENTORY:							$193,500.00					$167,100.00			

MASTER | Annual | Wk end 10.5 | Wk end 10.12 | Wk end 10.19 | Wk end 10.26 | Wk end 11.2 | Wk end 11.9 | Wk end 11.16 | **Wk end 11.23**

Fig. 39.1 Daily inventory spreadsheet.

A	B	C	D	E	F	G	H	I	Y	Z	AA	AB	AC	AD	AE	AF
Annual Inventory																
	UNITS	PRICE		January		February			March	November		December			7/10	Price of 2018
	Per box	Per box		Location1	Location2	Location1	Location2	Location1	Location1	Location2	Location1	Location2		Units	Inventory	
GALDERMA																
Restylane - L	1	$300.00		100	50	100	50	100	100	50				1650	$495,000.00	
Restylane - Defyne	1	$300.00		100	50	100	50	100	100	50				1650	$495,000.00	
Restylane - Refyne	1	$300.00		100	50	100	50	100	100	50				1650	$495,000.00	
Restylane - Lyft	1	$300.00		100	50	100	50	100	100	50				1650	$495,000.00	
Restylane - Silk	1	$300.00		100	50	100	50	100	100	50				1650	$495,000.00	
Sculptra	2	$300.00		100	50	100	50	100	100	50				3300	$495,000.00	
Dysport	1	$300.00		400	200	400	200	400	400	200				6600	$1,980,000.00	
ALLERGAN																
Botox 100 cosmetic	1	$300.00		400	200	400	200	400	400	200				6600	$1,980,000.00	
Juvederm - Ultra XC	2	$300.00		100	50	100	50	100	100	50				3300	$495,000.00	
Juvederm - Ultra plus XC	2	$300.00		100	50	100	50	100	100	50				3300	$495,000.00	
Voluma XC	2	$300.00		100	50	100	50	100	100	50				3300	$495,000.00	
Volbella XC	2	$300.00		100	50	100	50	100	100	50				3300	$495,000.00	
Vollure XC	2	$300.00		100	50	100	50	100	100	50				3300	$495,000.00	
Kybella	2	$300.00		10	5	10	5	10	10	5				330	$49,500.00	
MERZ																
Belotero	1	$300.00		100	50	100	50	100	100	50				1650	$495,000.00	
Xeomin	1	$300.00		400	200	400	200	400	400	200				6600	$1,980,000.00	
Radiesse volume advantage	2	$300.00		100	50	100	50	100	100	50				3300	$495,000.00	
ADDED NEW INVENTORY																
TOTAL COST OF INVENTORY:															$12,424,500.00	

MASTER | **Annual** | Wk end 10.5 | Wk end 10.12 | Wk end 10.19 | Wk end 10.26 | Wk end 11.2 | Wk end 11.9 | Wk end 11.16 | Wk end 11.23

Fig. 39.2 Annual inventory tracking.

physicians at location #2 clearly use twice as much Brand Y for the same price?" This intelligent purchasing keeps the inventory on the shelves fresh, and the overhead cost reduced as you eliminate waste.

Promotions from your brand/partners should always be assessed in conjunction with your intelligent purchasing. Promotions may provide you with an opportunity to reduce your price on certain products, but if you do not use that product often, there is no point in purchasing excess. Educate your brand partner on the products that are most important to your practice, and see if you can negotiate the reduced pricing on the products that you do need more than the products they'd like you to purchase. This negotiation process should be presented to all brand partners every time you purchase. Speak to other physicians about their systems, down to the details of these types of conversations. Remember, sales representatives have every interest in the success of your practice. You need to build a strong partnership with them and utilize their resources to help build and sustain a strong and intelligent financial practice. It is a triple win for patients, your practice, and your brand to use the products you like the most.

39.3 Patient Participation in Brand Loyalty

Patient input can be a factor when it comes to brand specificity. With advertising, media, and word of mouth, patients are becoming more educated about specific products and brands. Patients might participate in certain "Brand Loyalty Reward" programs which lead them to ask for specific brands based on a promotion that the brand may be offering at a certain time. Many brands are heavily investing in direct to consumer (DTC) marketing and advertising with TV and even old-fashioned radio, plus other forms of influence on social media ads. This presents another reason why becoming brand specific may not help, but hurt your practice. In short, diversification has many benefits.

In my practice, most patients trust my decision of what to use, where to inject it, and do not request specific brand or products. However, in different markets and for new physicians starting out, these reward programs may help bring patients back to the practice.

The Brilliant Distinctions program from Allergan and the Aspire rewards programs from Galderma both claim brand and physician loyalty in high percentages of patients enrolled. If, in fact, their claims are accurate, that still does not present an argument for single brand loyalty but again opens up the possibility of capturing patients with preferences across brands by offering all of your brand partners' products. While some physicians are vehemently against these loyalty programs, in my experience, even the wealthiest patients love discounts and dollars back. These programs require a little extra work for your office staff at all touch points so if your front desk staff is inefficient, ask for further training from the representatives.

39.4 Conclusion

In conclusion, after making many mistakes over the years, my advice is simple. Buy what you need only when you need it; do not stockpile excess inventory when you can receive your orders within 1 to 2 days; begin a simple tracking system with invoices, inventory counts, and reconciliation of all products. Analyze your average usage of products monthly and begin to anticipate your inventory needs. At this point, you will be able to make better informed decisions when faced with discounts or pressures to order in bulk. Be direct and transparent with your company representatives regarding which products you want and ask what they can do for you—perhaps they can swap products or propose something that works well for you. Finally, if a tier or loyalty program sounds confusing, then it might be purposely confusing as a means to coax you into ordering what the company needs to sell more than what is best for your practice. Keep it clear and simple so that your team, your patients, and your brand partners can continue to benefit and grow your practice successfully.

Acknowledgment

I wish to thank Ms Colleen O'Brien for her help with creating the example inventory table.

Section V

The Nitty-Gritty

V

40 Essential Instruments

Aleksandra G. Florek MD, Eileen L. Axibal MD, Mariah R. Brown MD

Abstract

When setting up a dermatology practice, physicians must purchase a large volume of surgical instruments. Selecting the number and type of instruments should be guided by the expected nature and volume of performed procedures. In general, higher quality instruments last longer and perform better. Knowledge of surgical instruments and their handling will improve surgical technique, increase safety from sharps injury, and enhance the lifespan of the instrument. The following instruments will be covered in this chapter: curettes, scalpel holders, blades, needle holders, scissors, forceps, hemostats, and skin hooks. It will also include a brief review of instrument sterilization techniques.

Keywords: surgical instruments, dermatologic surgery, essential instruments, cost effective, economical, scalpel, scissors, blade, hooks, hemostats, sterilization

Top 10 Things You Need to Know

1. High-quality, high-cost surgical instruments lead to greater efficiency, precision, and improved patient outcomes during dermatologic surgery.
2. Reusable surgical instruments are economical and will save money in the long term, but careful monitoring is required for potential dullness or misalignment.
3. Surgical instruments made of tungsten carbide will last up to five times longer than stainless steel instruments. The additional length of service makes tungsten carbide instruments more cost-effective than cheaper models.
4. When setting up a standard surgical tray, the most essential instruments are the following: blade handle, blade, forceps with teeth, skin hooks, curved hemostat, curved iris scissors, needle holder, and suture scissors.
5. Needle drivers with serrated jaws hold suture needles more securely and may prevent larger needles from twisting; however, they may damage smaller needles and shred fine sutures.
6. Disposable curettes cut through all tissues in an essentially identical manner. As a result, dermatologic surgeons often prefer to use reusable curettes for increased precision.
7. Skin hooks are the least traumatic instruments for tissue handling, but pose an increased risk of sharps injuries.
8. Tissue scissors should not be used to cut sutures due to the risk of instrument dulling.
9. Steam autoclave is the most popular, easiest, and safest method of sterilization, but it may lead to dulling of instruments.
10. The final decision on selecting essential instruments should be based on the surgeon's personal preference and the type of procedure being performed.

40.1 Introduction

Surgical instruments are essential to the practice of dermatologic surgery and may represent a significant start-up cost for new practitioners. Ideally, dermatologists should make an investment in high-quality instruments that offer the best performance and longevity. A high-quality instrument will more than offset its initial cost. Low-quality instruments should be avoided, if possible, as they are more difficult to use, lack precision, and require more frequent replacements.

40.2 Disposable versus Nondisposable Surgical Instruments

Surgical instruments come in two forms: disposable and reusable. Disposable instruments are advantageous in that they are always sharp and, with their one-time use, do not require the time or cost of sterilization. Reusable instruments, on the other hand, are of a higher quality but require ongoing care to maintain optimal function. For example, using delicate instruments such as Gradle or iris scissors to cut sutures may result in dulling, and rough handling of delicate forceps or needle holders during surgery or sterilization may result in instrument misalignment. Disposable instruments should be reserved for basic surgical procedures or situations in which instruments cannot be sterilized.

40.3 Curettes

In dermatologic surgery, curettes are used to treat and debulk a wide variety of benign and malignant tumors. Curettes are available in several disposable and reusable forms. Disposable curettes are sharp and cut through tissue relatively indiscriminately, making the distinction between neoplasm and normal skin more difficult. For this reason, most dermatologists prefer reusable metal curettes. Curettes can be straight with a round head or have an oval head at an angle from the stem. They are labeled by size, correlating to the width of the opening, and range from 1 to 10 mm in dermatologic surgery. Curettage is a helpful tool in defining tumor margins prior to excisional or Mohs micrographic surgery. Generally, larger curettes are used for gross tumor debulking and smaller curettes for removing focal areas of residual tumor.

40.4 Scalpel Handles and Blades

The choice of scalpel handle and blade depends on the surgical site and surgeon's personal preference. The most frequently used scalpel handle in dermatology is the Bard-Parker (No. 3), which has a flat handle and can accommodate the most commonly used scalpel blades. It is available with an optional

imprinted ruler (▶Fig. 40.1). The Bard-Parker is long-lasting and inexpensive. The No. 7 handle is most commonly used in plastic surgery. Another common scalpel handle is the Beaver, which is either round or hexagonal, has a groove, and holds smaller and sharper Beaver-specific blades (No. 64 and No. 67). These blades insert into a collet, which tightens by rotating around the handle. The Beaver provides better grip and more precise control in delicate surgical sites, particularly around the eye.

The most frequently used blades in dermatologic surgery are the #15, #10, and #11 (▶Fig. 40.2). Of these, the #15 blade is the most popular. It is gently curved and appropriate for the majority of surgical sites. A narrower version of the #15 blade with a smaller belly, the #15C blade, can be useful in areas where a smaller cutting surface is beneficial. The #10 blade is similar in shape to the #15 blade, but has a wider convex belly; it is primarily used for larger excisional procedures on the back. The #11 blade has a sharp point which may be used for incision and drainage procedures, removal of milia, and cutting sharp angles. Scalpel blades are made of either stainless steel or Teflon-coated carbon steel; the latter is sharper and more expensive but dulls more quickly. After completion of a procedure, a scalpel blade should be removed carefully from the handle using a commercially available blade remover to minimize the

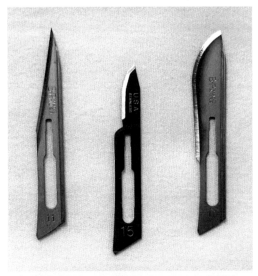

Fig. 40.2 Most commonly used blades in dermatologic surgery (#11, #15, and #10—from left to right).

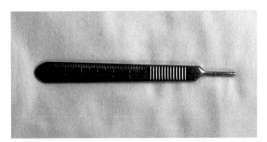

Fig. 40.1 Bard-Parker (No. 3) blade handle with imprinted ruler.

risk of sharps injury. Disposable scalpels attached to plastic handles may also be used in dermatologic surgery, but these instruments are less sharp and not weighted.

40.5 Needle Holders

Needle holders may be either light and narrow with fine jaws or large and broad with wide jaws; the latter are used for thicker surgical sites such as the trunk and proximal extremities. The jaws of needle holders are either smooth or serrated. Needle drivers with larger, serrated jaws hold the needle more securely and prevent needle twisting, but may damage delicate needles and shred small sutures. Smooth jaws are less damaging to fine-caliber needles and will not tear fine sutures, but the needle may slip and twist if not grasped carefully.

Alloy inserts of tungsten carbide serve to increase the strength of the jaws and improve the grip on needles in smooth-jawed needle holders. Instruments with tungsten carbide inserts can generally be identified based on their gold handles (▶ Fig. 40.3). Large needles should not be used with fine needle holders, as this may damage the instrument's insert. Popular models such as the Webster and Halsey needle holders, which have smooth or delicately serrated jaws and tapered tips, are ideal for the small needles and fine suture materials commonly used in cutaneous facial surgery. The use of these instruments for procedures on the trunk, however, will quickly lead to their misalignment. Castroviejo needle holders, with their unique spring and locking mechanism, are used most frequently for the very small needles in ophthalmology and

microsurgery. The Crile-Wood needle holder has a gently tapered blunt tip; it is designed to hold larger needles and is useful for skin surgery on the trunk and extremities. Baumgartner and Mayo-Hegar holders are durable, strong drivers with short tips and serrated jaws, providing a mechanical advantage for handing larger needles in thicker skin.

40.6 Scissors

Surgical scissors are used for cutting and undermining tissues, cutting sutures, and cutting bandages. Scissors may have short or long handles, straight or curved blades, smooth or serrated blades, and blunt or sharp tips. Scissors with short handles are useful for delicate work and those with long handles are useful for reaching far and undermining wide. Curved blades are optimal for undermining and straight blades for cutting sutures and trimming tissues. Serrated blades result in less tissue slippage, as they grasp the tissue while cutting. Sharp-tipped scissors puncture tissue easily and are considered best for dissection, while blunt-tipped scissors are believed to be the best for delicate undermining.

Iris scissors are sharp-tipped and short-handled. Of all the standard tissue scissors, iris scissors have the sharpest edge and is the most commonly used instrument for dissecting and undermining on the head and neck in dermatologic surgery. These scissors may be straight or curved and are available with either two smooth edges or one serrated edge. When one of the blades has a razor edge, they are specified as "supercut" and denoted by black handles (▶ Fig. 40.4). Iris scissors and other tissue scissors may be composed completely of

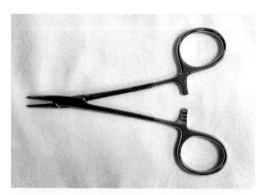

Fig. 40.3 Webster needle holder with tungsten carbide alloy insert, as indicated by the gold handles.

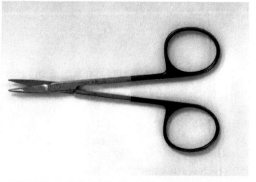

Fig. 40.4 "Supercut" iris scissors, as indicated by the black handles.

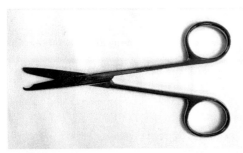

Fig. 40.5 Northbent suture scissors, with half-moon hook to prevent skin trauma.

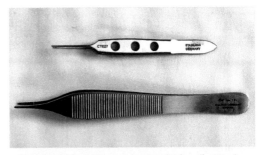

Fig. 40.6 Bishop-Harmon (top) and Adson (bottom) forceps.

stainless steel—which is most popular and least expensive—or have tungsten carbide inserts to strengthen the blades.

Undermining scissors, not including iris scissors, are blunt-tipped for the purpose of safety and have long handles for comfort. They are available in different sizes to accommodate the various anatomic regions in which cutaneous surgery is performed. Baby Metzenbaum scissors have a high handle-to-blade length ratio and, with the resultant small blade arc, are effective for sharp and blunt undermining. Larger Metzenbaum scissors are appropriate for extensive undermining in areas that require long reach, such as fascial planes on the scalp, trunk, or the extremities. Gradle scissors are small, delicate instruments that taper to a very fine point with a gentle curve. They provide great precision and are regarded as the best for dissection of delicate tissue such as periorbital skin. Gradle scissors must be used with care, as they are quick to dull and may misalign with improper use. Both Metzenbaum and Gradle scissors are also available as "supercut," again denoted by black handles.

Sutures should be cut with large, less expensive, non-tissue scissors. Specially designed suture-removal scissors with a half-moon hook on the lower blade (Northbent) are available (▶Fig. 40.5); the hooked tip easily grasps the suture loop and prevents accidental skin trauma. Lister scissors are commonly used for bandage cutting. They have angled blades and large blunt tips that easily side under a dressing without damaging the underlying skin. The Universal scissor is also a popular choice; the serrated edges and larger rings provide greater cutting power.

40.7 Forceps

Forceps allow for delicate, safe handling of tissue and suture needles during cutaneous surgery.

The most useful forceps in skin surgery are lightweight and fine-tipped. The tips may be serrated, toothed, or smooth. Serrated forceps enable the surgeon to easily grab the needle, but they may exert excessive pressure on tissues and result in crush injury. Toothed forceps have opposing fine teeth and exert less overall pressure, resulting in gentle tissue handling and decreased risk of crush injury. Only toothed forceps should be used to grasp the epidermis and superficial dermis. The Adson forceps (▶Fig. 40.6) are deemed the most useful for cutaneous surgery on the trunk and extremities. Some forceps have both distal teeth for tissue handling and a proximal raised platform for firmly grasping suture needles, allowing the surgeon to avoid manual handling of suture needles. Bishop-Harmon forceps (▶Fig. 40.6) are small, fine-tipped instruments that are useful for tissue handling in more delicate areas on the face. They have three holes in the handles, making them lightweight and easy to grip. Finally, Jeweler's forceps have sharply pointed ends and are most useful for suture removal.

40.8 Hemostats

Hemostats are used to grasp bleeding vessels prior to ligation with electrosurgery or sutures. The most popular hemostat is the Halsted Mosquito model, which is available in 3.5- or 5-inch lengths, curved or straight tip, and regular or delicate tip. A modified instrument known as an Allis clamp is particularly helpful during cyst or lipoma removal. It comprises finger grips and a locking mechanism similar to the hemostat, but the jaws have opposing sharp teeth that grasp tissue firmly. Since these teeth can devitalize tissue, the Allis clamp is only used to provide traction on tissue that is being excised such as a cyst wall.

40.9 Skin Hooks

Skin hooks enable the surgeon to handle tissue with minimal trauma, and they are particularly useful for elevating flaps and reflecting skin edges during undermining. They are an integral part of the least traumatic way to handle tissue during electrosurgery and suturing, but unfortunately are a common cause of sharps injury. Skin hooks may be single, double, or multi-pronged. The multi-pronged skin hooks are used mainly for rhytidectomies and larger truncal procedures in which large flaps or margins of tissue are being elevated. Single-pronged hooks are used most frequently on delicate skin. The single shepherd hook has a circular shape and holds tissue better than the single standard hook, but it does not release easily.

40.10 Sterilization Methods

Instrument sterilization can be achieved by either physical (heat, pressure, or steam) or chemical (gas vapor and disinfectant) technique. Steam autoclave, which is the use of steam under pressure, is the most popular sterilization method in the office setting due to its high-efficiency, low-cost, and favorable safety profile. The main disadvantage with steam autoclave is that it may dull and corrode instruments. Chemical autoclave involves the use of a heated chemical vapor mixture (formaldehyde, methyl ethyl ketone, acetone, and alcohols) to achieve sterilization. Due to the low humidity associated with this technique, there is less risk of instrument dulling. Chemical autoclaving requires protective gear and ventilation to prevent dangerous exposures. Dry heat, or oven sterilization, is an inexpensive method that does not result in corrosion or dulling. As instruments need to be heated at a high temperature (1 hour at 171°C, and 6 hours at 121°C), there lies the risk of burn injury. Gas sterilization is good for large instrument volumes, such as in the hospital setting, and requires expensive equipment. Finally, cold sterilization using 2% glutaraldehyde, formaldehyde, or orthophthalaldehyde solution is inexpensive but irritating to the skin, eyes, and nasal passage. This method has minimal to no efficacy against bacterial spores.

40.11 Conclusion

An understanding of essential instruments in dermatologic surgery will allow the new practitioner to invest in high-quality, durable tools necessary to optimize surgical technique and patient outcomes.

Suggested Readings

Bogle MA, Joseph AK. Instruments and materials. In: Robinson JK, et al., eds. Surgery of the Skin: Procedural Dermatology. New York: Elsevier; 2005:59–66

Burge S, Colver GB, Rayment R. Simple Skin Surgery, 2nd edn. Oxford: Blackwell Science; 1996:5–9

Cartee TV, Travelute CR. Wound closure materials and instruments. In: Bolognia JL et al., eds. Dermatology. Spain: Mosby Elsevier; 2018:2450–2461

Davila M, Nguyen TH. Surgery and anatomy. In: Ali A, ed. Dermatology: A Pictorial Review. New York: McGraw-Hill; 2007:175–204

Diwan R. Instruments for dermatologic surgery. In: Lask GP, Moy RI, eds. Principles and Techniques of Cutaneous Surgery. New York: McGraw-Hill; 1996:85–100

Grande DJ, Neuburg M. Instrumentation for the dermatologic surgeon. J Dermatol Surg Oncol 1989;15(3):288–297

Johnson TM, Tromovitch TA, Swanson NA. Combined curettage and excision: a treatment method for primary basal cell carcinoma. J Am Acad Dermatol 1991;24(4):613–617

Leffell DJ, Brown M. Manual of Skin Surgery: A Practical Guide to Dermatologic Procedures. New York: John Wiley & Sons, Inc.; 1997

Melissa BA, Joseph AK. Instruments and materials. In: Robinson JK, Hanke WC, Sengelmann R, Siegle D, eds. Surgery of the Skin. London: Elsevier-Moby; 2005:59–66

Rutala WA, Weber DJ. Disinfection and sterilization in health care facilities: what clinicians need to know. Clin Infect Dis 2004;39(5):702–709

Sebben JE. Sterilization and care of surgical instruments and supplies. J Am Acad Dermatol 1984; 11(3):381–392

Sebben JE, Fazio MJ. Sterilization of equipment for dermatologic surgery. In: Lask GP, Moy RI, eds. Principles of Techniques of Cutaneous Surgery. New York: McGraw-Hill; 1006:47–56

Weber LA. The surgical tray. Dermatol Clin 1998;16 (1):17–24

41 Essential Stock to Start a Practice

Michael T. Goldfarb MD, Jeffrey S. Orringer MD

Abstract

As a physician begins to stock a dermatology practice, the task may initially seem overwhelming. However, the essentials for performing the most frequent procedures are still surprisingly affordable. It is important to make sure your budget is adequate to purchase high quality items to provide the best care possible. Once you have established your basic setup, you can fine tune it as you determine the specific needs of your patient population. This chapter will outline the necessary equipment and supplies one must obtain, from larger one-time purchases including examination tables and an autoclave to single use supplies including sutures and syringes. With the increasing focus on cosmetic services in dermatology, planning this early in your initial setup is important. Initially, a patient survey can determine the demand for aesthetic treatments in your practice. Dermatologists often start by offering procedures with minimal risks to the patient and minimal financial risks to the practice, such as superficial chemical peels. Ultimately, more expensive procedures with higher upfront expenditures can be provided, including neurotoxin and soft tissue filler injections, if demand for such procedures justifies offering these services. Finally, if one pursues the energy-based devices, including lasers and radiofrequency systems, it is often advisable to rent these systems and cluster patients on a specific date until demand justifies the necessary initial outlay of tens of thousands of dollars needed to purchase such a device for the practice. Although beginning your practice is a significant undertaking, this chapter will demonstrate that most standard dermatological care and procedures can still be performed without spending an exorbitant amount of money.

Keywords: stock, supplies, setup, budget, examination rooms, cosmetic procedures

Top 10 Things You Need to Know

1. Determine your budget, that is, exactly how much are you willing to spend.
2. Decide how many examination rooms you need to be cost efficient.
3. Determine what type of tables you need.
4. Plan how best to incorporate your electronic medical records technology.
5. Prepare your rooms to best handle your most important services.
6. Determine how many instruments and supplies you require.
7. Establish your method of sterilization.
8. Have an inviting waiting room.
9. Be prepared to send patients home with appropriate supplies.
10. Sell and stock products if it fits your personal model for patient care.

41.1 Introduction

When a physician first decides to start a dermatology practice, the task of acquiring all the necessary equipment may seem overwhelming and expensive. However, to perform the most frequent procedures, the amount of capital needed is still reasonable, even in these inflationary times. If you are truly beginning from scratch, you can add to your equipment, as the demand for your services increases.

41.2 Step One: Your Budget

Make sure your resources are adequate to purchase what you need. Always buy the most high-quality item that you feel you and your patients need to provide the best care possible. It is far better to accrue more debt than have suboptimal equipment. As you begin your medical practice, you have already determined you will be a success, and the expense of setup is a single event. However, this does not mean you cannot add to your basic setup, as the demand for your services increases. Also, you will fine tune your needs, as you determine what the specific demographics of your dermatology practice requires.

41.3 Step Two: Examination Rooms

You must first decide how many examination rooms you require. Even for a new practice, we recommend at least three examination rooms. At any given moment, one room will have a medical assistant taking in the patients' initial medical history, or providing the postoperative instructions to the patient, you will be in the second room providing patient care, and the third room will have a patient dressing or undressing. Every day, small complications arise from an area of hemorrhage that needs five minutes of pressure to a patient feeling faint who must lay supine for 10 minutes, putting an examination room out of commission. Without three rooms, this can disrupt your ability to continue to attend to patients and keep you on schedule.

41.4 Step Three: Tables

Your examination table is one of the most important pieces of equipment you need to buy. There is certainly an opportunity to save money by buying a beautiful manual table with storage space and an attractive appearance for under 1,000 dollars. However, we are telling you not to fall for that apparently easy decision, but rather spend 5,000 dollars for an electric power table. The benefits of this more expensive option are numerous. First, many of our encounters with dermatology patients involve sitting. From care for acne, eczema, and psoriasis to many of our procedures of cryosurgery and intralesional injections, the patient and physician prefer the sitting position. The manual tables do allow for the patient to be upright, but in a far less comfortable position than the power table. Also, it allows special positioning to treat lesions on the foot to the top of the head. More importantly, if a patient becomes faint, it is the quickest way to get them in a flat or even Trendelenburg position. In addition, it can allow the elderly and patients with disabilities to be placed on the table without effort, as the power table can be brought down very low for easy access. Finally, it allows physicians to be able to perform any procedure on the patient without straining themselves.

One may consider buying one power examination table for the procedure room and have manual tables in the others. If your budget only allows for one table, so be it, but I see this as a short-term solution. Eventually you will want power tables in all your rooms, and the manual tables will be nothing but a donation to charity or an item you sell for pennies on the dollar.

41.5 Step Four: Incorporating Your Electronic Medical Record (EMR)

On the day of EMR, your examination rooms must be ready for patient intake, consents, note production, photography, and postoperative and postvisit instruction. What you purchase will be dependent on the requirements of the particular EMR you purchased. The bare minimum, as I have experienced with my practice, is a portable notebook for each of your medical assistants and yourself, two desk top computers at the front desk for patient intake and payments with a third in a separate office for billing, and two printers in a central location. Many practices prefer desk top computers in each room, but that often proves to be an extra expense with the additional wiring required.

41.6 Step Five: Prepare Your Rooms to Best Handle Your Most Important Services

Upon completing residency, you must determine what medical and surgical services you are most comfortable with and are willing to furnish. Medical dermatology often only involves writing or escribing an appropriate therapy with no special equipment required. Most items for medical dermatology are not needed in every room. We use a portable blood pressure cuff, stethoscope, and thermometer as required. We keep a scale for measuring patients' weight in a private area down the hallway. Every room must have patient gowns. We have used paper gowns without any patient complaints and avoided the expense of laundry. We do keep a stool in keep every room, so we can sit down and give the positive impression that we are not rushed and have time to listen. All my stools consist of wheels, so that I can move easily while we work on the patient. There is a disadvantage to this type of stool, as we have encountered many close calls wherein a very young and playful child or an elderly person with balance issues were almost on the verge of sustaining serious injuries when they fell off the stool. It is best to keep a stable chair for patients' friends and families in the room and ask them not to use the stool. Extra lighting and magnification lights are also a necessity for every room and can be affordably obtained. It is important to have cupboards with all your essential items in every room. It is imperative that it is kept locked until you arrive at the room, so no harm can come to the curious patient. Each room must have a container for medical waste as well as a trash can.

The daily routine of a dermatologist involves numerous procedures. As cryosurgery is an integral part of most dermatology practices, every room must be prepared to offer this service. We do recommend a liquid nitrogen sprayer in each room but here is an opportunity to save money. As it is easily transported from one room to the other, one sprayer can could certainly service all your rooms when getting started. Installing one sprayer in each room should be the practitioners' goal. Also, one needs a central container for the liquid nitrogen, the Dewar. Our Dewar is 30 liters and lasts for approximately three weeks, but this will vary according to your usage and patient volume. Filling the q tank costs approximately 100 dollars. This is variable depending on your vendor, and we have seen the same service cost 250 dollars in the exact same city, so you must get more than one bid.

Having a hyfrecator in every room for hemostasis and destruction is essential for office efficiency. The expense of under 800 dollars per room is well worth the versatility this small piece of equipment provides the dermatologist with to perform multiple procedures. The disposable hyfrecator tips are a nominal expense. Every office requires only one smoke evacuator to prevent the plume from being inhaled by the patient or staff. This item can easily be wheeled to wherever it is needed and is not a necessary fixture of every room.

41.7 Step Six: Determine How Many Instruments and Supplies You Need

What you purchase, as far as instruments and supplies are concerned, will again depend on your training and interests as a practicing dermatologist. It also will depend on the demographics of your population. If you are caring for younger patients, medical dermatology may prevail, but if you have an older, fair-skinned population, as in my practice, surgical dermatology prevails. However, one must be prepared to offer their services in an efficient, cost-effective manner.

Intralesional steroids is a procedure often performed daily in a dermatologists' office. We prefer my steroid vials which is in a tray that is passed from one room to another. The reason this is important to me is once a vial is opened, it must be used in a timely method. By using only one vial at a time, we ensure that a vial will be completely used and not have to be discarded. I use this same philosophy for any perishable therapy. We only open one bottle of cantharidin at a time to insure it maintains its high-quality. Any item that is not used frequently, should be placed in a central location and not in each room.

Depending on the practice, a variable number of sterile biopsy and excision kits need to be on hand. We will frequently perform a combination of 10 excisions or punch biopsies on a given day and feel the bare minimum for us would be 20 surgical kits. Therefore, the purchase of 20 needle holders, scalpel handles, forceps, and hemostats would be essential to my practice. It takes a day to sterilize your instruments, so a two-day supply is necessary. One set for the current day and another set that is being sterilized. My punch biopsies are all disposable, and we have all sizes from 2 to 5 mm, but what you carry depends on your practice habits. Also, suture is highly variable, according to each dermatologists' preference for type of needle and suture material. We have no problem ensuring we have a month's supply of suture, as we know it will be used. One tip is that the 10-inch biopsy suture, as opposed to the standard 18-inch, is significantly cheaper and more than adequate for closing a punch biopsy site.

Dermatologists need a host of additional instruments including curettes, suture removal kits, nail clippers, and any instrument you may need for special procedures you offer. The exact count of each item may take some time to determine. Whenever you are purchasing instruments, always buy those of the highest quality, as this is not the place to save money. If you were happy with the instruments you used in training, by all means, reproduce it; if not, determine what would be the best for your practice.

It is essential to have an adequate supply of your daily use items. The type of gloves you buy depend on your preference as well as that of your staff. Make sure you have the appropriate sizes and types of gloves at all times. We use both boxes of clean gloves and individual sterile gloves daily. We also make sure every staff member has a pair of gloves that fits them comfortably. I do like latex gloves for the comfort and dexterity over other materials, but these gloves must be avoided in a latex allergic patient. If we cannot use latex for a specific patient, we will move to vinyl gloves which are still reasonably priced and durable. However, vinyl gloves have a looser fitting and, for me, less desirable for performing procedures. Finally, we also stock the more expensive nitrile gloves for higher risk situations, as these gloves are the most durable and offer the best puncture resistance.

In addition, make sure you have gauze, Q-tips, bandages, and any other items you use for patient care. At the beginning of every day, we approximately prepare all the lidocaine syringes that will be needed; this is a tremendous time saver. We prefer a 3 mL syringe with a luer lock tip. Although more expensive than larger bore needles, we use a 30 gauge needle, as the additional patient comfort is worth it. I also stock a 1,000 count bottle of cephalexin and clindamycin for premedication when needed. Be prepared for any and all contingencies. We keep an AED on hand as well as a facial mask for CPR, but fortunately, in 33 years, we have never needed either. Finally, other considerations include a refrigerator for medical perishables and a separate one for staff lunches, microwave, staff table for lunches and breaks, as well as numerous other items that will be necessary for your practice to run smoothly.

41.8 Step Seven: Establish Your Method of Sterilization

Many of your medical instruments will need to be sterilized. One must follow a protocol for sterilizing all the equipment to fulfill this task. We first place my instruments in a container with a neutral pH holding/presoak enzymatic solution directly after patient use. We will then proceed with disinfecting and cleaning. We do use an ultrasonic cleanser as the most effective method of removing blood, dried body fluids, and tissue prior to sterilization. We then place the instruments in pouches and place them in the autoclave. We recommend purchasing both an ultrasonic cleanser and autoclave to ensure your instruments are

properly sterilized. Also, make sure you have a testing spore kit to determine your autoclave is completely effective.

41.9 Step Eight: Have an Inviting Waiting Room

An adequate waiting room is essential. You must determine how many seats you need to accommodate your patients and their families. We attend to approximately 40 patients a day; I have 10 waiting room seats and it is on rare occasions that I run out of seats. My only form of entertainment is an extensive collection of magazines that appeal to my patients. As one of us is next door to a major car company, I carry all the car magazines, so customize your collection to your demographics. Also, my patients enjoy golf magazines, homemaking magazines, children's magazines as well as the standard People and Time magazines. It is important to keep your magazines up-to-date. Before you purchase numerous subscriptions, pharmaceutical companies will often supply you with the standard waiting room subscriptions. Please make sure the magazines you put out are not offensive. Some standard magazines will have inappropriate content listed on the cover and must be identified and discarded. Many offices will have a television monitor for daily news and television shows, highlighting the services you offer. Depending on your location, you may prefer a stereo that plays a local music station. This was a personal choice of my staff and patient population. We do avoid a clock in the waiting room. A large clock seems to accentuate the waiting time and makes for anxious patients.

41.10 Step Nine: Be Prepared to Send Patients Home with Appropriate Supplies

After a procedure, we do like to send the patient home with the supplies they require. It may be something as simple as packets of Vaseline for use after a surgical procedure to more extensive supplies for a larger procedure. However, if it is affordable, we prefer to provide the supplies as a complimentary service included in the procedure price. It is usually inexpensive and greatly appreciated by your patients.

41.11 Step Ten: Sell and Stock Products If It Fits Your Personal Model for Patient Care

It has become common for dermatology practices to carry products for both the medical and cosmetic needs of their patient population. Many patients find this convenient as this allows them to obtain exactly what their physician recommends. On the other hand, many physicians do not sell products, as they prefer to be able to make recommendations without any possibility of being biased.

41.12 Building a Cosmetic Component to Your Practice

The following section serves as an overview of this subject which will be dealt with in greater detail in the subsequent three chapters.

41.12.1 Step One: Assess the Demand

Unless you are joining a large, established, cosmetically-oriented practice, most physicians will have to gradually build a cosmetic focus in their practice. Whether yours is primarily a medical or surgical dermatology practice, the first step involves assessing your current patients' interest in aesthetic treatments. This may be conducted informally or via patient surveys. After this initial step, one can begin to determine the potential demand for cosmetic treatments by investigating the demographics of the area near the practice location and the saturation or lack of clinicians offering these treatments in the local market. Mean income data for various areas is usually available for public consumption, for example, and a simple search of local practices' websites may also prove to be very informative.

41.12.2 Step Two: Assess Your Knowledge and Preparation to Provide Aesthetic Treatments

If you become convinced that there is a desire for cosmetic services among your patients and/or in the surrounding area, and you believe that patients are likely to have adequate disposable income to support this, careful thought must next be given to honestly evaluating your own preparation to provide such care. Have you gathered adequate experience in the context of your residency and/or fellowship training? If not, one must consider the time and expense necessary to become trained in these procedures, such that it is possible to deliver high-quality care. There are myriad options for didactic and hands-on education in cosmetic dermatology provided at the annual meetings of several dermatology organizations, and some companies who manufacture devices for use in cosmetic dermatology also offer extensive training options. The important thing is to be certain that you have been adequately trained in a procedure before offering this to your patients, as bad outcomes may jeopardize your reputation while you attempt to build your practice.

41.12.3 Step Three: Which Services to Offer?

Once convinced that your patients want cosmetic services and confident in your ability to provide them, the next step is to consider which types of procedures you wish to offer. Some procedures, such as superficial chemical peels, come with minimal risk to the patient and minimal financial risk for the practice. As the complexity of procedures increases, so do the costs generally. Injectable products, such as neurotoxins and soft tissue fillers, require an upfront expenditure by the practice, so initially small quantities should be purchased. On considering energy-based devices like lasers, radiofrequency systems, ultrasound devices, or others, the practice is potentially looking at an initial outlay of tens of thousands of dollars, so the stakes become higher when calculating a potential return on investment. Some practices have found it preferable to initially rent devices and cluster appropriate patients on specific dates. Once demand is established, it may be appropriate to transition to purchasing or leasing a device.

When deciding which devices to prioritize, it is helpful to think in terms of categories such as lasers that target vascular lesions, lasers that target pigment, lasers used for hair removal, devices used for cutaneous textural irregularities including scars and wrinkles, devices for body shaping, or devices for skin tightening. Most medical dermatologists see plenty of patients with photodamage, which includes both issues of hypervascularity and dyspigmentation, so it might be wise to initially consider devices that target hemoglobin or melanin as an easy transition for medical patients into the cosmetic aspect of the practice. Laser hair removal is also a frequently performed procedure and consideration might be given to purchasing or leasing a laser system for this indication. For this device, make sure you assess the prices nearby competitors are charging, as, in many states, this is a delegated procedure and priced lower than physician time. In addition, energy-based devices are often highly complex and require specialized maintenance and care. Staff must be trained on day-to-day routine care of each device, and plans must be made for how inevitable repairs and preventive maintenance will be handled. In addition to freelance or health system-based biomedical technicians, who offer laser repair services, many companies offer extended warranties and service contracts. These vary widely in terms of cost and duration, and this issue must be fully addressed at the time of purchase or lease (see, Chapter 37).

41.12.4 Step Four: Consider Supplies and Stock

Many energy-based devices are large pieces of equipment—too big to conveniently use in a standard-sized examination room. Therefore, one must choose wisely while planning where to place these systems, and consideration must be given to whether demand and logistics require a dedicated space for these treatments. Beyond the physical space, there are various safety requirements that must be addressed with regard to cosmetic treatments. For example, some laser treatments produce a plume that contains viral particles, necessitating the purchase and use of a smoke evacuator. If light-based treatments are to be offered in a room with windows, protective covers must be purchased and placed. Wavelength-specific goggles are required to protect the eyes of all medical personnel, and patients generally wear special opaque laser eyewear during treatment. In addition, some lasers require nonstandard plugs and power sources which should be taken into consideration when purchasing them.

As noted, neurotoxins and soft tissue fillers are expensive to purchase in large quantities, yet when offering these treatments, it is preferable to have an adequate supply in the clinic at all times. Some manufacturers provide bundled discounts for purchasing both fillers and neurotoxins from the same company; similarly, volume discounts are often available for loyal customers of given brands. It is absolutely worth taking the time to consider the actual after discount costs to the practice in various scenarios. In addition, one should have a clear sense of how quickly, from the time of order, a company is able to replenish your supply. It is, of course, also vital to use products with which you are comfortable from a safety and efficacy standpoint, and most companies are willing to provide samples for you to "test drive" with friends, family, or staff serving as patients.

Cosmetically oriented patients sometimes appreciate or even expect certain amenities beyond their medical care. For example, some patients request access to over-the-counter skin care products. While the efficacy of such products appears to vary greatly, each clinician must consider whether he or she wishes to enter into the retail aspects of aesthetic care.

41.12.5 Step Five: Consider Staffing

While the question of which, if any, cosmetic procedures are appropriate to delegate to other staff is beyond the scope of this discussion, state rules vary with respect to regulation of this issue. Physicians must be aware of the state laws governing their practice. Regardless, patients undergoing cosmetic treatments frequently expect a high-level of personalized service, including those offered during procedures, and the ability to quickly and easily reach staff with any questions about pre- or post-procedure care. One must consider the adequacy of staffing to support these expectations. Ongoing training related to the practice's devices is critical and may often be accomplished with regular in-service sessions provided by the manufacturer, physician, or other experienced personnel.

With respect to finances, aesthetic services are, of course, an out-of-pocket expense for patients, and they must know up front about the practice's fees and collection policies. Many physicians prefer not to address the financial details with patients, so the practice must develop a system whereby designated individuals discuss pricing with prospective cosmetic patients prior to patient scheduling for treatment.

41.12.6 Step Six: Consider Advertising

Broadly speaking, advertising simply signifies methods to raise awareness of services among potential patients. Often this may be as simple as flyers in the reception area, email blasts to established patients, or, perhaps most ideally, via word-of-mouth. Increasingly, an online presence in the form of a user-friendly website, search engine optimization, and, perhaps, social media outlets has become common for cosmetically focused practices. While a full discussion of such options is beyond the scope of this chapter, it is important to consider the degree to which you are or are not comfortable with advertising your practice. If you do pursue standard advertising methods, remember that each contact with the public is a reflection on the practice and on the physician himself or herself, so it is recommended that all advertising materials be reviewed and approved by the physician. Advertising can be very expensive and a substantial commitment of financial and staff resources is necessary for it to be productive.

41.13 Conclusion

Beginning your practice is a significant undertaking, but do not be discouraged. Most of the standard dermatologic care and procedures can still be performed without spending an exorbitant amount of money. You must be prepared to efficiently and safely provide the care your patient requires from day one, but you can always add additional and more specialized services, as your patient base and their needs expand. We always stress that it is best to buy the highest quality instruments or equipment that you require.

42 Essential Stock for Cosmetic Procedures: How to Determine What to Carry, and Control Inventory and Costs

Elizabeth L. Tanzi MD

Abstract

Embarking on a new dermatology practice is an exciting, yet potentially daunting endeavor. If cosmetic procedures will be offered, it is helpful to develop a thorough list of necessary items to deliver the most popular services while minimizing waste. Careful attention to a camera system, pain management, small items needed for procedures and larger device purchases is the foundation of the list. Creating a comprehensive list of essential stock is time-consuming, but it is an important task for a successful launch of a new dermatology practice.

Keywords: essential inventory, photography system, vascular occlusion kit, device consumables

Top 10 Things You Need to Know

1. Beyond large items such as surgical chairs and medical lights, a master list of smaller items that are necessary for the delivery of cosmetic procedures is useful when stocking a new office.
2. A quality camera system is indispensable.
3. A smoke evacuator and good ventilation system are mandatory requirements for any procedure that generates a plume.
4. Appropriate pain management is paramount for a successful cosmetic practice.
5. Although low-tech, electrosurgery and cryotherapy are excellent treatments for many common cosmetic concerns.
6. As injectables are the cornerstone of any cosmetic dermatology practice, a readily available, well-stocked vascular occlusion kit and well-defined protocol are essential.
7. Consider ancillary costs of lasers and devices such as consumables and maintenance contracts when calculating overall costs to the practice of device-based procedures.
8. The "best" device to purchase is based on individual practice needs; consider those devices that compliment treatments already offered (such as laser skin resurfacing if injectables are already part of the practice).
9. Add devices based on practice needs, not flashy marketing or trends dictated by industry.
10. A well-curated offering of medical-grade skin care products can complement in-office procedures and enhance patient satisfaction.

42.1 Introduction

Dermatologists embarking on a cosmetic practice, either initially after residency or as a new venture after years as an established general dermatologist, face numerous challenges. Initial capital costs, finding and securing a favorable office location, furnishing and staffing the practice, regulatory concerns, information technology and marketing decisions are but a few major considerations at the outset. For inventory, beyond medical chairs and surgical lights, an autoclave, waste management, sharps removal and linen services, there are hundreds of smaller items that are necessary to obtain prior to offering cosmetic services. It is useful to have a thoughtful list of these small items to purchase in order to be efficient when stocking a new office (▶ Box 42.1). The goal of this chapter is to provide a rough outline of essential inventory to establish a nonsurgical cosmetic practice that is able deliver many of the most popular services as requested by patients. Services including benign lesion removal, injectable neurotoxin and dermal fillers, chemical peels, microneedling, laser- and energy-based treatments, and skin care recommendations are among the most popular.

In general, there are a few universal requirements for the best implementation and delivery of

Box 42.1 Author's list of small supplies

Kenalog 10 mg/mL
Kenalog 40 mg/mL
5-Fluorouracil 50 mg/mL (if applicable)
Lidocaine 1%
Lidocaine 1% w/epi
Lidocaine 2%
Lidocaine 2% w/epi
Bacteriostatic water (30 mL)
Bacteriostatic NaCl 0.9% (30 mL)
8.4% Sodium bicarbonate (50 mL)
NaCl for irrigation (1, 000 mL)
Sterile water (10 mL)
Bandaid 1 × 3 inch
Bandaid 2 × 4.5 inch
Coverlet spot bandaids
Telfa pads 3 × 4 inch
Liquid Bandaid
Kerlex Bandage roll
Ultra-gauze sponges 4 × 4 inch
Ultra-gauze sponges 2 × 2 inch
Tongue depressors
Cotton-tipped applicators
Transpore surgical tape
Paper surgical tape
Webcol alcohol preps
Chux underpads
Scrim examination towels/drapes
Disposable razors
Disposable paper bikinis
Disposable paper bras
Disposable male boxers
Sanicloth germicidal wipes
Lens/laser wipes
Disposable ice packs
Isopropyl rubbing alcohol
Aquaphor healing ointment
Mupirocin ointment
Proparacain ophthalmic solution
Aquasonic ultrasound gel
Triamcinolone 0.1% cream
Latex examination gloves (small and medium)
Latex-free examination gloves (small and medium)
Dermablades
Disposable curettes
Disposable #11 surgical blades
Disposable #15 surgical blades
Mastisol vials
Steri-strips

4.0 Ethicon black sutures
5.0 Ethicon black sutures
6.0 Ethicon black sutures
4.0 Vicryl sutures
5.0 Vicryl sutures
6.0 Vicryl sutures
Forceps with teeth
Forceps without teeth
Gradle scissors
Iris scissors
Comedone extractors
Needle holder
Blade holder
Benadryl-generic 25 mg
Ibuprofen 800 mg tabs
Tylenol 500 mg tabs
Benocaine oral gel
Betadine surgical scrub
Sterile gloves sizes 6, 6.5, 7, 7.5, and 8
Sterile table cover
Sterile drapes (fenestrated and nonfenestrated)
Curity sterile 4 × 4 gauze
Laser plume masks
Needles 18 gauge 1 ½ inch
Needles 20 gauge 1 ½ inch
Needles 25 gauge 5/8 inch
Needles 25 gauge 1 ½ inch
Needles 27 gauge 1 ¼ inch
Needles 27 gauge ½ inch
Needles 30 gauge ½ inch
Subcision needle 18 gauge x 1 ½ inch Nokor
Dermasculpt 25 gauge 1 ½ inch cannula
Dermasculpt 27 gauge 1 ½ inch cannula
TSK 25 gauge 1 ½ inch cannula
TSK 27 gauge 1 ½ inch cannula
Syringe 30 mL
Syringe 1 mL
Syringe 3 mL
Luer-lock syringe 1 mL
Luer-lock syringe 3 mL
Disposable biopsy punch 2 mm
Disposable biopsy punch 3 mm
Disposable biopsy punch 4 mm
Disposable biopsy punch 5 mm
Sterile indicators for autoclave
Sterilizing pouches 3.5 × 5.25 inch
Sterilizing pouches 3.5 × 9 inch
Sterilizing pouches 9"x 15"
Sterilizing pouches 5 ¼ × 10 inch

(Continued)

Box 42.1 Author's list of small supplies (*Continued*)

Maxitest spore culture tests
Autoclave cleaner
Cidex plus sterilization solution
Cidex plus test strips
Cidex OPA
Hibiclens
Acetone
Chemical spill kit
Mayo stand
Sharps container (small and large)
White ointment jars (small and large)
Plastic eye shields (small, medium and large)
Metal eye shields (small, medium and large)
Suction cups to remove metal eye shields

Aluminum chloride
Electrolase blunt blades (for electrodesiccation)
Skylar Instrument soak
TCA 20%
TCA 25%
TCA 90% (for CROSS method)
Compression hose (if sclerotherapy is performed)
Buffalo filters (for any device that creates a plume)
Ice masks (full face and eyes)
Disposable red fluid connectors (to mix dermal fillers, if applicable)

Note: Quantities of some listed items are dependent on the number of practicing physicians and the number of rooms that need to be stocked.

cosmetic treatments. An established photography system with good lighting to allow the capture of reproduceable baseline and follow-up photos is essential for all cosmetic procedures. Not only is a good camera system indispensable for medical–legal purposes, but good clinical photos also help guide future treatment recommendations. Several cosmetic treatments such as electrosurgery, ablative laser resurfacing, laser tattoo removal, and laser hair removal create ultrafine particles in the plume generated during treatment. Potentially harmful chemicals are released when tissue is vaporized during these treatments; therefore, the plume should be considered a biohazard. Therefore, a smoke evacuator, good ventilation system, and proper respiratory protection with masks is mandatory for a cosmetic practice performing these procedures.[1]

Smaller items such as disposable headbands and robes allow for full visualization of areas during treatments. Washable, salon-quality robes are preferable to paper disposable robes, as they allow the patient more modesty and create a more aesthetic (rather than medical) experience. Likewise, washable blankets for each room are appreciated by patients as they await their treatments. Handheld mirrors are important to allow patients to identify their areas of concern. Ice application prior to and after injectables or laser treatments is helpful. Cost of disposable ice packs can be kept to a minimum by using ice cubes in a single 4 × 4 inch gauze for use during and after treatment.

Management of pain during procedures warrants special consideration. As the tolerance for pain varies between patients, do not assume patients are "overly sensitive" when they articulate discomfort. The negative connotation between many cosmetic procedures and the pain associated with them can have significant impact on the bottom line of the practice if not managed adequately. It is well known that although patients may desire certain cosmetic procedures such as injectables and laser resurfacing, they may be unwilling to commit to a procedure (or return for a second treatment) if there is pain involved. Therefore, proper pain management is paramount for a successful cosmetic practice. Beyond commercially available 4% topical lidocaine preparations, many practices purchase customized topical anesthesia through a compounding pharmacy. Higher percentage lidocaine ointment (up to 30%) or betacaine–lidocaine mixtures can provide more comfort to patients during procedures. However, customized topical anesthesia products are expensive, so consider regular comparing prices between compounding pharmacies. Although customized anesthesia can add a considerable expense to the practice, in the authors' opinion the cost is justified, as even a single lost or dissatisfied patient due to inadequate pain management is likely to eclipse the cost of the topical anesthesia. With customized anesthesia products, caution is warranted as excessive application to large treatment areas by improperly trained staff can lead to lidocaine toxicity. Other helpful tactics to improve patient comfort that add little or no additional expense to the practice include a slow and steady injection technique, talking to patients during each step of the treatment to lessen anxiety (particularly during laser procedures where eyes will be covered), distraction by using a small vibratory device applied to an area adjacent to the treatment area, and fanning the patient during treatment.

42.2 Benign Lesion Removal

Seborrheic keratoses, sebaceous hyperplasia, skin tags and other small, benign lesions are very common cosmetic concerns. Excellent cosmetic results can be obtained for many of these common concerns with either cryotherapy or electrosurgery. For cryotherapy, the costs can be kept to a minimum with little wasted liquid nitrogen by using a Styrofoam cup and cotton-tipped applicator. However, a cryogen-can delivery device is best to improve efficiency when treating a large number of lesions. Electrosurgery is an extremely useful tool in a cosmetic practice, as it can treat many common, unwanted skin growths and be combined with other treatments such as laser skin resurfacing or chemical peels on the same visit. Although the initial and operating cost of a hyfrecator unit is relatively low, cost to purchase and maintain a plume evacuation system must be factored into the overall costs.

42.3 Injectables

Injectable neurotoxin and dermal fillers are the cornerstone of any cosmetic dermatology practice. Injectables are becoming increasingly popular for rejuvenation and soft tissue augmentation. Other than a dedicated refrigerator for medications, insulin or regular 1 mL syringes and 30 gauge needles, the delivery of neurotoxins requires little else. However, a well-trained staff experienced in the reconstitution and handling of neurotoxins is important to minimize risk to the patient and loss to the practice via over-delivery of product or spillage. When offering soft tissue augmentation with hyaluronic acid gel (HAG), calcium hydroxyapatite, or poly-L lactic acid products, there are additional technique and safety concerns to consider. Achievement of desired cosmetic outcomes is largely dependent on technique, appropriate filler product based on the indication, and thoughtful approach to treatment. Furthermore, preferred techniques for placement through cannula or needle (or a combination of both depending on facial area) will vary among injectors. Variability in preferred technique and filler selection is common among dermatologists and these considerations are well beyond the scope of this discussion. However, a thorough understanding of anatomy, side effects, and complications is crucial to all dermatologists who perform soft tissue augmentation to optimize clinical outcomes and safety with dermal fillers. Hyaluronidase can be used to dissolve HAG fillers and reverse undesired outcomes such as nodules, asymmetry, and over-correction.[2] Reversibility of HAG's by hyaluronidase has also proven effective for severe complications of vascular occlusion due to compression or embolization.[3,4] As the most serious vascular occlusion complications such as impending tissue necrosis and visual compromise require immediate treatment for the best possible outcome for the patient, a readily available, well-stocked vascular occlusion kit and defined protocol is essential in any cosmetic practice that injects facial dermal fillers (▶Box 42.2). Hyaluronidase has a relatively short shelf life; therefore, expiration dates should be checked routinely to ensure the emergency kit is up-to-date.

42.4 Chemical Peels

Chemical peeling agents have been the mainstay of a cosmetic dermatology practice for decades. Low in cost and versatile, a series of chemical peels can effectively treat early photodamage, melasma, and acne. There are several commercially available chemical peels that typically blend a mixture of lactic acid, salicylic acid, resorcinol, and retinoic acid. These superficial peeling combinations are simple to administer with no neutralization required and little downtime for the patient. However, the ease of use is offset by increased cost to the practice, as these chemical peel kits are more expensive than simple glycolic acid solutions. Medium-depth peeling agents include Trichloroacetic acid and Jessner's formulations. For little cost, medium-depth peels can deliver more impressive results; however, they require more training for the dermatologist to deliver optimal results with few side effects and incur additional recovery time for the patient.

Box 42.2 Dermal filler emergency protocol

If vascular compromise is suspected, immediately initiate the following:

- Discontinue injection and ice application
- Injection of hyaluronidase (roughly 10–30 units per 0.1 mL of HA injected) with repeat injection, as required for severe vascular compromise
- Give patient aspirin 325 mg po x 1
- Massage and warm treatment area to promote blood flow
- Nitroglycerin paste: after obtaining baseline blood pressure reading, apply ½ to 1 inch of paste to the affected area with massage; observe for headache and/or blood pressure changes (Note: not all patients will require or benefit from nitroglycerin paste; therefore, clinical correlation is required)
- If the above protocol does not result in improvement of vascular compromise, consider hyperbaric oxygen treatments (#xxx-xxx-xxxx)

If there are signs or symptoms of visual and/or neurologic change:

- Injecting physician to alert the staff to an emergency situation in order to secure the help of a registered nurse, medical assistant, and administrative assistant
- Physician to quickly access visual acuity, visual fields, and pupillary reactivity
- Cursory neurologic evaluation including bilateral strength assessment
- Staff to call and text local ophthalmologist (mobile #xxx-xxx-xxxx) to notify of arrival and assist in transferring patient to their practice with retrobulbar hyaluronidase kit that includes hyaluronidase (2,000 units to be available in office at all times), 27 gauge 1 ½ inch needles and 3 mL syringe. Consider ocular massage en route to the ophthalmologist
- Inject high-dose hyaluronidase throughout treatment area (while waiting for, not in lieu of, ophthalmology consultation)
- If applicable, contact stroke team (xxxxxx Hospital Stroke Team at #xxx-xxx-xxxx) and arrange for transportation to the ER

42.5 Microneedling

Microneedling offers an effective, inexpensive option for a variety of indications such as aging skin, atrophic scars, and surgical scars. Microneedling procedures are satisfying to patients due to minimal downtime and a relatively small amount of discomfort. For physicians, microneedling represents an economical option for the practice, as the devices and disposable tips are far less costly than laser- or energy-based devices. A series of treatments are required for the best cosmetic response, with additional treatments on a regular basis to maintain the results. Microneedling is particularly helpful when treating skin of color, as the incidence of post-inflammatory hyperpigmentation is lower than when using laser- and light-based devices to stimulate neocollagenesis. However, in the authors' experience, microneedling techniques have yet to consistently deliver the impressive clinical results seen after fractional or fully-ablative laser skin resurfacing for scars, photodamage, and aging skin.

42.6 Cosmetic Devices

A solid noninvasive cosmetic dermatology practice can be initiated with a few basic services such as injectable neurotoxins and dermal fillers, cryotherapy, electrosurgery, chemical peels, and microneedling. However, in order to deliver a comprehensive selection of nonsurgical cosmetic services, laser- and energy-based cosmetic devices are required. There are many factors beyond the initial capital cost of the device to keep in mind when considering such a large expenditure for the practice. Consumable treatment tips and pricey maintenance contracts must be factored into the overall "cost" of acquiring a new device. Do not be afraid to ask for a reduction in maintenance contracts or free treatment tips when negotiating for a new device. If the practice is considering the purchase of several devices concurrently, a company may be incentivized to "bundle" their technology together to offer a lower cost option. Finally, there are several good financing options available if purchasing a device outright is not feasible. Laser and cosmetic device companies often have good financing partners for support.

Although the discussion of the "best" laser to purchase is beyond the scope of this chapter and dependent on the unique patient population of each practice, in general, give the highest consideration to those devices that compliment treatments already offered. For example, laser skin resurfacing and broadband light treatments will address many of the signs of photodamaged skin and work together with injectables to deliver more impressive antiaging results. In the authors' experience, the three most utilized devices include a nonablative fractional resurfacing laser and broadband light source to address photodamage and lentigines, and a pulsed dye laser for the treatment of telangiectasia and rosacea. Beyond these well-established devices, each subsequent decision to bring on new technology should be based on a thoughtful and realistic review of the practice patient population, cosmetic needs, sustainable goals, and the support (such as additional staff, marketing, space) that is required to make the additional device a financial success. Adding devices to a practice based on the relative popularity of common cosmetic procedures, rather than the hottest new "toy" based on industry marketing, is a sound strategy. For example, the addition of a nonsurgical body contouring device is likely to be more successful in a dermatology office than a tattoo removal laser, based on procedural surveys.[5]

42.7 Skin Care

A thoughtful and well-curated offering of medical grade skin care products can complement in-office procedures to increase both patient and physician satisfaction. At the very minimum, quality sunscreen with excellent cosmetic properties are appreciated by cosmetically minded patients. Beyond sunscreen, skin care does not have to be complicated to be effective for the vast majority of cosmetic concerns. With little capital outlay and a small amount of storage space, an initial order can include a retinol, glycolic acid cream, anti-oxidant serum, and moisturizer that supports the protective barrier of the skin. Growth-factor serums, peptide lotions, and sulfur-containing products also top the list of popular skin care products. As many patients already have a few favorite products in their routine, a thoughtful product recommendation to help improve their current regimen is usually appreciated. Consider dispensing both self-labeled skin care and well-established, physician-only skin care lines to deliver a truly customized approach to each patient.

References

[1] Chuang GS, Farinelli W, Christiani DC, Herrick RF, Lee NC, Avram MM. Gaseous and particulate content of laser hair removal plume. JAMA Dermatol 2016;152(12):1320–1326

[2] Sclafani AP, Fagien S. Treatment of injectable soft tissue filler complications. Dermatol Surg 2009;35(Suppl 2):1672–1680

[3] Chesnut C. Restoration of visual loss with retrobulbar hyaluronidase injection after hyaluronic acid filler. Dermatol Surg 2018;44(3):435–437

[4] Fagien S, Carruthers J. Commentary on restoration of visual loss with retrobulbar hyaluronidase injection after hyaluronic acid filler. Dermatol Surg 2018;44(3):437–443

[5] The American Society of Dermatologic Surgery. 2017 Survey on Dermatologic Procedures. Data Bank Statistics;2018

43 What Devices Does Your Practice Need?

Jordan V. Wang MD, MBE, MBA; Nazanin Saedi MD

Abstract

Determining which devices your practice needs can be an important, yet complex, decision for many aesthetic practitioners. This often depends on the needs of the patients and local market, level of training of yourself and staff, space and finance of the clinic, and how established and equipped the clinic is. This chapter will help to guide aesthetic practitioners when making this decision.

Keywords: aesthetics, business, dermatology, lasers, medical devices

Top 10 Things You Need to Know

1. Perform your market research: Evaluate your personal skillset, consumer demand, and competitive opportunities prior to purchasing new devices or offering new procedures.
2. Decide if you should rent, lease, or buy: Know the terms offered for each option and perform break-even analysis to predict future profitability.
3. Determine if used or new devices are right for you: Purchasing used or demonstration devices can be more affordable, but ensure they come with a warranty and service contract from the device company.
4. Purchase at the right time: Prices may be more negotiable near the end of quarter or end of fiscal year due to quotas and the need to unload inventory.
5. Search for your best financing options: Compare the rates available to you, including from the device company, local or national banks, and online lenders.
6. Understand the profitability of your devices: Know the overhead, profit margin, break-even point, and time demand for each device to better determine its profitability.
7. Build working relationships with your device companies: Befriending company representatives can lead to increased access, discounted equipment, speaking engagements, and offers for new, cutting-edge products.
8. Master your devices and develop your own niche: Recognize all of the conditions that your devices can treat and master them prior to purchasing other devices that can treat the same conditions.
9. Familiarize yourself with your own limits: Avoid purchasing devices or offering procedures that you feel uncomfortable with in relation to personal skillset, equipment, clinic space, or staff training.
10. Grow your practice slowly and steadily: Master your devices one at a time before jumping in to purchase new devices all at once in order to prevent overextending yourself.

43.1 Introduction

Over the past several years, the field of dermatology has flourished. In particular, dermatologic and cosmetic surgery have experienced exponential growth with regard to both volume and variety. What had originally started as a small subspecialty based on the surgical treatment of skin cancers, has now expanded to encompass an assortment of procedures, including neuromodulators, soft-tissue fillers, lasers and light-based devices, and energy-based devices for body contouring and skin tightening. The list continues to grow with each passing year as new devices are brought to the market.

According to the American Society for Dermatologic Surgery (ASDS), members performed nearly 12 million procedures in 2017 alone, which increased from 7.8 million in the previous year.[1] The top procedures were skin cancer treatments, injectable neuromodulators and soft-tissue fillers, and laser, light, or energy-based procedures. In the last six years, there was a 79% increase in soft-tissue filler treatments, 63% increase in laser, light, or energy-based procedures, and a nearly 300% increase in body contouring.[1] Consumers also voted dermatologists as the top physician of choice for many of these procedures.

Due to the large variety of devices, it is important for clinicians to understand which ones are essential to his/her practice. Whether starting a new practice or joining an existing one, this information is beneficial to operating a successful business.

43.2 Market Analysis

Prior to purchasing new medical devices or offering new surgical procedures, clinicians should take the necessary time to thoroughly evaluate the current market that they are working in. This can allow for adequate research and planning, proper prediction of demand and estimation of profitability, comprehensive evaluation of competition and saturation in the marketplace, and sound decision-making. Preparation is essential in order to avoid any impulsive purchases and potentially extending yourself in terms of time, space and, perhaps most of all, budget. This is the most crucial step for any important business decision and can ensure highly profitable, marketable, excellent quality, and safe care for patients and consumers alike. The three key components to consider are your personal skillset, consumer demand, and competitive opportunities (▶Fig. 43.1).

43.2.1 Personal Skillset

Your personal skillset is the most important of the components, since it will be you who will be performing or overseeing the procedures. This should account for your comfort level with various

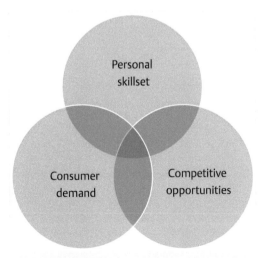

Fig. 43.1 Three key components to consider when analyzing the local aesthetic market.

procedures in addition to your already established abilities. Practitioners should never feel forced, enticed, or coerced to offer a procedure that they feel uncomfortable or unsafe performing. Of course, skillsets are dynamic and can evolve with additional experience and training. Over time, clinicians may feel more prepared to trial advanced techniques or experiment with newer devices. However, early on, it may be best to stay within your own comfort zone as your practice and confidence builds.

43.2.2 Consumer Demand

Consumer demand should be carefully studied prior to the purchase of any device. While a new device may seem trendy and in vogue, either from persuasive marketing material provided by the company or on social media, it may be unwise to make such a purchase if there is simply no local demand. It would not be financially prudent if it remains unused, occupying space in the clinic that could be utilized by a more profitable device. Performing consumer research can easily be accomplished by surveying your own patients either in person, through email, or on social media. This can ensure that you capture your own local demand and not that of a geographic market located hundreds or even thousands of miles away. Staying in touch with the needs of your local market's consumers is critical to your clinic's successful operation.

43.2.3 Competitive Opportunities

Uncovering competitive opportunities can help your office emerge as a leader in your local market. Searching for procedures that are high in demand is only the tip of the iceberg. Determining which devices competing practices own and which procedures they offer plays a substantial role in influencing your business decisions and, subsequently, your bottom line. It may be imprudent to purchase an expensive device that is only modestly demanded if many other local practices offer the identical service and are performing it well. Finding underexploited demand can make your practice more competitive in the marketplace. You should strive to create a targeted and in-demand niche.

43.3 Purchasing Timeline

The decision to purchase new equipment for your clinic can be an arduous task, but it can be rewarding if done properly. It is important to take your time and make the correct decisions in the beginning. A poor decision can set you back financially for an extended period, depending on how ownership and payment of the device are structured. Purchasing the right device at the right time can make a world of difference. Appropriate planning and preparation can help to avoid acquiring the wrong device for your clinic in terms of patient demand, scheduling availability, clinic space, overhead costs, and level of staff training.

43.3.1 Early On

Early on, the best devices to purchase are those that have stood the test of time (▶ Fig. 43.2). They have long-term safety data readily available and a proven track record of success. This can help in maintaining a high-level of patient satisfaction as your business and reputation grow. The devices should ideally provide in-demand treatments and serve multiple purposes in terms of having the ability to treat various conditions. This can avoid the need to purchase multiple devices and potentially overextending yourself financially. Just be sure that you are not sacrificing quality for efficiency, convenience, and cost. Some devices that do a bit of everything, do not do anything particularly well. Low-cost devices should also garner special attention. For example, purchasing an inexpensive microneedling device may prove to be profitable with low upfront costs and high return.

Two of the most versatile devices that should be considered when starting out are the intense pulsed light (IPL) device and the pulsed dye laser (PDL). Each can be used to treat a variety of skin conditions and together can treat many basic cosmetic concerns. IPL, the most versatile technology in cosmetic dermatology, can be used to treat small vessels, facial redness, rosacea, vascular lesions, dyschromia, pigmented lesions, unwanted hair, and acne. The unit serves as the main power source, while specialized handpieces are utilized for various treatments. Additional handpieces that treat skin texture and scars can also be added to most of the sophisticated IPL systems.

The PDL can be used to treat a variety of vascular lesions, facial redness, rosacea, erythema and texture of scars, epidermal pigmented lesions such as lentigines, verrucae, and psoriasis. Vascular lesions can include hemangiomas, telangiectasias, and port-wine stains. Both devices offer the treatment of a broad range of common dermatologic conditions. If cost is an issue, practitioners may choose to purchase the IPL first due to its broader range of treatments and versatility. However, it is also important to note that other available inexpensive options exist to treat some pigmentary disorders, such as chemical peels.

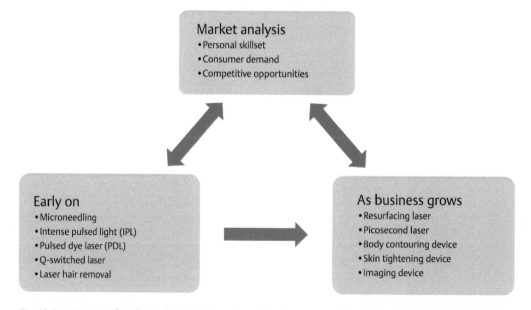

Fig. 43.2 Integration of market analysis for determining which devices to purchase both early on and as business grows.

Another consideration is the Q-switched lasers. They can be used to treat pigmented epidermal and dermal lesions, dyschromia, some vascular lesions, tattoos, and even onychomycosis. While most laser and light hair removal is now done in non-medical facilities and more tattoos are going that same route, patients still seek expert treatment from dermatologists for both of these conditions. This is especially true if they have had poor experiences previously, experienced untoward side effects from these other settings, or encounter a less than straightforward issue.

43.3.2 As Business Grows

As business grows, you may find that you are already maximizing your current devices and are now in the market for newer ones (▶Fig. 43.2). In order to determine which devices may be the best fit, you should again perform market analysis with specific interest in which treatments your own patients are either asking for or would benefit from. It is often easiest to survey your own patient population. What do they routinely ask of you that you and your practice do not provide? You may also find that newer technology has become available or trendier treatments have become popular. If this is the case, be sure to properly vet the devices to ensure that they will still be heavily favored and utilized in the future as well as the present.

Resurfacing lasers are an ideal purchase when expanding your collection of devices. They can include non-ablative fractionated lasers, which can treat acne scars, fine lines and wrinkles, various surgical and traumatic scars, striae, and some forms of hyperpigmentation. They have a proven track record with predictable results and minimal downtime. While they may be more expensive than some of the other devices, they can be frequently utilized in the right patient population.

Newer picosecond lasers are helpful in treating pigmented lesions and tattoos. They have been shown to be more efficacious for tattoo removal than traditional nanosecond pulse duration Q-switched lasers due to shorter pulse durations. They have also been used for photorejuvenation and the treatment of acne scarring and slight textural imperfections, which further expands their use. However, picosecond lasers may not be as versatile as other devices, which can limit their overall utility.

Non-surgical treatment options have experienced a recent surge in demand by consumers. Two burgeoning areas are non-invasive body contouring and skin tightening. In terms of body contouring and fat reduction, cryolipolysis first became popular, while devices using laser light, ultrasound, and radiofrequency energy are gaining more traction. While each has their own nuances, treatments have overall demonstrated moderate efficacy in the right patients. These procedures offer little to no downtime with minimal risks and can be delegated to nurses or other allied health personnel in the dermatology office (depending on the state in which you practice). Non-surgical skin tightening can be performed with unipolar radiofrequency and microfocused ultrasound. Non-downtime procedures that are also frequently delegated by the dermatologist are worth considering as you expand your practice offerings.

Finally, good photography is essential to the cosmetic practice. More devices have become available that offer imaging systems. These can be used to take before and after photographs and also serve the purpose of pre- and posttreatment analysis to aid in patient discussion. The technology has advanced and led to the development of both two-dimensional and three-dimensional models that can quantify cosmetic concerns, such as rhytides, pigmentation, erythema, and scars. While these devices are helpful, they may not add significant upfront revenue to your practice.

43.4 Financial Considerations

When purchasing a new device, be sure to perform your due diligence regarding its financial impact. The first things to consider are its price and purchasing terms. While devices can be expensive, they can occasionally be cheaper when purchased near the end of quarter or end of fiscal year due to quotas from the company and their need to unload inventory. Always consider the different terms between renting, leasing, and buying, especially leasing with the intent to own. Know the terms for each option and perform break-even analysis and calculations for return on investment to predict future profitability. This is described elsewhere in another chapter. Be sure to shop around at local or national banks and even online lenders, since terms may be lower than those offered directly by the device company. If your practice has an open loan from a bank for capital expenditures, consider extending this, rather than opening a new account or switching lenders.

Another consideration is the comparison between used and new devices. Used devices can be more affordable, but it is best to find those that come with both a warranty and service contract from the company. Maintenance of devices can be costly, and no one knows its nuances better than its own company, which should trump any discounts a third-party may offer as enticement. Negotiations for service contracts are different for each company. A service contract can cost upward of $10,000 to $15,000. Practitioners can often negotiate with consumables such as tips for the lasers. For older devices that are no longer in use, companies can often buy them back or offer credit to be used toward the purchase of newer devices.

The final consideration is the financial analysis of the device. For each device, you should know the overhead, profit margin, break-even point, return on investment, and time demand to determine its profitability. Some procedures naturally take longer to perform, so it would be reasonable to calculate its amount of profit per unit of time and compare this to other devices.

Reference

[1] American society for Dermatologic Surgery. https://www.asds.net/Medical-Professionals/Practice-Resources/ASDS-Survey-on-Dermatologic-Procedures. Accessed on December 1, 2018

44 Loyalty and VIP Programs

Daniel I. Schlessinger MD, Joel Schlessinger MD, FAAD

Abstract

Loyalty reflects on the success of a medical practice. There are numerous ways to accrue and reward loyalty, and these are discussed below.

Loyalty is earned via reputation and a patient's personal experience over time. It is important to work with all staff members to ensure patient satisfactory. To reward patients for loyalty to a medical practice, a variety of "programs" may be employed, including but not limited to: gift certificates, discounted products or procedures, or exclusive events. Although insurance-based rules often restrict medical patients from being rewarded for procedures which are covered by insurance, these patients can serve as important referrals for cosmetic patients who can participate in loyalty programs. Before starting a loyalty program, it may be important to work with an attorney to set the terms and conditions and ensure that the loyalty program is ethical and compliant with the Health Insurance Portability and Accountability Act (HIPAA).

Keywords: business, loyalty programs, VIP programs

Top 10 Things You Need to Know

1. Loyalty isn't bought, it is earned.
2. Look for opportunities to partner with cosmetic companies, but don't always trust them to keep your data or patient relationships secure. They may co-market other cosmetic procedures or practices to your patients once they are involved.
3. There isn't one perfect time to start a program, but it is important to consider what you might wish to do from the beginning of your practice and carefully manage data accordingly.
4. Data on these patients is crucial to keep safe. Lists are power and the loss or sharing of these lists could entail huge ramifications.
5. Staff can make or break a loyalty program and must be on board with the concepts.
6. Loyalty programs can be built around any number of procedures or product sales.
7. VIP patients are very heterogeneous. Realizing this early may allow you to cultivate either low- or high-maintenance patients.
8. Events can be beneficial or detrimental to a steady-paced stream of cosmetic patients; while fun, they can also train patients to purchase only at that time of the year.
9. Consider checking with an excellent attorney before starting any loyalty or VIP program in order to save yourself from potential legal and "lost property" problems in the future.
10. Don't focus on the nuts and bolts of loyalty as much as the nuts and bolts of running a successful practice and having fun while doing so. The rest will come naturally.

44.1 Introduction

Like trust, loyalty cannot be bought—it must be earned.

Before any attempt to explain and illuminate loyalty programs, it is essential to define "loyalty" in the context of any and all practices. Although it is important to have adequate customers to make a loyalty program worthwhile, which may be something that a smaller or beginning practice wouldn't even initially think about, loyalty is something that should be considered from the moment you "hang your shingle." We would argue it is the most important business aspect of your entire practice.

Loyalty reflects on the success of your practice and is an instantaneous measure of you, your staff, your environment, your marketing, and every other soft or hard measure of the overall feeling your current and prospective patients have about your practice. Although counterintuitive, loyalty can be accrued without ever having touched the product and this accrual often occurs via reputation. For example, consider the countless fans who are deeply loyal to sports teams whose games they have never attended. The same reality applies to dermatology: reputation directly correlates with loyalty (and trust) of a practice, and the ambassadors (you, your staff, patients, and vendors) impact the "word on the street" about you and your practice. This is why the term "loyalty program" is clearly about more than simply crafting a set of rules and a card or Internet-based "program."

Imagine a loyalty program for a brand that clearly doesn't value the customer– consider one of the no-frills, no customer service airlines, or one of the many now extinct car companies that delivered shoddy products. Such a loyalty program would be laughable, if not oxymoronic. The same could be stated about a loyalty program for a dermatology practice without a patient-centric culture. For the purposes of this article, we will assume that you pride yourself on hiring only friendly and caring staff; that you care deeply if a patient has an issue with the front desk or billing department (or *even* yourself); and that patient satisfaction is paramount. It simply isn't worth creating one of these programs if the concept of quality and patient satisfaction isn't already part of your practice paradigm. If those descriptors don't apply to your practice, you need more than a loyalty program. Although it is outside the scope of this article, you may want to consider a revamp of your practice and/or staff to achieve the ability to go to the next step: a loyalty program-ready practice.

Each loyalty program should reflect the nature of the practice and the level of complexity of the practice. For reasons that are elaborated later, most programs are based on cosmetic-related services. As a rule, when starting out, if you are offering only one procedure (e.g., neurotoxins and/or fillers), your loyalty program will be built around that one procedure (in this case, injectables). As your practice grows, you will probably incorporate other procedures, so it is important to be flexible when initially crafting a loyalty program. One way to imagine a loyalty program is via dollars spent in the practice. This could conceivably encompass both medical and cosmetic procedures, but it would normally only apply to cosmetic procedures. Alternatively, a loyalty program could be procedurally-based, with various incentives based on how many times or how many units a particular patient has acquired from the practice. This is particularly common in many medspas and, for this reason, the senior author doesn't use a procedurally-based loyalty program in his practice. The same thing goes for cards or other low-quality instruments such as plastic cards to be attached to keychains. Clearly, this is something that is used by shopping stores and tanning bed shops, but it

doesn't seem to be a "quality" feature. The hallmark of your practice should be quality and its consideration should influence every measure of your program.

In contrast to cosmetic procedures, medical procedures are, too, price-variable, making it difficult to determine the actual reimbursement for the actual procedure and/or visit. In addition, insurance-based rules often restrict patients from being rewarded for procedures which are covered by insurance. It should be noted that the concept of the actual monetary worth of a patient is highly dependent on the availability of accurate data and a willing-and-able billing staff or office manager to continually analyze it. Without careful analysis of trends and utilization of the program, there are few ways to effectively harness new options for patient acquisition and retention. While this isn't essential in order to develop and maintain a loyalty program, it bears significant importance in the practice and should be a part of any sophisticated cosmetic-dermatology practice.

With that being said, medical patients may still be a huge referral source with other benefits that accrue to the practice from their presence. This is why the senior author maintains that every cosmetic dermatologist ought to first and foremost be a medical dermatologist. In the case of the senior author, the medical to cosmetic ratio is 60:40, which, interestingly, has remained constant through more than 25 years of practice.

The question of referrals and whether to "reward" them often arises when considering loyalty programs, because a referral is so very valuable to the practice. The challenge with this is that it may not always be immediately clear that a patient has been referred rather than coming as a *de novo* patient. When greeted with a number of "how did you hear about us?" options on a dropdown menu (e.g., Google, billboards, social media, etc.), people often choose the most expedient referral choice, yet the fact that one single person may have made the difference in their choice of your practice is not noted or given its share of weight. Therefore, the provenance of the new patient in your waiting room is often unclear. In addition, the person in your office may not necessarily want the referring patient to know, and HIPAA rules may be violated by writing the referring patient a simple note saying, "thank you for your kind referral." In times when physician referrals were more common, this was less problematic (as were HIPAA-related concerns), but in certain cases, it may be reasonable to consider a thank you note to the referring patient or doctor. At the very least, make a mental note when significant numbers of patients are referred by one individual person, whether it be a physician or a nonmedical individual. Again, rules have changed significantly, and gifts to physicians or any medical individuals for referrals could be considered illegal. Therefore, the wisest course of action is to thank them and perhaps write a note but not include this in any standard loyalty program.

44.2 Outside Loyalty Programs and How They Relate to You and Your Patients

Several cosmetic companies offer outside loyalty programs. These programs have evolved over several years to often integrate cosmetic products, such as neurotoxins and fillers, alongside other procedures and skincare lines. Both the practice and patients benefit, but the programs don't always single out and maintain uninterrupted connection with the doctor's office that initially enrolled the patient; therefore, patients are free to change practices and might even be encouraged by the program to try other procedures that a particular doctor's office might not offer. This is one unintended consequence of patient enrollment in these programs. On the other hand, there are countless opportunities to interact with the patient that don't come directly from your office, such as a reminder of the need for services or an incentive to obtain such services. In addition, while addresses and emails may change and be unrecorded by your office, this once again allows for a third party to market to the patient and potentially keep a relationship, and the opportunity for future services, alive.

These programs are ubiquitous, and they clearly have their own pros and cons. In the senior author's opinion, the benefits to the patient will always outweigh the risks of extraneous marketing of potential procedures not offered by your office. This wasn't always the case, and there is still a case to be made for going without these programs, but the calculus seems to have changed to be in favor of participation. Unfortunately, these same programs are often used by anyone with a practice and are widely available to medspas and other, noncore specialty offices. This is part of the decision as to whether it is a consideration for your practice.

44.3 VIP Programs

Once your office has obtained a critical number of cosmetic patients, there will be some who are VIP in nature. This doesn't always equate to notoriety or sophistication as much as value to the practice. Most physicians starting out tend to expect that overall wealth correlates with VIP status, but the reality in (at least) the senior author's experience is that the "soccer mom" and everyday nice patient (whether they are a waitress or CEO) is a much better VIP than the demanding, fickle, and mercurial patient who lets you know they are special from the moment they enter the office. Therefore, it is much more rewarding to cultivate and "feed" those patients than the ones who will potentially end up being challenges to you and your staff. Depending on how you react to and "coddle" these higher maintenance patients, you could end up with a clinic full of them, a stressed-out staff, and a less fulfilling daily experience. Choose wisely as you "create" your practice and determine reward structures.

In some practices, VIP patients are given parties and events that range from wine and cheese parties to lavish, all out extravaganzas. Huge dollars are often generated at these events (often touted with questionable veracity by the various companies who produce such events), which usually seem to correlate with the end of the sales representatives' fiscal year. We have never hosted such events, as it is unclear whether the profits gleaned from the events are any more than having well-designed and announced "specials" through the year. Clearly, this approach is able to generate some "buzz," but the flip side is that patients are incentivized to purchase only at the time of an event and save up their purchases for this one season. One season or event does not make a practice and this sort of approach essentially trains your patients via classical conditioning to look to one season for their higher purchases.

A constant discount is both problematic, yet essential, to some practices. It is unfortunately part of our culture in the cosmetic world to "shop" for a better deal due to the other players we compete with on a daily basis. They work off of a discount and our patients have no way of comparing us other than via price.

While quality is a soft measurement, people don't generally suffer deadly consequences from our competitors, so in most peoples' minds it is a fair comparison. Therefore, we have to offer some value proposition.

This can include a free syringe of filler from time to time, a little extra neurotoxin, gifts with visits (GWPs can be obtained from many of the companies that supply our products), or other things. We have the occasional event that offers food, drink, and access to our staff in a more social environment.

Staffing can be a huge determinant. By offering a patient coordinator, you can offer a "white glove" experience that outweighs the other competitors. Having said this, many of our competitors are doing as well as we are, if not better, to offer a delightful experience. This is where we have to excel in the future.

We don't often encourage two visits at the same time as it tends to be messy and challenging from a staffing issue, but when they do occur, we try to offer a little extra to the new patient (e.g., a gift, extra syringe of filler, or more neurotoxin for free). On the other hand, it tends to put us in a difficult situation from the beginning as two people are now in a room together and that alone can slow down the process as one patient has to be taken care of initially and then the changing of the patients and cleaning of the area has to occur. It isn't optimal, but the idea of having two patients instead of one is definitely optimal!

44.4 Ethics and Legality of Loyalty and VIP Programs

It is essential to develop and maintain these programs with the utmost of attention accorded to ethics and legality. Rules in some states may determine how you enroll patients and, in particular, how you must reward them. Gift certificate rules in some states may result in huge payments to patients (or the state) in unclaimed dollars, depending on subtle wording of your rules and regulations. For this reason, it is incumbent on you and your legal team to assure that the verbiage of any such program is carefully scrutinized by an attorney thoroughly versed in this matter. This alone could be the most important lesson in this chapter!

As for the ethics of rewards programs: while unlikely to result in monetary loss, it could lead to a loss in reputation if done incorrectly, which

is much worse! Be careful to consider the implications of your program. Are you doing something that is unethically enticing someone to purchase unnecessary services from your practice? Are you encouraging someone to purchase services as the result of "peer pressure" by friends or other staff? Are you offering alcohol to patients and then asking for a commitment to a series (or any) treatment? All of these situations could be construed as unethical in certain analyses. Be careful and consider checking with your attorney or an impartial and well-intentioned individual about any questionable areas. It could save your practice and your name from a ruinous episode.

Finally, the referral process is also a challenge from the patient privacy and HIPAA perspective. It is extremely important to handle this deftly and with great care as the opportunity for problems occurs immediately, when one person knows that the other person is coming in and they are not family. This can be dealt with, but it is something to be aware of in this situation.

44.5 Conclusion

The end result of loyalty and VIP programs is to craft a practice and sustain a practice. If there is one parting word of wisdom that we can give to the reader, it is to have fun in practice. In many ways, dermatology (in particular, cosmetic dermatology) is more of an avocation than a job. Your advertising, staff approach, and overall practice "vibe" will either lead to overall happiness or misery for you and your staff. Therefore, you should make it something that you actually *want* to do, and be careful whom you attract. Thankfully, you can use loyalty programs to cultivate the sorts of procedures and patients you enjoy spending your day with. While this is intuitive in the context of this chapter, it isn't always immediately obvious when a speaker on a podium encourages a complicated and potentially unsuccessful procedure or approach to a problem and it is quickly (and occasionally disastrously) incorporated into your practice with much ballyhoo. Loyalty programs may either incorporate these procedures or leave them out initially. Be wise and make the right decisions to prepare for happiness.

The following personal anecdotes reflect the senior author's experiences with loyalty and VIP programs.

Personal Anecdote 1

Our first "event" for the practice occurred in 1995. It was centered around a new laser procedure at the time, the full-face CO_2 laser. The practice was fairly new at the time and we had spent a seemingly huge amount, $56,000, on the latest technology and rented a ballroom at the local Marriott for the event. We advertised in newspapers and radio and, with approximately 200 individuals preregistered, we were fully subscribed for the event. On the day of the event, another 100 individuals called to make a reservation, but the hotel didn't have space for more than 200 in the room we had reserved.

This led to the dilemma of whether to add another date, which would have been costly and possibly less successful, or try to add them in somehow. The senior author made the decision to do an "early" and "late" event on the same day. We started the early event at the advertised time of 6 pm and then started the late event at 7:30 pm. This worked out wonderfully, as we were able to serve a group of working individuals at the later time who may not have been able to otherwise attend. In addition, a few attendees who had signed up for the initial earlier time ended up coming to the later event. While the event did not end up converting many of the attendees (most weren't even close to candidates for full-face laser resurfacing), these same individuals remembered us over the years and quite a few became loyal patients. They appreciated the warmth of the staff and the fact that we tried to accommodate their needs instead of turning them away.

Interestingly, we tried this same approach in a hotel in a city 50 miles away from our office a year or so later and received a mediocre response. Not only was the response significantly less than our first event (with similar advertising and preparation), but the results were less impressive both in the short- and long-term. This goes to show that marketing is not always logical, and that repeating a prior successful strategy may produce variable results.

Personal Anecdote 2

When I first started my practice in 1993, the most important asset I could imagine was goodwill = loyalty. This is still the same case with any starting practitioner—goodwill begins at zero when starting your practice and only builds with the proper care and maintenance of your patient base. This is where loyalty begins and ends. A loyalty program as such need not be a card, an app on a computer, or another fancy system, but it must contain some methodology for "appreciating" patients. This is the essence of loyalty and how it builds.

For example, after the first year of my practice, every cosmetic patient was sent a flower and candy on Valentine's Day. These were hand-delivered by our then fledgling staff to the patients' houses. The next year, we did this yet again and it took nearly the whole day for the entire staff during a blinding snowstorm in Omaha, Nebraska, with many wilted roses along the way. The third year, we realized we were unable to cope with the rising number of cosmetic patients in our practice and hired a delivery company. Unfortunately, the company cancelled on us the day before Valentine's day, leaving us to, yet again, hand-deliver both flowers and Godiva Chocolates to every cosmetic patient who had frequented our practice. At this point, we realized that as much as we wanted to reward loyalty in a personal manner, we could no longer do it this way and moved onto a different method of rewarding it.

From that point on, we sent a card in the mail with a discount for future cosmetic services and a special, hand-signed note from the senior author to his patients. Over the years, we have adapted and currently send a gift to all of our cosmetic patients around Thanksgiving, depending on their total yearly spend in the office. Data is easily tabulated with our NexTech billing system. In addition, we include those who have spent significant sums in previous years but who may not have returned to the practice. This is overall a fluid list, and for the past several years, it has been sent to approximately 1,500 to 2,000 of our best patients every year. Various metrics can be used on a yearly basis to determine the point of inclusion in the list, but there are clearly benefits of rewarding individuals who continue to return and refer to your practice.

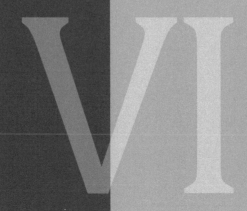

Section VI

Your Image

VI

45 The Most Important Components of a Successful Website

Kavita Mariwalla MD, FAAD

Abstract

A successful dermatology website is dynamic and ever-changing. Those that are successful have a clear look and feel to them extending from color and photos through to the actual design and layout. Most patients these days do not access the entirety of a website but typically visit it for key information like location, phone number and hours of operation. For this reason, it is important to display this prominently on each section of the website. There are basic items every website should have like an "About Us" tab and a section detailing specialties of the practice as well as access to patient forms. If you spend most of your time building this out, your website will be a success. The added components such as a retail store or online bill pay can improve the bottom line of your practice and should be considered as add ons to the site with time.

Keywords: website, URL, search engine optimization, website hosting, patient portal, online patient appointments

Top 10 Things You Need to Know

1. Your website is essential to your practice.
2. On day 1, own two parts of the process: the license for your uniform resource locator (URL) and where the website is being hosted.
3. From the start, know that a website will cost you a few thousand dollars and will entail ongoing expenses to maintain it. Expect this and be prepared for it.
4. Concentrate on your "About Us" tabs, as patients are interested in knowing who they are coming to see before their appointments.
5. Build essential components before adding bells and whistles.
6. Reassess your website, at least, every 6 months to make sure it is updated and reflects new procedures and changes to the practice.
7. A mobile version of your website is *essential*, as most patients access the Internet on a device other than a computer.
8. Highlight your phone number and address on all pages of your website.
9. Cross branding: Pick a color scheme that matches the color scheme and fonts of your office logo and design. Cross pollinate your website with content from your social medial channels.
10. Use your website as a patient education platform and a way for patients to access forms and policies, and potentially message you through a patient portal.

45.1 Introduction

In the age of Internet, it is essential for a practice to have a web presence. "Googling" is the new Yellow Pages and without any web presence, it will seem as if your practice does not exist. The problem with this mandate is that while you may be able to get away with a simple thing like claiming a Google Business listing, most roads lead to operating a practice website which can be a costly endeavor. Several companies that exhibit at national meetings promise to make the creation of a website hassle free for you, but knowing what you *need* versus what you *want* is an important first step.

45.2 Who Are You?

The first part of any successful website is the URL address. In other words, what do I type into my search bar to find you? Ideally, you want to come up with a name that will communicate who you are and what you do. You also need to do this with as short a name as possible, so that patients will be able to remember it.

Is your website going to have the name of your practice or you as an individual? If you work in a large group or at an institution, it may actually be worth your while to set up an individual website, so that your patients can find you without navigating through a large university web page for your department (if there is one). If your practice has a long name, do you intend to abbreviate it for the URL? If so, how will patients know to look for you in that way? Hint: The abbreviation will not only have to be part of your practice marketing materials but also your business cards and appointment cards.

There is a solution if this question alone makes you unsure. You can claim all of the options. What does that mean? When you decide on your practice web address, you must register that address, so that it is not used by anyone else. Several companies allow you to do this on your own for a licensing fee. One of the most popular domain name registrars is GoDaddy.com. Why do this if you have hired a website developer? I believe there are some parts of the process that you should personally own and be aware of. If you have a falling out with your website developer and the registration of your website name expires, you may never know. While you are purchasing names of websites, I suggest purchasing various commonly misspelled versions of your name, so that people who use that will still be directed to your website. I also recommend purchasing the various extensions of your website like .net and .tv in case someone tries to buy those and is able to redirect web traffic to a site that has your name but is clearly not you (see also, Chapter 11 and Chapter 45).

Case One

My name is Kavita Mariwalla and my practice is Mariwalla Dermatology, but I wasn't sure what I wanted my website's main address to be when I was building it. The result? I purchased drmariwalla.com, mariwalladermatology.com, and kavitamariwallamd.com. I also purchased these names as .net in case someone tried to copy my website. The final product is hosted on mariwalladermatology.com, but in case someone types in drmariwalla, they will still be directed to my main website.

Case Two

You have been in practice for many years and have a website URL that was created before social media was a thing. Now the name seems outdated, or you have brought on partners and decided the website address needs shortening. This is a relatively quick and free process. Choose the new URL that you want to use (keeping in mind that, by now, most short URLs have already been taken). You can then configure the new URL to connect to your website and the old URL to redirect to your new URL address. Most URL renaming services will do this for you, but a website developer can also do this for relatively little cost.

45.3 Find a Host

Although the start of this chapter is about the technical components of a website, registering a URL and finding a place to host your files for your website are the two most essential parts of designing a website. A host is the place that keeps all of your files and the URL points to these files. Hosting can range widely in price. For the average medical practice, the less expensive option is fine unless you feel you will have thousands of visitors a day, so that the host must be able to accommodate an extremely large amount of traffic. Most domain registrars will offer a hosting option and this is what I recommend in the beginning. Why? If you decide to hire a website developer, they will likely want to host your site. This is fine, but you must make sure that in your contract, you have it very clearly specified that in the event of a termination of the agreement or services, your website can be transferred back to the host of your choice without delay or without additional incurred cost. In other words, you don't want to fire someone only to realize that they can hold your website ransom, because they own the URL license and are hosting the site.

45.4 Create the Website

45.4.1 Step One

You have your web address and you have a host. While you decide whether you are going to have your cousin build your site or the best website developer in town, it is worthwhile to put up a basic homepage which you can construct yourself. Most domain registrars that offer hosting services will also offer a very basic and templated homepage design. While the real website is being built, it is important to put up the contact information and office hours of your practice. The key thing is you don't want to end up with a blank page if people start looking for you before you are ready. A simple "Under Construction" image can be effective as long as your information is prominently displayed.

45.4.2 Step Two

The design itself. The content of your website is what drives search engine optimization, and the initial feel and look of your landing page can give a patient a clue about what kind of practice you have. While writing copy takes a lot of time, I would suggest investing your time primarily in figuring out the design and what it looks like. To that end, spend time surfing the web and looking at websites of colleagues. Look at the websites of large established groups, but also look at individuals who are relatively new as they often have interesting layouts and ideas. Think about color schemes, background imagery, and fonts. Are there certain images you want to stay away from or are there ones that speak to you? Is it important for you to have photos of people on your site, and if so, do you want them to be stock photos? Understanding how many pages you want, and the basic feel of the landing page, is good to have in your mind before approaching a website development company. That way, when you review their portfolio, you will know whether they inherently understand your vision.

45.4.3 Step Three

Choosing a website developer. This does not have to be complicated but it can be expensive. And because it is digital, you don't even necessarily need to go with someone in your town. When you interview a website design company, make sure you understand the length of time building a site is going to require. Also, assess whether they are going to be using one of the templates they have on hand just with different color variations. While that may make economic sense, in the future, your website may end up looking the same as a competitor in the same town. However, if your goal is simply to put up a website for patients to find you and know your hours, then a template, low-cost approach is absolutely fine.

Whenever you interview a website developer, I recommend asking to see their previous work and if they have built medical websites before. Try to get a sense of how responsive they are to changes you want made (which will happen inevitably the day after your website goes live). Find out if they have a graphic designer who can customize things for you and edit videos, and how long their average turnaround time is.

The words search engine optimization ("SEO") are batted around a lot. This is how your website ranks during searches for particular words like, for example, "Dermatologist on Long Island." The most frequently used search engine is Google and the "rules" Google has to rank your site change often. In my opinion, it is best to leave SEO to a professional. While this can be costly, it is widely considered a necessity in today's Internet age. What happens if you don't manage your SEO? Probably not a lot if your goal is just for the patients who know you to be able to find you because they can just type in your URL. But, if you want people who are searching for a dermatologist in general in your area, your website may not rank highly and thus not be found by prospective and new patients. This is particularly important for a cosmetic practice as you will want your website to be listed prominently if someone were to search for a particular procedure provider.

45.4.4 Step Four

Now that you have chosen a website developer, write out the timeline with fixed deadlines for specific components of your site. When I built my website, the part that surprised me the most was how much time it required of me. The hold-up was not on my developer's side but rather me in getting copy to them. By being clear on who was responsible for which step, it made communication much easier and also prevented frustration.

If you are in medical dermatology, your website should be clean and easy to navigate. If you are a Mohs surgeon, information about the procedure and answers to common questions should be easy to find. Aesthetic dermatologists must have a website that reflects their aesthetic and can draw patients in. Know the most common things your patients ask you and see if you can preemptively put that online. There are some universally necessary components, however, and this has changed with time.

45.5 The Essential Components

Location, Phone Number, Fax Number, Parking details, and Hours of Operation

According to widely available data, most patients access a physician website primarily to find out the address and hours of operation and phone number. In addition to claiming your Google Business page and listing, it is important to make sure this information is prominent on every page of your website; more so on the mobile version. I recommend this information not only be placed in a separate tab but also on the footer of each page or on an informational bar.

45.6 About Us

This is an often forgotten about page, but when new patients are assessing a practice online, they click this tab to find out who you are. Here are the dos and don'ts of an "About Us" page.

Dos:
- Include a photo of yourself that is somewhat recent, standardized, and professional. This does not mean that a professional needs to capture it, but it should not also be a cropped photo of you from your last family vacation.
- Include your schooling, degree, honors, and awards.
- Include information about your staff and extenders, including aestheticians along with their titles and schooling.
- Make sure you proof the text carefully and are mindful of the designation of board certified.
- Detail your special areas of interest within dermatology and end with a line or two that is personal.
- Do consider linking areas of your bio to other areas of your website like your blog or Instagram account.
- Update it frequently, including when people leave your practice.

Don'ts:
- Make it in the form of a book that a patient has to scroll through multiple pages.
- Make your bio significantly longer than anyone else's.
- Forget to include everyone in your practice who is responsible for attending to patients.

45.7 Access to the Patient Portal

In order to meet requirements of the merit-based incentive payment system (MIPS), one of the components is that patient portals in your electronic medical record are "opened" and available for patients to use within four days of their visit being made. While this can be burdensome to engage in (creating a patient username and unique password and then communicating that to them), it is pointless to open the portal and then not have the patient actually use it. I recommend a separate tab on your website for this subject alone. On that page, include the instructions for how to log in to the portal as well as a link. Then, patients should be able to fill out all of their new patient paperwork online before coming into the office.

45.8 Access to Patient Forms

Although the doctor expects that everything is recorded electronically, for many of our patients, this is cumbersome. I recommend housing a paper copy of your patient intake forms on your website for patients to download and fill out prior to their visit. Let them know that this will save them time at registration. Although some practices house patient consents online, keep in mind that informed consent implies you have not only given the patient adequate time to read the consent but have also reviewed key portions of it with them in person, thus it may not be efficient to keep them on your website.

45.9 Access to Privacy and Policies

If you have specific policies in your office, it is helpful to have these outlined on your website. For example, deposits for booking certain cosmetic procedures, no show fees, or charges for copies of medical records. It is helpful if patients have access to this and can refer to it in case they misplace a paper copy of it. It is also helpful to state your Health Insurance Portabilityand Accountability Act (HIPAA) compliance in this section as it is a requirement.

45.10 Access to Online Patient Appointments

With the rise of companies like ZocDoc, a segment of the population truly looks to make appointments online rather than wait on hold to talk to a receptionist. Finding an "app" that you can insert in your website, which then connects to your appointment scheduler, is difficult but ultimately the most ideal way to go about this. Most companies that offer this "widget" charge a significant amount for integration with your electronic medical record. Others waive this fee if they can then host your website and manage other electronic components of your office like credit card storage. This may be worth looking into, especially if you are starting out. It becomes more difficult when you are wedded to certain preexisting programs.

Websites like ZocDoc are already online and new patients can find you and make appointments through the site. All you then have to do is put up a link to their site from your page. Anecdotally, this has been very helpful for practices in saturated urban markets. One of the downsides is that there is a monthly fee, and in recent months, depending on your state, a move to charge a fee per patient who books with you through them. Another is that no show rates of these patients are very high. In my opinion, this is a costly endeavor and must be investigated carefully before signing up. Questions about whose patients they are once they book through ZocDoc are chief among the items you should make sure before you understand. Other online booking companies include Acuity, PetalMD, and PatientPop, and all are worth assessing and receiving quotes from before choosing one.

Offering online patient appointments is also very popular among those who access your website electronically on their mobile device. Again, make sure you do this, you actually have appointments available for patients to book. When a live person answers the phone, the advantage is that they can "squeeze" a patient in, depending on the acuity of the problem. With online appointments, it can seem as if you are never available when the reality may be different. The other downside is that patients who book online may be expecting a total skin check but booked a routine follow-up visit, thus throwing your schedule off. If you are going to put an online appointment widget on your site, make sure you have careful templates in place for appointments and that this feature is on your landing page for patients to clearly see.

45.11 "Message Us"

This is a feature that I find particularly helpful in our practice. We use a HIPAA compliant texting service called Klara. The advantage is that patients can set up a username and password and then text us questions, concerns, and book appointments. The communications are stored by the patient name and are easily accessed. Although they do not integrate with my electronic medical record, I am able to access Klara at any time on my mobile through a desktop and also on an iPad. This also facilitates communications with specialty pharmacies; in addition, the app records all voicemails, so that they are stored by patient and can be documented as answered. This feature alone has helped us tremendously, as patients who tell us they have "called and never get a call back" are able to be politely reminded that the office records all messages and that there is no record of such calls or that the call was returned and a voicemail left.

Some practices use the Facebook business page and the messenger app as a method for patients to send them quick communication. Beware that this may not be HIPAA compliant.

Depending on the electronic medical record, there may be a built-in messaging feature. Again, this is ideal, so long as staff can access it regularly and the messages are returned in a timely manner. The downside to a "message us" button is that, in today's marketplace, patients often expect a text message back immediately. If this is not the case, then an automated reminder that the message will be returned before a certain time of the day can enhance the patient experience.

45.12 Services Offered

Detailing what services you offer is important, especially for cosmetic patients. I do not recommend publishing the pricing of your procedures. If you decide to publish before/after photos, make sure you write a disclaimer that these are not intended as a guarantee of results. It is also critical that you have patient consents and that the photos are watermarked, so that they cannot be copied and used by someone else.

In today's digital age, it may also be helpful to include short videos of what the procedures actually look like being performed, and in the case of long procedures that require significant wound care or downtime, what a day-to-day expectation should be. This will allow patients to utilize your website as a trusted resource for information and their questions.

45.13 Mobile Accessibility

It is known that half of Internet users access the web via mobile phones or tablets. Therefore, it is more likely that a patient is viewing your website from their mobile device rather than their desktop. What this means for you is that while your desktop version of your website is beautiful and dynamic, if it doesn't translate to a 3 × 5 inch screen or a larger tablet, your visitors will be frustrated and leave the site. Look at each section of your website on your phone and make sure it is updated each time new technology emerges in the mobile market. On a mobile device, for example, it is probably most important that your address and phone number are visible clearly on the landing page as opposed to the desktop version. Under this same umbrella, make sure that, while you are focusing on the mobile experience of your web site, you keep in mind other ways patients can find you on their mobile like via GPS. It is helpful to plug in your office address into common direction apps like Google Maps, Waze, Garmin, TomTom Map Share, and HERE Map Creator. If they direct people to an incorrect location, you can hire a company to fix it or visit https://www.gps.gov/support/user/mapfix/devices-and-maps/ and fix the location yourself.

45.14 Online Bill Pay

Collecting balances from patients is difficult, so any way to make payment fast and easy will be helpful to patients. Many practices offer online bill pay. To do this, you must make sure that your vendors are secure and that this data cannot be breached, as you will ultimately be responsible for any loss of information.

45.15 Bells and Whistles

If you have the basic components listed above on your website, you will have created the content that most of your patients will access. The next step in thinking about a successful website is how to distinguish it from others. I call this the "bells and whistles." Key to determining what extras you need is asking yourself what you expect from your website. We have already established that the majority of people who access your website will be established patients looking for specific information. New patients and potential patients, however, will also click it once they have found your listing or perhaps read a review of you or even seen a magazine quote attributed to you. So, what are these added sections? Here are some examples:

45.16 An Online Retail Store

Patients who buy cosmeceuticals from you may want refills or refer friends. Instead of having them come to the office, you can offer an online store. The downside to this is that it is costly to build and maintain, as payment information must be securely taken and then you have to deal with shipping. However, if you have in-house branded products, this may be a nice way for patients to be able to access the goods.

45.17 Join a Mailing List

People who are not your patients may nonetheless want to be part of your audience when it comes to practice newsletters or specials. While promotions are typically driven through social media, it is helpful to have a mailing list to reach more patients via individual email. This can be a pop-up window when patients land on your home page or a separate tab.

45.18 Start a Blog

Dermatology and lifestyle brands tend to go hand in hand for many patients and consumers. If you write a blog or want a way to communicate your thought process to patients, blogging is a common way to achieve this. If you have one, keeping it on your website allows patients to access it as a repository of good advice.

45.19 Videos

In addition to written content, patients are drawn to video content. This can easily be shared across platforms like Instagram and Facebook and then housed on your website. It may also be a place to keep TV interviews or any other videos you feel will be helpful to the patient experience.

45.20 Publications

Patients like to know their doctor is well-educated. If you have written articles or abstracts, housing links to them adds legitimacy to your credentials and education.

45.21 Clinical Trials

If you are a practice with a clinical trials unit, let patients know, as they may want to enroll in a study, and it is a good way to signal to patients that you are on the cutting edge of your field.

45.22 Conclusion

Building a practice website can seem like a herculean task but keep in mind that it does not have to be everything on day 1. By design, your web presence is always changing and needs updating. Start with the basics and as your practice grows and changes, add additional components. I highly recommend looking at websites of physicians you admire to see what you like and don't like, so that you are not reinventing the wheel. Finding a good website developer is key, but laying out the ground rules and what is expected of each of you is most important to a successful end product.

46 Social Media

Kavita Mariwalla MD, FAAD

Abstract

Social media is a requirement of dermatology practices today. But what does that mean? The first requirement of social media is to be social and that means creating a platform that is comfortable for you to interact with patients. The platforms that have shown the most success for patients are Facebook and Instagram. Understanding how to post, what to post and when to post will allow new patients to find your practice but also allow a medium through which you can educate patients of your views on products, skin care and showcase all that you do in your practice. There is not one proven formula to be successful on social media, but as the number of 18- to 29-year-olds continue to use these platforms multiple times a day, it is becoming clear that future patient populations will be targeted through a digital medium.

Keywords: social media, Instagram, Facebook, Twitter, SnapChat, YouTube, digital marketing

Top 10 Things You Need to Know

1. When entering the realm of social media, it is important to define your goal for each medium you choose to use.
2. Look at the data available for each platform; for most dermatologists, the current best platforms are Facebook and Instagram.
3. YouTube users and followers continue to surge; video is the most difficult content to produce but also likely to be viewed often.
4. Do not become obsessed with numbers of "likes" or "followers." Key performance indicators to consider are reach of your posts as well as engagement by your target audience.
5. You do not need to be an expert at Photoshop or video editing; however, it is important to have tools available to you to edit and refine.
6. If you are unable to spend the time social media requires, consider hiring an outside agency and have definable goals for this agency.
7. If you choose to outsource your social media, have defined objectives, measurable targets to achieve, and make sure the voice of your account is what you want to put out on the web.
8. Being on social media should be considered part of a dermatology practice business plan, as it can increase patient engagement and also prove to be a great way to market services.
9. Do not post on a daily basis, however do have some consistency of posting on a semi-regular basis (2–3 times a week for example).
10. Take photos of interesting cases, good results and even interesting places as you never know when a photo in your camera reel may inspire information to create a post with.

46.1 Introduction

Twitter, snap, insta. So many words, so many hashtags, what's a busy dermatologist to do? You have patient calls to return, charts to finish, and sometimes the last thing you think about is constructing a post for your social platforms. Increasingly, patients are finding doctors through two main avenues—search and social. Having a strong website nowadays is not adequate, especially for aesthetic patients. And though it seems overwhelming and easier to abstain from social media than be consumed by it, there are ways to successfully navigate social channels if you plan and think about them strategically. Dipping your toe in the water is easier than you think.

If you are new to social media, here is a quick recap of the social media landscape most relevant to physicians currently:

Facebook: A user-to-user connective platform, Facebook has changed the way people communicate and receive their news. It is also an interesting platform for a business trying to grow and for health care practices to reach patients in order to showcase what the practice offers. It is an essential component of a marketing program, especially for small dermatology practices. A business page can be created with administrator rights given to a third party or to the practitioner.

Instagram: Originally, it was intended as a unique social networking platform that was entirely photo and short video based, but it has changed to be more of a messaging, information-based one. Tools within the app and editing apps are available to enhance imagery posted to the site. Similar to Twitter, hashtags are used to create searchable content. It is a very popular medium for dermatology and plastic surgery practices (It is owned by Facebook). Recently Instagram has added IGTV (Instagram TV) which allows users to create video that is in a longer format than a regular Instagram post allows for.

YouTube: Original video content is the cornerstone of YouTube. It is the fastest growing brand in social media. To use it, the medical practice has to create a channel for itself and populate it with videos. The videos can be as simple as those taken on a mobile phone or GoPro device or as complex as a professionally shot and edited film (It is owned by Google).

Twitter: Frequently used by opinion leaders, Twitter allows the poster 140 characters or less to express a thought. It is truly a mobile device-friendly platform since the ability to write at length is limited. In a medical practice, it is a way for followers to engage in discussion with you. Hashtags allow the content to be searched.

Pinterest: Boards based on subject are available for users to "pin" their favorite images. For a dermatology practice, it is a platform to engage patients with visual images of products and treatments. Multiple pins can be created with backlinks to your office website.

Snapchat: A messaging app intended to send pictures and messages that are available for a short time before they become inaccessible. Originally designed for person-to-person photo sharing, it currently features "stories" of 24-hour chronological content. The focus of Snapchat is user interaction; however, with regard to dermatology practices, the brief availability of its content may not be helpful for patients.

Tumblr: A microblogging website that allows users to post multimedia content to a short-form blog. It is used less frequently for medical practice marketing but if you choose to use this, it gives you the flexibility to customize almost everything.

Although some may recommend opening an account on each platform (if for no other reason than to prevent someone for using your practice name), keeping active on all these sites would be a formidable task. Doing it well is not something an individual would likely be able to do while also maintaining an active office. Now that you know the names of the major players, it's time to decide which ones you will toss out and which ones you will want to grow (see also Chapter 50).

46.2 Step One: Who Is This For?

The first question to ask yourself is who are you doing this for? In other words, is your social media account meant to be a reflection of the personal you or a reflection of your practice? To help guide this answer, ask yourself the following questions:

- Is your goal to increase patient volume?
- Is your goal to promote yourself individually?
- Are you looking to gain thousands of followers in order to parlay your social media presence into the level of being a micro-influencer?
- Do you plan to showcase patient before-and-after photos or are you more interested in having an account that people can follow to learn more about you?
- Are you trying to use the platform to gain followers, so that you are noticed by industry or media?

There is no one right answer. But once you decide, you have to stick with your goal. It is best to keep one account that is your personal self and the other that is for your practice, so vacation photos and dinners out with friends don't end up on the same site as your lip filler results.

46.3 Step Two: Name It

Once you establish whether your social media persona will be inward facing or outward facing, it is time to choose a name.

Choosing a handle name can sometimes be trickier than you think. On Instagram, your personal name is unlikely to be taken which is why most doctors choose their own name. This works well if you are using your account for personal promotion, but may not work if it is meant to represent the practice as a whole. It is easy to fall into the trap of picking "cute words" like skindiva or fillergod, but remember that if you plan to promote these channels to patients, professionalism is key.

Often times, the name itself can dictate the type of content a follower can expect. For example, the handle @saysmyderm may be confusing until one sees the posts of that account and realizes that they are filled with memes about life as a dermatologist and short quips that end with @saysmyderm. The poster is unknown and chose a handle in which he or she can remain so. The handle is easy to remember and with good content, that account has a loyal following and grows quickly.

In my case, I chose @mariwalladermatology. In retrospect, not a handle that rolls off the tongue; however, my account is meant to attract patients, showcase what we do in the practice, and coincides with my practice name and website address. Looking back, however, I would have shortened it, so that it was easier to type in and find. I specifically chose not to use @drkavita or @mariwalla because my social media platforms are not about me but rather the practice as a whole.

46.4 Step Three: Which Platform to Choose

Social media is defined by its constant changing nature. Increasingly, aesthetic patients shop for doctors via Instagram which is a picture-heavy platform. Facebook tends to be geared toward a different demographic but continues to be a popular driver for patient visits, especially existing patients. In choosing where to be present, perhaps the best driver is data. In social media, there is no one right answer, so as a physician, when I made my decision, I looked to the numbers.

In 2019, Facebook had 1.62 billion active daily users compared to Instagram's roughly 500 million active daily users. Compare this to Twitter, which has 330 million monthly users, and Pinterest, which has 291 million active monthly users. According to the Pew Research Center, which began surveying social media use in 2012, Facebook remains the primary platform for most Americans, with roughly 69% reporting in 2019 that they are Facebook users. YouTube is also becoming very popular; 90% of 18- to 24-year-olds use it. This highlights the reality that your choice of social media platform should be tailored to the demographic you want to reach. Different social media platforms have shown varied growth. Other than YouTube and Facebook, none of the other apps measured by Pew Research were used by more than 40% of Americans (▶ Fig. 46.1).

In looking at the data, the other thing that stands out is the frequency with which users visit these social media sites. Many do so on a daily basis with younger demographics sometimes using apps like Snapchat multiple times a day. What does this mean for you? Posting frequently (e.g., more than once a week) is key for capturing a good audience (▶ Fig. 46.2).

Although the numbers seem to point to Facebook and Instagram, what is important to note is that cross-posting is key...and possible. What that means for you as a practitioner is that you don't need to come up with entirely new content for each post necessarily. For example, I can post on Instagram and share that post to Facebook and Twitter with the click of a button. There are times when I want to post only to Facebook or Twitter– the content and audience reach is different for each. When looking at the most recent data from Pew, it becomes clear that most users also use YouTube, but it is the most underutilized of sites by physicians because of the time and effort it takes to produce quality videos.

The bottom line is that these demographics change as new platforms arise; however, clear leaders have emerged. So, if you were to start with social media, Facebook comes out as the winner for overall views and general patient reach but Instagram should be given equal weight as it is particularly popular in the 18- to 29-year-old age bracket.

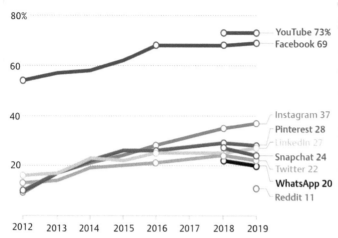

Fig. 46.1 Survey showing percentage of U.S. adults following online platforms or messaging apps online on their cellphone. Source: "Share of U.S. adults using social media, including Facebook, is mostly unchanged since 2018." Pew Research Center, Washington, D.C. (April 10, 2019) www.pewresearch.org/fact-tank/2019/04/10/share-of-u-s-adults-using-social-media-including-facebook-is-mostly-unchanged-since-2018/

Note: Pre-2018 telephone poll data is not available for YouTube, Snapchat and WhatsApp. Comparable trend data is not available for Reddit.
Source: Survey conducted Jan. 8-Feb. 7,2019.

Roughly three-quarters of Facebook users visit the site on a daily basis
Among U.S. adults who say they use __, the % who use each site...

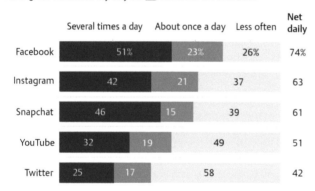

Fig. 46.2 Survey showing percentage of U.S. adults who visit various sites on a daily basis. Source: "Share of U.S. adults using social media, including Facebook, is mostly unchanged since 2018." Pew Research Center, Washington, D.C. (April 10, 2019) www.pewresearch.org/fact-tank/2019/04/10/share-of-u-s-adults-using-social-media-including-facebook-is-mostly-unchanged-since-2018/

Note: Respondents who did not give an answer are not shown. "Less often" category includes users who visit these sites a few times a week, every few weeks or less often. Source: Survey conducted Jan. 8-Feb. 7, 2019.

46.5 Step Four: How Do I Do It?

Time and Money. Unfortunately, time is the thing physicians have the least, and money is the thing we most hate to spend on social media engagement. While it is true that social media does not necessarily have a direct return on investment (ROI), it is important to establish key performance metrics for your posts. What does that mean? Well, in the beginning there will be a lot of trial and error. You will put up a post and see how much engagement you garner and how many views you obtain. Comments are always better than just likes or views, but do not chase them. Quality content will allow your account to grow organically. One golden rule: never ever buy followers. Bots can lead to the closure of your accounts and become obvious to true followers, who will see that you posted five times and have 1,000 followers. Unless you are Beyonce, those followers are typically purchased and do not result in meaningful engagement.

The silver lining in the social media world is that while you may have to spend money, you can do very well if it's wisely spent. First things first: establish a social media calendar. Decide the tone of your account. Will you be someone who posts a patient skincare tip every Sunday in order to be found by those who search for #selfcaresunday? Will you create your own #tiptuesday? Content is king so while you may be inclined to mainly post about promotions, this will not build a following or draw visitors. Sometimes, the content can be as simple as a quippy meme or an inspirational quote. Reposting infographics can also be an easy way to draw attention to certain months like May which is melanoma awareness month or October which is eczema awareness month. In a given calendar month, it is always helpful to try to create some Instagram Instastories which have now surpassed the Snapchat app by a wide margin. Once this roadmap

is planned, you can then build on your promotions around holidays or even contests. The list of what you can do is infinite for a creative mind.

If you are creating a post with patient photographs, remember to obtain patient consent even if the photographs are not identifiable. These consent forms should not only be reviewed by your attorney or malpractice provider but a customizable photo consent also has to be published by the Journal of Dermatologic Surgery. Remember that patient photographs can be lifted and repurposed by others. To prevent this, create a watermark that is placed on all of your photographs before you post them to deter such activity.

Many apps are available to help you enhance the look of your posts. Popular Instagram apps are listed in ▶ Table 46.1.

Table 46.1 Examples of commonly used apps to enhance Instagram posts. Many exist and are constantly being updated—this is just an example of a few.

Category	App name	Function
Instagram photo editing	BeFunky	A web-based photo editing tool
	PicMonkey	Editing of selfies, particularly removing blemishes or imperfections
	Adobe Aviary	One touch photo editing; the app will even suggest edits for you
Instagram photo design	Canva	Allows the creation of social graphics from scratch; contains templates for images and announcements
	Piktochart	Attractive templates to create infographics
	Framatic	Multiple adjustable layouts, borders, and effects to apply to photos
Instagram photo resizing	Insta Size	Allows users to import photos from personal albums to be optimized for Instagram and edit the newly sized photos
	No Crop and Square	Allows posting full-sized pictures on Instagram without cropping
Instagram collage	Layout	Instagram's own collage creator, which allows collages from photos taken on your phone's camera roll
	LiPix	Used across multiple platforms, it has adjustable templates, borders and photo effects
Intagram videos	Boomerang	Native to Instagram, this functionality creates small videos that appear like GIFs on repeat
	InShot	An editing tool that allows you to place borders, filters, and voice-overs
	Video Editor	A comprehensive video editing system with features that allow adjustment of brightness, contrast, exposure, and saturation; also, contains several filters to use
VideoDesign	Hyperlapse	Allows time-lapse videos with built-in stabilization technology
	Lapse it	Another time-lapse app that provides a variety of editing options to enhance the visual effects
Video resizing	Crop Square	Allows video position adjustment to resize and rotate videos and fill with background colors

So far you may be asking okay but where does the money come in? For a fee, you can boost your Facebook posts to reach a certain demographic. You can also promote certain posts to gain more visibility based on terms people may be searching. These investments can be as little as $10 to allow you to understand what these functionalities do for your practice.

46.6 Step Five: Gaining a Following

The rule of thumb in social media is that users tend to follow other users they know and like, and who follow them and engage with their content. Best practices for connecting with other users involves following people you know both directly and peripherally, and they are more likely to follow you back.

- **Follow users who know you:** To build a base of followers to market to, it helps in engaging with others in your own field as well as related fields to cross-promote your social media efforts. Following colleagues around the world is a great way to promote collaboration, get ideas, and show support for their practices too. They are more likely to follow you back, share your content, and like your posts as well– and as a courtesy, you should plan to do the same for them.
- **Follow users with a bigger following than yours:** Aim for alliances with like-minded users who have more followers than you have, but with a similar target audience of consumers with common interests. Avoid celebs and large scale media outlets, as they are not likely to follow you back. For example, don't assume that any Kardashian is going to like your content, and CNN is too busy keeping up with world news to be interested in your new laser or filler treatments.
- **Follow local businesses and entities:** The local golf resort, gyms, restaurants, shops, and hotels are ideal fodder for social media connections. Think about your community and expand from there to grow a larger network. Your local media outlets should also be added to this target list—start hyperlocal with print, individual anchors, reporters, bloggers, and writers.
- **Follow vendors you work with:** Follow brands and vendors you work with, including all laser, filler and skincare companies you may be a customer of. Tagging them in your posts will likely result in reposts by that brand.

- **Follow professional organizations and institutions**: Follow all the organizations you belong to, and institutions where you have trained. For example, AAD, ASDS, WDS, and ASLMS. Add to that list national and regional arms of these organizations, and also look for international organizations in the same categories. Finally, every major meeting or conference in your area of practice and market segment can also be found on social media; find them and follow these too.

While gaining followers may seem slow at first, this organic growth will pay off in the end, as it ultimately leads to a more engaged community interacting with you. Remember to put your social media handles on your office communications, including your business cards, so that people know where to find you. In your aesthetic space, encourage patients to tell their story on your channels.

The one warning is that if you engage in social media interaction, one has to remember to be social. This means if patients can interact with you on that platform, they will likely expect a response or acknowledgement. Unless you are able to dedicate time to this yourself, choose a staff member who is responsible for it on a daily basis or consider some automatic replies (like in Facebook messenger), directing people to call the office, thanking them for the message, and letting them know someone will be in touch with them.

46.7 Great, but I Am Already Overwhelmed

You may have come to realize that you simply don't have the requisite extra hours in a day to manage Facebook, Instagram, YouTube, and more. At some point, most dermatologists are faced with figuring out the best way to outsource their social media to keep up with the pace and volume of creative content needed. There are three basic choices to consider.

1. Hire an intern, employee, or community manager in-house to do it all.
2. Enlist a social media agency or PR firm to take it off your plate.
3. Let your SEO company do it.

In many cases, the best choice may be to hire a professional; however, if you do so, be sure to ask for the definable goals of your accounts. One option involves creating the content, having them post it, and managing engagement and decisions about who to follow. The belief that hiring someone and never having to think about what he or she does on your social media channels is false– all relationships require a back and forth and a social media manager will be no different. If you decide to hire someone, remember that they will still need photos, videos, content, and direction from you, which you will need to make time for or else you will end up wasting your money and in the long run, time.

If you decide to hire an intern, it may not be easy to find someone who has experience. We often hear doctors saying that they will look for a millennial from the local college to take care of their social media interaction. While this sounds compelling, it may not be ideal. Social media management is an important component of your marketing plan and should dovetail with all your other marketing tactics, including website updates, special offers, blogs, etc.

If you decide to outsource this to a current employee, your needs may not require 40 hours a week for social media. And it will take time to make sure this person understands your brand, specialty, and your goals for your target audience. Social media marketing requires someone who possesses digital experience and who can actually create good content. A keen aesthetic eye is important, and more than just a basic understanding of social media is required.

If you decide to hire a firm, the costs can vary. Some include it for an extra fee as part of managing your website. Typically, on the East Coast for example, a social media manager will cost anywhere from $125 to $175/hour. Usually, the brands and doctors, which you see doing well on social media platforms and producing daily content, have more than one staff member and/or agency on board and are actively involved in the process.

46.8 Pitfalls

It is easy to get frustrated when you do not see a daily increase in follower counts and likes. One helpful resource I found in educating myself was the blog from one of the authors in this book: Wendy Lewis (wendylewisco.com). She describes the following common errors:

1. Sporadic, irregular, and inconsistent social media engagement.
2. Not following the right target audience to gain new followers.
3. Putting too much focus on pushing out discounts, deals, and "Buy Now" messages that serve as a turn-off for users.
4. Lack of originality and creativity in your content.
5. Not working off a formal content calendar and just posting randomly with no strategy.
6. Not posting adequate or high-quality content to make an impact.
7. Not including any video.
8. Not allocating a sufficient budget for sponsored posts, boosted posts, and social ads to get your content seen.
9. Creating wordy content—think in phrases, short strings of impactful words, rather than long run-on sentences.
10. Not using the right hashtags—both popular ones (like #dermatologist) and some ownable ones for your brand (like #AskDrKavita or in my case #mdderm).

46.9 Conclusion

Not every dermatologist is meant to master the social media game. However, don't give up on it easily. The very traits that have allowed you to excel in dermatology, namely, creativity, ingenuity, patience, and determination are the exact traits that will enable you to obtain a basic knowledge of digital content. Even if you are an introvert and hate having your picture taken, you can outsource this and still make sure that your ideas are available for your patients to learn from.

It seems strange that, as a physician, there is now the added task of being on social media; however, as times change and patients look for doctors through both social media and search engines, it is a necessary component of the practice business model.

47 Creating and Nurturing a Brand/Logo

Heather D. Rogers MD

Abstract
This chapter outlines the key steps required to identify and strengthen a brand that can accurately and consistently represent your dermatology practice.

Keywords: brand, pillars, mission statement, slogan, trademark

Top 10 Things You Need to Know	
1. Identify the goals of your brand.	6. Pick web address and social media handles.
2. Identify the pillars of your brand.	7. Design your logo.
3. Create a mission statement for your brand.	8. Design your website.
4. Create a tag line.	9. Protect your brand.
5. Pick a name.	10. Design the office to reflect your brand.

47.1 Introduction

Like all great ideas, a brand starts as a seed of an idea that requires a great deal of attention to flesh out. This chapter will take up the daunting process of creating a brand and breaking it down into bite-sized pieces that build on each other until the seed of your idea becomes a well-formed and resilient plant.

The desire to build your own practice may emerge from life experiences or from an entrepreneurial spirit. For me, it was a little of both, and as we work through the 10 steps of building a brand, I will share examples from personal experience to help provide further insight into each of the steps.

I completed my dermatology training at Columbia University and followed it up with a fellowship in Mohs and aesthetics, also in New York City. During my 5 years in Manhattan, I was lucky enough to spend time in a few successful, boutique dermatology practices. These practices were beautiful, well-designed, and featured brilliant dermatologists at the helm. But it was clear that they were NOT just about the physician. These practices were successful because the reasons that brought them to life were clear in every aspect of the practice.

When I returned to Seattle, I decided to join a small private practice that reminded me of these boutique practices in New York. It was a beautiful practice where great importance was placed on patient care, but the office goals were often lost in personal issues, which squelched the team spirit. I worked there for 6 years, learning what kind of doctor I was and how I wanted to run a dermatology practice if ever given the opportunity. When it became clear that the practice was no longer the correct career choice for me, I knew I had to forge my own way. I needed to build my own dermatology practice with that desired boutique feel, where equally high emphasis was laid on patient experience and outcomes and the work experience of the office team.

As you already know, if you are reading this book, starting a practice involves more work than you could ever imagine. Months are lost learning and worrying about topics you knew nothing about before starting this journey. I tell every person who is considering starting their own practice that it is a decision that should be taken as a last resort. Do not do it if you can be happy in any other situation; however, if you are one of those people who will not be happy with anything less, then take the plunge and open your own practice! Bring your concept to fruition and enjoy the ride.

47.2 Step One: Identify the Goals of Your Brand

So, you have decided to start a private practice. Despite this having been done thousands of times, each time this decision is made, it requires the founders to recreate the wheel. Yet, if you are going to make the same old wheel, why go down this long and challenging road? Don't! Only go down this road if you can improve the wheel, or in this case, the way you practice dermatology.

Creating your brand needs to be a very early step in the process of starting your practice. I believe it needs to be the first step. Your brand is what you are selling. It is what will make your practice special and why patients will choose to come and see you... or not. Once you have identified the essence of your dream, then you can build your brand around that core, with each step building on the core concepts of your brand.

Once I decided to start my own practice I had to identify what would be the special and essential characteristics of my practice.

I wanted medical care to be provided by only board-certified dermatologists.

I wanted a practice that emphasized quality care over quantity.

I wanted a referral-based, word-of-mouth practice with minimal advertising.

I wanted a well-designed, beautiful office.

I wanted long-term, happy employees who were proud of where they worked.

I wanted to care for educated patients who could go anywhere, but who were choosing to come to me because of the added value we offered in customer experience and outcomes.

I wanted to be the go-to practice for dermatology in Seattle.

I wanted to have partners.

An additional person complicates things, but if you find the right person, they also can make things better and so much more possible. I am a younger sister. In high school, I played doubles tennis, and in college I raced two-person sailboats. I like having a teammate. After identifying what I was trying to do, I had to sell the concept to a future partner. This was an important and useful exercise because it made me solidify what I was attempting to do before I could convince someone else to do it with me. I found a partner in Dr. James Collyer, who is a brilliant, kind, eagle scout-turned-dermatologist and agreed these were worthy goals; together, we took these goals and used them to build the core pillars of our brand.

47.3 Step Two: Identify the Pillars of Your Practice

Once you have identified the goals of your brand, you need to distill the core values of the practice, which you can use as guidelines to reach these goals.

The guiding pillars for the practice we wanted to build were condensed as follows:

- Dermatologist-only practice
- Staff and patients are on the same team, working towards the same goal of outstanding patient care
- Beautiful and functional work space
- Ethical and supportive employment environment

As another example, I also created a skin care brand in the saturated beauty market. I developed the Doctor Rogers RESTORE out of necessity. I needed products I could recommend to my patients in their time of need, like when their skin was inflamed, irritated or healing; something safe and effective, as well as good for them and the world we live in. I could not find them, so I decided to create them based on the following pillars: All products had to be safe, smart, selective and sustainable.

- Doctor Rogers RESTORE products are safe for you, your family, and the world. They are made to help every skin type at every age.
- Developed by a dermatologist after years of studying and caring for the skin, Doctor Rogers RESTORE is the better solution for your skin's everyday needs.
- The RESTORE products are only made with safe, effective, and premium ingredients in the USA at a Food and Drugs Administration (FDA)-certified facility to ensure the highest quality and consistency.
- Every step in creating Doctor Rogers RESTORE strives to minimize our impact on the world while maximizing outcomes for our patients. We offer natural skincare without sacrificing efficacy or safety.

Pillars are like street lights, as they highlight the road you have picked and help you to stay true to your brand.

47.4 Step Three: Create a Mission Statement for Your Brand

The goal of your mission statement is to constantly remind you and your team members about why your office exists. It takes your goals for your brand and the pillars of your practice, and works them into three or four sentences that explains your reason for being. This message should be honed and then framed in your office as your guiding light. For our practice, the mission statement is as follows:

To provide excellent dermatologic care for our patients, which is tailored to their individual needs.

To hire and train team members with the skills they require to ensure all patients at Modern Dermatology are well cared for.

To be a warm and welcoming environment where team members feel appreciated, challenged, and fulfilled by their work.

47.5 Step Four: Create a Slogan

The goal of a slogan is to ensure your staff, patients, and potential patients know what your practice is all about. It is cutting down the pillars and mission statement to a more easily shared tidbit. For our practice, the slogan is "Excellence in Medical, Surgical, & Aesthetic Dermatology through Physician-Driven Care." This tag line explains that we are striving to provide superb dermatologic care in all aspects of dermatology.

For my skin care company, the tag line is "Skin Care Made Clean" because Doctor Rogers Skin Care is all about creating effective products that are clean—meaning good for you and the world. They are made with the fewest, plant-based, hypoallergenic ingredients, and come with 100% recyclable packaging.

47.6 Step Five: Pick a Name

I realize the first thing most people who are starting a practice do is pick a name. I would like you to try to delay the final decision on this until you are done with the preparatory work outlined above. You want your name to reflect your practice's reason for being, but that name may not be an available option. Picking a name becomes a process of elimination, as it will be dictated by a number of factors that are out of your control. Do you want to use your surname? Do you want to use the location of your practice in the name? Do you want to start with the letter A to be at the top of alphabetical searches? Once you think you have a good name picked, you will need to scour the Internet to see if your name is being used. If it is, does it matter? Is there another dermatology office with a similar name nearby, or is it on the other coast? Will it cause confusion? Is it trademarked, so that you cannot use it? Do not be deterred if this happens a number of times. This is where having your

pillars and mission statement clearly defined can be incredibly helpful in aiding you get creative in finding the right name. When we set up shop in Seattle, we knew we would have multiple doctors, so we did not want to use our last names. Seattle was already in the title name of several dermatology practices, and we did not want that to contribute to confusion in finding us. We are on Mercer Street, but there is also Mercer Island with a Mercer Island Dermatology, so our street name was out. We settled on Modern Dermatology which felt right as we were building a state-of-the-art facility where all the medical care would be provided by physicians, and Modern Dermatology could be abbreviated to MD. In our Internet research, there was one other Modern Dermatology in Texas that was a new and small practice. Although not ideal, we decided Texas was far enough away to avoid significant confusion. We love the name but, as we age, we do wonder if some day we will have to be Midcentury Modern Dermatology!

47.7 Step Six: Pick Your Web Address and Social Media Handles

Once you have the practice name selected, you have to find and own your website address and social media handles. Again, you have no idea what is already claimed in these arenas until you start hunting. For us, ModernDermatology.com and modernderm.com were already owned by the practice in Texas. We wanted our website and social media handles to be consistent, so after a day of typing different options into the Internet, Instagram, and Twitter, we were able to claim mdinseattle.com for everything. For my skin care line, we decided to spell out Doctor versus Dr to be able to own DoctorRogers.com and doctor.rogers on Instagram.

Again, once you have engaged in adequate research to ensure you can have a web address and social media handles that match, it is time to start buying websites. There are several resources available. I used GoDaddy, and for a very reasonable price (typically $15 a year), you can purchase web addresses. I encourage you to buy your selected web address, name web address, and other web addresses that are similar to yours. For example, for our practice, we use www.mdinseattle.com but we own HeatherrogersMD.com, JamescollyerMD.com, moderndermatologyinseattle.com, southlakeuniondermatology, and about

10 others which we own to ensure they are not used by another practice, thus causing confusion.

47.8 Step Seven: Design Elements of Your Branding

Once the name is decided, you need to determine how you want your name and logo to look. I strongly encourage you to spend a bit of money on a good artistic director to help here because you will get a much more professional end result. Give her/him your mission statement, name, and any gut feelings you have about how you want things to look and feel. The more information you provide, the happier you will be with the end result, and the less back and forth it will take to get there. My two logos can be seen in ▸ Fig. 47.1 and ▸ Fig. 47.2. For Modern Dermatology, we want to make a medical cross and highlight the MD. The three lines symbolized the three layers of the skin (epidermis, dermis, and subcutis) and the

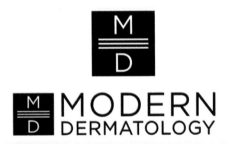

Fig. 47.1 Modern Dermatology logos.

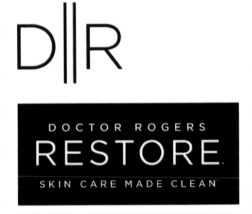

Fig. 47.2 Doctor Rogers Skin Solutions LLC logos.

three fields of dermatology (medical, surgical, and aesthetic). My skin care line is remarkably similar, as we are highlighting the fact that it was created by a doctor with the DR, and the two lines symbolize the first product which I made with only two ingredients.

Once your logos are finalized, the art director will provide you with a branding deck, with all the dos and don'ts of your branding, including sizing, fonts, and logo markups. Referencing this document will allow your look to be consistent and professional, as you create all the required paper documents for your practice, including stationary, patient handouts, and business cards.

47.9 Step Eight: Design a Website

Now that you have done all this work, the daunting task of creating your website will be much easier. You have your mission statement, tag line, name, logo designed, and a web address purchased. Now you just need to get them on the Internet. Yes, you will want a beautiful, well-designed website with great visual appeal, before-and-after photos, and search engine optimization, but that may take a year or two to get done. While you hunt for the right designer to create your forever page, get a basic page up as soon as possible. Use a website design service that is easy to edit by you or someone in your office. There will ALWAYS be updates, and it is remarkably handy to be able to make little ones in-office as opposed to waiting for your designer to get around to it. You want to get your website up as soon as possible, so everyone who is interested will know what you are doing, as you get closer to opening day.

47.10 Step Nine: Protect Your Brand

Now, that you know exactly what your dream practice is about and you have created the word and images to represent it, you need to protect your work. Another of the many excellent reasons for getting your website up as soon as you can, is that it allows you to lay claim to your name, logo, and slogan publicly. From the first moment, these are used in the public sector, you want to have a "TM" next to them. The TM mark is used to protect an unregistered brand by alerting potential infringers that the term, slogan, or logo is being claimed as a trademark. If there were ever a conflict over your branding, the person who used it first with the TM will have a significant advantage in laying claim to the brand. In addition to adding a TM next to your work, you will need to work with a patent attorney to get your brand items registered with the United States Patent and Trademark Office (USPTO), which may take 6 months to a year. Once you are formally registered with USPTO, then you switch your TM for ®, which is the mark used for brands that are officially registered.

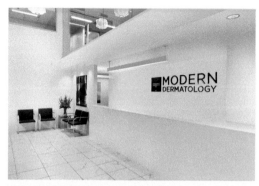

Fig. 47.3 Office design with branding.

47.11 Step Ten: Design Your Dream Office

Again, with all this heavy lifting behind you, you will be able to add lovely brand-specific details to your office, making the patient experience all the more memorable: the signage behind the front desk (▶ Fig. 47.3), your logo on the windows, and your color scheme in your furniture. Voila! Congratulations on building the brand of your dreams.

48 Managing Your Online Reputation

Wendy Lewis BA

Abstract

Social media platforms and review sites have created the need for dermatologists to carefully monitor their reputation online. Reputation management has emerged as a critical success factor for running a medical and aesthetic dermatology practice. Patients will rule you out or choose your practice based on the information that they find when searching online. This chapter offers some essential strategies for managing negative reviews and controlling your online presence.

Keywords: reputation management, maximizing social media, dealing with negative reviews, defining your online brand, reviews and ratings, social media monitoring

Top 10 Things You Need to Know

1. Become well-respected: Trust should be the ultimate goal for every dermatologist. Never take it for granted because it does not come easily. Making people respect you and your work is more important than any other reputation management commandment.
2. Be part of the conversation: You have to be social to understand how social media works. Join relevant conversations and establish your presence on the platforms that matter to your practice, and in the way you are comfortable.
3. Monitor what people are saying about you: Assign a staff member to follow comments posted on relevant sites and social platforms, and enlist a monitoring service to alert you to new developments so you can be proactive if negative information turns up.
4. React respectfully to comments when appropriate: Online audiences have short attention spans. Therefore, a prompt and straight forward reply may be better than a late more detailed reply.
5. Address critiques carefully: Avoid the temptation to be defensive or snarky in your responses and try not to take comments personally that it colors your good reasoning and logic.
6. Treat the first page of Google as your landing page: First impressions count. If words like "overpriced" or "cold and impersonal" are associated with your practice, turn these critiques into an opportunity to make improvements.
7. Listen to your detractors: Criticism can offer a chance to learn about your audience and do better in the future. It can be humbling some dermatologists, who may be out of touch with how they are perceived by patients.
8. Keep it real: Consumers relate to practitioners who are approachable and down-to-earth, so so try to strike a conversational tone and show empathy; let your caring and compassionate side shine through.
9. Don't get mad, do better: A negative review can be a real ego deflater, but a few unflattering comments will not destroy the brand you have built through hard work and dedication.
10. Always keep your license in mind: It may be tempting to emulate what rappers, influencers, and reality stars do, but as a licensed health care practitioner, be mindful of how you come across so you are taken seriously as a practitioner.

48.1 Introduction

People are talking about you.

Yes, it's true. They are talking about your brand and posting about you online, whether you like it or not, and you have very little control over it.

If you're not listening to what is being said on these platforms,

Not long ago, if a patient had a bad experience from an office visit or treatment, they may have told a few close friends in their innermost circle. Today, they may go on YELP and broadcast their displeasure to thousands of people in the blink of an eye.

So, if you're not proactively building and managing your brand online, it's time to start. In today's climate, all professionals need to take control over how they are perceived to protect their most important asset—their reputation. Once that is tarnished, it is difficult to get it back.

48.2 Online Reputation Management Pearls

Until the rise of social media, practitioners were not really engaging in a two-way conversations with patients, but rather selling to a passive audience. Today, everyone has the right to express him/herself, and you really have no choice but to listen.

If you are just starting out in practice, colleagues, patients, and everyone you interact with may be blogging about their latest treatment, commenting on your Facebook page, posting on Instagram, or writing a review on RealSelf. You cannot build a thriving practice anymore without taking into account people's opinions, ratings, and reviews. This can be frustrating if your brand is the target of an attack by competitors or their webmasters.

Patients can connect with you via email, chatbots, and social networks, and they expect a response in real time. Practices of every specialty, size, and stage will benefit from having accurate listings, building their online presence, and increasing positive reviews to protect their reputation.

48.3 Track Mentions of Your Name and Brand

If you don't monitor what people are saying about your practice online, you are unable to prevent future damage or intervene swiftly to turn things around. Negative comments travel quickly and can affect how people view your practice for years to come.

To help make sure you never miss a mention of your brand or name, set Google and Yahoo alerts for your name, common misspellings of your name, and your practice name and variations of it.

Do remember that Google is also a verb.

If someone leaves a negative review, first determine if it is from a real patient. If so, rather than responding in an open forum, attempt to take it offline to resolve the situation. If you let it go, it can gain momentum and get out of control if others join the conversation. The best outcome is often if a happy patient posts a glowing commentary

about you on the thread to negate the negative remarks. Effective reputation management entails acknowledging mentions of your brand, so you can minimize negative comments and amplify the positive ones. Another point to keep in mind is that your online reputation can also affect your website's rankings on search engines making it harder for prospective patients to find you.

Tools You Can Use

Check out Brand24.com as it monitors mentions across social networks to help you keep track of what is being said about you and your competitors.

48.4 Claim Your Brand on Key Social Media Platforms

Do remember that the Google+ of today could be the Instagram of tomorrow.

Even if you're not ready to jump on every social network right now, register on ALL major social channels with both your practice name and your name to secure ownership on platforms where you may become active now or in the future. Ideally, aim to use the same username across all your social channels whenever possible. Twitter is the only platform that has a character count name limit, that is, 15 with no spaces. Don't risk letting someone hijack your brand name whether intentionally or unintentionally, especially since it is free to claim an unlimited number of names.

Tools You Can Use

Use Knowem.com to check for the use of your brand name through social media and register your user name on every relevant channel.

48.5 Proactively Track Your Online Reviews

In the online world, your brand ambassadors as well as detractors have equal opportunity to voice their opinions. Consumers hold all the power and they can use it to shape others' perceptions of you. Rather than avoiding negative reviews, adopt a proactive approach to monitoring sites that are relevant to your practice. If you do choose to respond to negative reviewslet your practice manager respond for the practice and offer a solution such as *"We pride ourselves on taking exceptional care of our patients and welcome the opportunity to invite you to our practice…"*

Don't acknowledge, whether directly or indirectly, any doctor–patient relationship in an online forum, which could be a HIPAA violation. HIPPA has been known to regularly scan review and rating sites to monitor whether practitioners are crossing a line, so don't let this happen to you.

48.6 Addressing Negative Reviews

There will always be a risk of getting negative reviews despite your best efforts, so devise a strategy for how to respond. It is important to listen to patients and help resolve any unfortunate experiences they may have had in your practice. When a negative comment appears, take time to decide on whether to reply. Don't take action when you are upset or stressed. Assess the nature of the comment and respond only in constructive phrases and not in the heat of the moment when you're angry. Look at the situation from your perspective and also that of the patient to obtain a good balance.

If you feel compelled to reply, proceed with caution. Anyone who is reading these reviews is judging whether you are the kind of physician they want to visit. A response should be short and nondescript like, "Patient satisfaction is our number one goal and we are committed to taking excellent care of all of our patients." Rather than responding in your own name, have a staff member be the point person and try to take the conversation offline. Showing your willingness to be responsive can demonstrate that you stand behind your reputation. It is often best to try to privately resolve the conflict, assuming that it is actually a real patient with a valid issue. This is the best and sometimes only way to have a negative review retracted or removed from a site.

Common complaints often center on waiting times, rushed staff and doctor, feeling that the practice was too busy, high fees, and bedside manners. Attempt to distill commentary about long waits and short visits with a statement like "We are among only a few aesthetic practices in the area, and we pride ourselves on providing quality

care to all of our patients." Don't be defensive, which can be misconstrued as arrogance.

When you see comments that address a genuine shortcoming, use it as an opportunity to improve. Work on an approach that instills trust and confidence with each patient visit.
Don't undermine your own brand.

48.7 Develop a Robust Plan to Generate Positive Reviews

A collection of favorable reviews by real patients will outweigh a few negative ones, so be vigilant about fostering goodwill with patients. Persuade them to write good reviews about your practice by showing that it matters to you. To many patients, it is counterintuitive that you need reviews for your practice. They are accustomed to doing this for hotels, restaurants, and salons, but may not realize its significance to a respected physician.

Foster a program to encourage 5-star reviews by including the best ones on your site and social platforms. Post a sign at the front desk that you value patient feedback, including in person, by phone or email, or via online forums.

Don't be shy to ask patients to give you a review but avoid incentivizing patients with freebies and discounts in exchange for positive reviews which is considered unethical. However, thanking a patient for a 5-star review, and rewarding them after the fact shows your appreciation.

It is often easier for staff to ask rather than the doctor. When a patient compliments their result, the staff may say *"It would make our day if you gave us a 5-star review."* This is common practice among all service businesses, including hotels, restaurants, salons, airlines, Uber and eBay, and consumers are accustomed to it. The doctor can also ask if he or she shares a comfortable relationship with the patient; however, be aware that just asking a patient may not be adequate, as the thought passes out of their mind immediately after they leave your office. Give them a card with the top rating sites as a reminder. Having patients write reviews in your office may not work because it will come from the same ISP address and not be considered legitimate. There are many automated services that can be implemented to send emails to patients to ask for reviews to help circumvent this.

Encouraging patients to post good reviews about your practice continuously is the goal. Then, if you get a 3-star rating, you won't have to scramble to get more 5-star reviews to push it down. The best way to counter negative ratings is to make sure they are buried under a slew of positive ratings from real, satisfied patients.

> **Tools You Can Use**
>
> Key ratings and review sites:
> 1. Google
> 2. Facebook
> 3. RealSelf
> 4. YELP
> 5. ZocDoc
> 6. Healthgrades
> 7. RateMDs
> 8. Vitals
> 9. Realpatientratings
> 10. Healthcarereviews
> 11. TripAdvisor
> 12. Google My Business

48.8 Create a Consistent Voice Online

Social networks play an important role in building your online reputation. Having a consistent voice and brand online helps people remember you and sends the message that your brand is reliable. For example, use the same color schemes, logos, layouts, and filters on photos, so your social media channels have a cohesive look and theme. Create a signature design to black out facial features or body parts on patient photos to protect their privacy, such as a circle in your brand color or your logo.

> **Tools You Can Use**
>
> BrandYourself.com lets you scan social media posts to find and delete any older posts that could affect your reputation.

48.9 Beware of Negative Search Engine Optimization (SEO) and Other Online Attacks

Negative SEO means using what is referred to as "Black Hat SEO" on other people's websites to get them penalized by Google. These nefarious tactics can work to diminish the effectiveness of a site's SEO properties by disabling or altering them. These strategies are often used by web companies who represent your competitors or hackers who are intentionally working to bring down how your site comes up in search results. Spammy links are another common aspect of a negative SEO campaign. If someone is creating poor quality links to your site, you need to regain control. The process of getting links removed should be managed by an SEO expert who may be able to send a link removal request to the webmaster of the site from where it was generated to have it taken off. If this doesn't suffice, you may have to escalate a plan to protect your site from further attacks.

> **Tools You Can Use**
>
> MonitorBacklinks.com can provide a list of all your site's backlinks and metrics that show how valuable or damaging each link is in order to decide which should be removed.

48.10 Build Your Influence Through Great Content

Great content can help to engage audiences, shape opinions, and impact purchasing decisions. By creating entertaining or informative unique content you can grow your authority as a thought leader in your field which, in turn, can help your search results. Content that Google deems to be of low-quality, duplicate, or just uninteresting, can work to your detriment.

Transparency is a critical success factor online. It can be very beneficial to embrace an open communications approach with your audience and establishing a direct dialogue with fans and followers. It can be risky to strike the right balance between too much vs. too little transparency. But in the long run, not being transparent can undermine your reputation and the trust factor you have built up with your audience.

Do Take Your Reputation Temperature.

48.11 Enlist in Social Media Monitoring

Smart online reputation management is not only about responding swiftly to what people say about you when appropriate, but also about whether to react at all. Sometimes a reaction is not necessary, and one that is too late can reignite negativity.

A proactive approach should involve monitoring on a regular basis, rather than only when you learn about a specific occurrence. Social media monitoring allows practitioners to gather public online content, such as from blogs, tweets, reviews and Facebook and Instagram updates, process it, and determine what is being said that may impact your reputation positively or negatively. This can be accomplished internally by setting Google alerts and monitoring your name on important review and rating sites. These efforts should be boosted by a professional web marketing firm with expertise in the health care field to monitor your reputation and report results on a monthly basis.

48.11.1 DON'T Set Up Reputation Roadblocks

There are two basic types of negative content to be aware of. The first is in the form of social network complaints, most often viewed on Facebook, Instagram, or Twitter. On Facebook and Instagram these should be addressed swiftly or removed, and the user can be banned so they do not pose a serious threat.

The other type may present a bigger threat that can cause long-term damage to your professional reputation. These may show up prominently in search engine results. Review sites allow users to express their opinion about your brand at will, and only some sites actually validate that the reviewer is an actual patient. Negative content on these consumer-facing sites can affect your practice. Sites like RipoffReport.com are natural fodder for angry patients eager to air their grievances and most of these boast a "no removal" policy.

In rare instances, a patient may go beyond simple negative reviews and create individual websites or blogs to air their opinions. These sites may be used to post defamatory and false information. Thus, a search result like "The truth about YOUR-NAME" or a site like "YOURNAMEsucks.com" or "IhateYOURNAME.com" could make potential patients run the other way.

The adage that there is no such thing as bad press no longer prevails in the era of social media. Unfavorable TV, print, and online media coverage can have a negative impact, especially since it is so difficult to bury now. Years later, these media hits can pop up on search engines when a patient Googles your name. Like a violation that appears for eternity on state board sites, scandals played out in the media can leave a black mark on your reputation.

48.12 How NOT to Sue or Get Sued

Don't let amateurs post or engage on social media for your practice. Everyone should be well versed in the guidelines that apply to health care professionals and patient privacy.

We all have the right to our opinions, according to the First Amendment to the U.S. Constitution which protects freedom of speech.[a] This means that everyone, including your competitors, former employees, partners, or ex-spouses, can exercise this right too.

Every time we go online, we leave electronic footprints. If you want to track down someone who has posted about you, you may be able to gather their personal information if they gave an ISP when they signed up (name, address, phone, email, etc.). Many sites only require an email to register, which can be easily faked. In that case, a subpoena to the ISP that hosts the email address will be necessary to obtain their true identity, but that doesn't always work.

Some practitioners have filed lawsuits against patients or rating sites over negative reviews. This is often an expensive experiment and the big winners are the lawyers. It is generally more prudent to address complaints by encouraging the poster to come back to your practice, rather than to risk escalating their rage.

Although everyone has the right to express their feelings about your brand, there are certain boundaries that must be respected. Negative content online may be deemed to be a violation if it meets any of these criteria:

- Includes defamatory language
- Contains false information
- Is aimed at damaging the reputation of the brand or business

To defend yourself against these behaviors, here are some remedies to consider.

---

[a] https://constitutioncenter.org/interactive-constitution/amendments/amendment-i.

48.13 SEO Tricks

Try Googling your name or practice name. If your website doesn't appear on the first page, you may be hidden from a high percentage of patients looking for a "dermatologist near me." Anyone searching for you by name will view the high-ranking online resources that are talking about you. If they display false or misleading information, consult with your webmaster to develop a digital marketing strategy in order to increase the ranking of positive content and move the content you don't want to get noticed down. It is widely believed in SEO circles that inbound links are a dominant ranking factor. These are hyperlinks that link back to your site from another site, and an ongoing strategy to get more backlinks is the key to marketing your website.

48.14 Review Removal

DO work hard to continually solicit 5-star reviews from happy patients to overcome any negative reviews.

Getting bad reviews taken down is often a fool's errand. If a poster has claimed something false about your practice, or you can prove that a review is clearly aimed at destroying your reputation or contains defamatory language, you may have a shot at getting it removed. Website owners possess a lot of discretion when it comes to taking down content, but most just won't do it. First read the terms of service on the site. If the poster has violated the terms, you may have some recourse. For example, YELP's terms of service states that you must be a customer (i.e., patient) to post a comment, so this would be a clear violation and you might have a case, but nothing is guaranteed.

If you can prove that a post is not factual or fake, such as the writer is talking about a procedure that you do not offer, and you can substantiate that, or you can prove that the poster is not an actual patient, you may have a case. If the post is just an opinion, you probably won't have standing to get it removed.

48.15 Conclusion

By vigilantly monitoring and constantly aiming to improve your online reputation, you will be in a better position to protect and grow your brand and drive a steady stream of new patients.

49 Tips for the Media

Doris Day MD

Abstract

Getting the call to appear on television is exciting and it is a great opportunity to represent your practice and our specialty. There are many ways to increase your potential for being selected to appear and once you get the call there are very specific steps you need to take to prepare for your appearance in order to convey the information in a clear and concise manner and to increase your chances of being asked back in the future.

There are specific steps you can take to have the best success in the interview and increase your chances of being invited back on, such as being available for the segment, over-preparing, having before and after's and talking points available for the producers, being on time and concise in your answers when you're on. It's important to understand that being on television will not jumpstart your practice and can be costly if you have to close your schedule in order to travel or block out time in order to be available for the show. It does however offer credibility for your patients and is a great way to represent all of us.

Keywords: media, television, TV interview, TV appearance, presentation

Top 10 Things You Need to Know

1. Make yourself visible by posting videos and photos in your area of expertise.
2. Participate in ASDS, AAD, WDS and other major organizations media committees.
3. Respond promptly to media inquiries.
4. Be available when called to be on radio or TV.
5. Show up early for the segments and be over-prepared.
6. Dress appropriately for your interview.
7. Share the link after your segment, they will notice and it will encourage them to have you back on the shows.
8. Stay in contact with producers and send them regular pitches with your ideas.
9. Create your own YouTube channel to share your content but beware trademark restrictions.
10. Remember it's not all about you. The more you inform and the less you "sell" the more you will succeed.

49.1 Introduction

It can be very exciting and even flattering to be invited as an expert on a television show. It is an opportunity to highlight a new treatment, increase awareness about important medical issues, and represent your specialty. What it won't do is make you famous overnight or have new patients knocking down your doors the next day.

Patients come in every day and ask me for my opinion about a device or treatment they saw on a television interview. I ask them: Who was the doctor in the interview? Their answer is nearly always: "I don't remember." That doctor just helped bring my patients, and the people they refer come in to see me and build my practice, but he or she did not benefit from being on TV themselves as much as they may have hoped or expected. Over time, as you develop relationships with producers and shows and become a regular guest expert, you may gain traction and recognition, but it takes time to become recognized as a go-to expert on the "short-list" of any given show, and it takes having a unique and compelling message when you're on. Also, it often requires cancelling patient hours, loss of income due to the travel and timing schedules of many of the shows, and no guarantee on a return on your investment (ROI) unless you are a regular or frequent guest on a show or various shows. This can take years to cultivate, and in today's competitive environment, it may require a media trainer and a publicist.

Producers from one show are watching other stations and shows to see what they're doing, who's on, and the rating that goes with it. If they see something or someone compelling enough, they will take note, pursue them, and try to get them on their show at some point. The shows often have a rating system of guests they have had on the show. At the top of this list is the "short-list," which is the people they consider to be camera ready and reliable and the first ones they will go to when they need a sound bite or quote about the particular topic at hand.

On the negative side, all the shows compete with each other, so if you do one show, like Good Morning America, then another show like the Today show will be less inclined to have you on within the next few months because they want the "exclusive" with their guests, and they want the "scoop," meaning they want that guest on their show first, unless you have reached a certain level of celebrity.

49.2 How to Increase Your Chances of Being on a Show

- Be available: This may require travel, adjusting your schedule, and canceling office hours, often with very short notice.
- Produce it for them
  - Send before-and-after photos and b-roll (background video).
  - Offer clear talking points and do the research for them.
  - Have product/devices, etc., on set and ready.
  - Bring in patients as models if required.
- Have visibility on social media and in publications: producers and show researchers look at publications, studies, and social media for the latest and most interesting information that they think are newsworthy.
- Increase your involvement with associations like the Skin Cancer Foundation, American Academy of Dermatology (AAD), and American Society for Dermatologic Surgery (ASDS). They all have media sections and many shows will contact them requesting recommendations for experts on a given topic.

49.3 Talking Points

- **Over-prepare:** It helps to know much more than needed, so you will feel comfortable with anything that comes up.
- **Keep it simple:** One of the most important lessons is that you can't impart all your knowledge

in the 3 to 5 minutes of your interview. Have three points you want to make, have them in order of priority, and feel very proud of yourself if you get to the first two!

- **Practice:** If you know what you want to say to start with, then you will be in control of the interview and it will help you be less nervous about being on live television.
- **Know the show and interviewing style of the show you will be on:** They may be sarcastic, contentious, talkative, or submissive.

49.4 Preparing for the Event

- **Before-and-after photos:** Send these ahead of time, so they can be approved by the producers.
- **Ensure patient permission:** Even if you have written consent, make sure to contact the patient to let him or her know about this individual use and obtain his or her permission for it.
- **Props:** Bring supplies, products, and devices.
- **Live patients:** Have models ready if you're performing demonstrations on set.
- **Cancellations:** Anything can happen and even after all your hard work they can cancel for any reason. They may decide the topic is no longer newsworthy, there may be breaking news, they may run long with other segments, and you get cut. I have had shows come to tape in my office, spend over an hour for a 3-second sound bite and then have that cut without explanation or apology. That's showbiz!
- It can take up to or more than 1-hour preparation time for each minute you're on the air.

49.5 The Interview

- **Arrive early:** This gives you time to get comfortable with the studio and rehearse with producers, so you're ready for your segment. It also gives you an opportunity to shoot behind the scenes video and photo for your social media (#BTS).
- **Dress appropriately**
  - It's all about how you look. We are professionals, we should look professional. If you're a woman, I think a dress is better than pants. Take into account that if you're sitting, the dress will ride up, so try to wear a longer dress to avoid over-exposure of thighs or

underwear. The reality is that if you're wearing a dress you'll get more camera time. No judgment, just facts.

- Solid colors or patterns that are not overly busy are better.

- **Hair/Makeup:** Some studios offer touch ups but go in hair- and makeup-ready. One time when I was on Rachel Ray, I arrived at the studio an hour and half early to give them plenty of time to get me in to hair and makeup, but things got mixed up and I ended up going on with only a blow-dry of the front of my hair and lashes added on to make the eyes pop a bit. All done in 6 minutes. Of course, my luck, the studio had a rotating stage and the back of my hair which was barely brushed totally showed as the stage moved from interview to demonstration sets, all on national television! Now, I get my hair done the day before or morning of the show if there is time.

- **Have your first line ready:** This gives you an opportunity to land back in your body once the interview starts and you realize you're on live TV. It also gives you an opportunity to control the interview. For example, if the topic is skin cancer, your first line could be: "skin cancer is more common than breast, colon, lung, and prostate cancers.... (purposeful pause) ... combined. The good news is, if found early, we can offer a greater than 98% cure rate." Now, the interviewer can ask anything at all. They can ask "what are the different types of skin cancer" or "we hear skin cancer is on the rise, what is basal cell carcinoma that Hugh Jackman had?" or "how does exposure to sunlight cause skin cancer?" It really doesn't matter what they ask, you have your first line ready; from thereon, you shape the interview and they will follow your lead. It's a dance. As long as you keep your answers short, so you give them time to talk too, they will be happy.

- **Smile when you talk:** Doctors tend to look very serious. Of course you don't want to smile when giving details about melanoma deaths, but when the interview starts and ends and when talking about new treatments, be conscious of your facial expressions and smile!

- **Don't overly nod or move your head:** To look engaged, lean forward, look at the interviewer, and be still. Overly nodding to show you agree or moving your head to show you're alive is distracting and makes you look nervous in interviews. Of course, you don't want to be a stiff mummy either.

- **Don't interrupt:** Let the interviewer finish their sentence before you begin to speak.

- **Don't have run-on sentences**: Make your point. Period. Try to limit your talking time to about 10 seconds. Give the interviewer a chance to talk and ask you questions as well.

- **Make your most important point early**: This gives you an opportunity to build on it, repeat it, and make sure you don't run out of time before getting to make it.

49.6 General Points to Consider during the Interview

- **You are the expert:** You know more than the interviewer or anyone watching, so take control, be patient, and educate the reporter—don't make the reporter work hard.

- **Bridge conversation:** Bridge conversations as needed and guide the reporter back to key messages—always take the lead.

- **Listeners/viewers must hear your excitement (verbally, expressions and body language):** Personalize the story and tell them what patients want to know...or really should know...or relay information through your own personal story/experience. For example: "I see patients every day who..." or "many patients come in complaining of..."

- **Less is more:** Be concise and memorable, too much information allows the reporter to choose what is most interesting, and reduces the chance of communicating a clear message.

- **Minimize negative phrases:** Do not repeat negative phrases. A reporter may say, "Isn't BOTOX a poison?" ... Instead of saying: "No, Botox is not a poison..." consider saying: "On the contrary, Botox is a purified protein, we know, down to the molecule, how it works and we place it precisely where we want it to work, like for the frown lines between the brows." Try saying that out loud, you'll see it takes about 10 seconds and makes a very strong point.

- **Do not be self-serving**: Give information rather than selling yourself. You will have a much bigger impact and will have a better chance of being invited back on the show.

Examples of Key Messages

For the holidays:
"Give yourself the best gift, and see a board-certified dermatologist for your next cosmetic treatment."
In the summer:
"Being sun smart is the best way to reduce your risk of skin cancer and premature aging of the skin."

Three Key Messages

- Primary Key Message Goals
  - New information
  - Timely
  - Useful to many
- Secondary Key Message Serves as Backup
  - Research
  - Statistics/data
  - Anecdotes
  - Patients experiences
- Final Message Call to Action
  - Website
  - Phone number
  - Visit a board-certified dermatologist

Key Bridging Phrases

- What I do know
- Most importantly
- Since then
- For example
- In addition
- Our main focus
- In fact
- What I can say
- Furthermore

49.7 Examples of Dos and Don'ts for Neuromodulators

Do	Don't
Natural	Poison, toxin
Smooth	Stone-faced
Relax, softer	Plastic face, freeze, frozen
Reduce fine lines	Paralyze
Safe, effective quick	Deadly toxin

49.8 Case Study

Several years ago, I was invited to appear on the Today show to talk about Botox. I was looking forward to the interview. I prepared, had my talking points, and was ready. The day before my interview, a story broke in the news and stole the headlines. A chiropractor had injected four people, including himself, with "Botox" and all were now hospitalized, intubated, and were near death. Within hours, it was on every network and it was all everyone was talking about. Patients were in a panic. It took hours for Allergan to be able to prove that it was not Botox but actually an industrial-grade botulinum toxin type A that was being offered to doctors. Some took the offer and figured they could dilute the product, inject it safely, and save money since the branded product was so expensive. My "fun" interview on how to age beautifully was now potentially a contentious debate on national television. My preparation had to adapt.

As expected, it was a difficult interview but in the end I used it to enhance the need to see a board-certified dermatologist or plastic surgeon. I spoke of Botox as a drug and like with any drug, if used or dosed incorrectly, it could lead to toxicity. I never used the word poison even though the interviewer mentioned it several times and even challenged my directly, asking me: "isn't Botox a poison?" I responded by opining that it was an Food and Drugs Administration (FDA)-approved drug, a purified protein, and if used properly and as directed it had an outstanding record of safety and efficacy. I had many other positive points and I led the conversation in that direction. She had no choice but to go along with me.

49.9 Challenges

- What would you do if you were asked to go on a show, a big show, but they wanted you to do something live or taped-live in studio which you didn't think was ethical? Would you do the show or pass on it. What would you do if the show was Wendy, Oprah (back when she had a show), or Dr Oz?

Years ago, when Oprah's show was in it's prime, they called and told me they had been following me from my other interviews and that Oprah wanted to invite me on the show. They wanted to discuss under eye filler and do injections live in studio. This is in the relatively early days before social media and way before everyone was doing fillers of nearly every body part on nearly every show on TV. I had extensive conversations with her team. I explained how this was a medical treatment with consequences and should be performed in a controlled medical environment, both for patient safety and comfort. I offered for them to come in to the office to pretape and then have the patient in studio to see the after. It was important to me to be true to my specialty. I didn't want to diminish the work we did or for the public to think this was anything but a medical treatment that we worked hard to create and perform for our patients in the safest and most appropriate of medical environments. End of story… They ended up using another doctor. It did not make her career and it did not ruin mine. Maybe I made a mistake, or, maybe they were considering her anyway and the outcome would have been the same even if I agreed to do the injections live in studio, but, at the time, I felt that standing up for my ethics and protecting my profession was more important even than being on Oprah. Years later, I would do injections under conditions I felt were controlled– sometimes pretaped in studio, and sometimes in the office with the patient on live to discuss their experience. Stay true to who you are, don't do anything you believe will compromise you, it is never worth it. I don't regret my decision.

- What would you say if the interviewer asked if you have these procedures performed on yourself?

I was on a show on CNN with Paula Zahn. The camera zooms in on me as she looks right into my eyes and asks "so, do you get Botox yourself?" Without skipping a beat, I responded "of course I do." She looks again and says "well, you're the poster child for the treatment! You can still move your face and you look very natural." I thanked her and then redirected the conversation back to the treatment and proper technique.

- What would you do if you were asked to say something you don't believe to be true?

Seems easy, but think about the slippery slope. I've heard doctors talk about how diet can help cellulite, sun exposure is good for your skin, or embellish information about procedures and minimize risk in order to meet the ever-increasing, sensationalized demands of the ever-insatiable audience who want dramatic instant results for everything they can think of. Don't give in to the temptation. It never ends well. Your reputation is built over time, producers will come back to you if they see that what you say holds true long after the interview has aired.

Suggested Readings

American Academy of Dermatology. AAD.org
American Society for Dermatologic Surgery. ASDS.net
Skin Cancer Foundation. www.skincancer.org/
The Interview Book: How to prepare and perform at your best in any interview

50 Marketing and Advertising Your Dermatology Practice

Michelle Henry MD

Abstract

This chapter will provide you with tools that will strengthen your marketing plan. There is no "one size fits all" or one budget that guarantees success. The best strategies are tailored to the individual practice's needs, with a clear goal that is set from the beginning and supported by a strong physical and virtual presence.

Keywords: marketing, social media, website, Instagram

Top 10 Things You Need to Know

1. Creating a concrete brand.
2. Website.
3. Digital media.
4. Search engine optimization (SEO).
5. Content.
6. Social media.
7. Newsletters, blogs.
8. Reviews.
9. Deals and offers.
10. Online shop.

50.1 Introduction

Launching, marketing, and advertising your new dermatology practice used to entail listing it in the yellow pages, meeting or calling physicians to generate referrals, and if budget allows, buying a TV or radio ad. In stark contrast, today with all the technological innovation in the world of communications, we are able to design a do-it-yourself multipronged approach to broadcast our message and mission to our prospective patients. From interactive websites with online booking options, social media channels, and a plethora of independent websites where we can gain cross-promotion by listing our practice (zocdoc.com, healthgrades.com, etc.), there is more than one way to get ahead of your competition and promote your practice. While some physicians are apprehensive in engaging in self-promotion, as it may dilute and affect the trust their patients show in them, it is the reality of establishing a practice. Whether your niche is in cosmetic, medical, or surgical dermatology, if you want to continue to treat patients, retain patients, and attract new, thus enjoy a long-standing career as an expert, marketing is part of the way to get there.

There is no shortage of marketing and public relations agencies that specialize in promoting medical practices. Retaining experts is a great way to propel yourself and accelerate your practices' growth. In this chapter, however, we describe the overarching failproof approaches and principles that your marketing strategy should be based on, regardless of its size and special area of interest. This way you can educate yourself, be attuned to your consultant if you end up seeking help, or customize the elements of marketing that you wish to outsource versus the one you will take upon yourself. It all depends on your energy levels, budget, and time constraints. In my experience, most practices outsource the design of their website and the setup of social accounts, and from then on, with the help of some capable staff members, who continue to roll out messaging independently on their own.

Finally, marketing is the art of persuading and enticing people to use a product and service. For the dermatologist, this means attracting new patients and keeping existing patients in one or more locations. The most successful marketing practices are those that adhere to the AMA guidelines which advise against aggressive advertising and deceptive claims. Focus on the value the practice brings to the patient and patient appreciation. On the other hand, from a business perspective, it's good to remember that quality is better than quantity, that is, more profitable patients are better than more patients alone.

50.2 Creating and Establishing a Brand

Creating a brand is the first step that defines and directs the marketing strategy. Branding is one of the most important and most often overlooked aspects of marketing as it influences nearly every consumer-purchasing decision. This includes prospective patients who are looking for dermatologic services. If they have a choice between several practices, they will gravitate toward the ones with a message that aligns with their own goals and preferences. Branding is about defining your practice and connecting with people. Creating a brand involves the following:

- Identifying the core values of the practice.
- Developing an identity that patients can recognize and connect to.

When trying to define your core values and subsequently your message, you should list what is the mission of your practice, who is your ideal patient, and what sets you apart from your competitors. Your messaging should immediately convey what do you specialize in and what you focus on. Distilling these core values can help filter out many patients who would not benefit from your services and attract those who would not only gain from being your patient but can also be retained for the long term; even more, refer other patients to your practice.

So, who is your target patient? No doctor or practice can be everything to every patient. One of the best ways to figure out your target market is by surveying you current patients. Consider their age, gender, ethnicity, and socioeconomic background?

Why did they choose you? My patients often say that I feel like their good friend who happens to be quite smart. I translate that to mean I'm approachable. As a young physician, I know that is a part of my appeal and I utilize that in my branding. Do they consume the same types of social media? Do they socialize in the same places? Do they watch the same television shows? What guides their decision-making process? Is it price sensitivity? Is it the promise of a luxury experience? Is it a natural result? Is it their confidence in your expertise?

Next, identify what you offer, and what is your core mission statement of the practice. Are you a boutique practice? Do you offer spa services? Specialize in quick, convenient, and affordable care? Focus on cutting-edge technology and unique treatments? Finding a particular niche will provide you with a competitive advantage. Many become anxious about carving out a niche as they believe it will limit the number of patients that they will attend to. Conversely, specialization gives the perception of excellence in that area. Instead of considering specialization as making your patient offerings smaller, think of it as making your practice sharper and better-equipped to provide a unique level of care. When you position yourself as an expert you must offer results and not treatments. It gives you more control over market factors affecting your pricing. Instead of competing with medspas that merely sell syringes or units of a treatment, an expert sells the end result. As our field becomes commoditized, we have to be certain not to price compete as this doesn't project expertise. On the contrary, it projects a lack of confidence that you are worth it and thereby diminishes your brand.

Knowing thy enemy, in this case other practices, can also help you refine the values you want to highlight. Assess your competition to get an idea for what models are successful in your space and determine what you could offer that they do not. Not being intimidated by your competition but solidly understanding your place in the market is important to developing your niche. No one is YOU but understanding the space you occupy is important.

Developing a brand identity is the second step in creating your brand and what the blueprint of your marketing plan will revolve around. Brand identify can entail unique words or visual clues that people associate with your practice and allows them to quickly recognize you, whether they are looking at a logo online, ad on a bus, or when listening to your employees on phone calls. It is consistent, memorable, and distinctive. It is communicated online and offline through materials or the voice of your staff. Adding a company logo to a giveaway can help build brand awareness, but not if the item is a label on something disposable like a water bottle. Consider putting a company name and logo on a tube of lip balm because it will last for a while and is relatively inexpensive. A brand identity can range from a few simple elements to a complex strategy outlined in a multipage manual. This will depend largely on the size of your practice and scope of your marketing activities. The most common and powerful elements of brand identity are usually the logo, slogan, and name; however, it also extends to how you present your brand. It may include elements such as the following:

- A signature color, or color scheme
- Symbols that or spokespeople who you want to associate with your brand
- Graphic design and layouts inculcating modern, elegant, or minimalistic styles
- Writing tone, style, and even specific fonts
- Key phrases, quotes, or words to be used frequently

Practices with a well-defined marketing plan usually outperform those without a plan. The most important part of a marketing plan is the goal, as it is the foundation for other critical decisions. To start with, develop 5-year goals for your practice, and your 1-year goals will fit within the context of a 5-year plan. A 5-year plan is not only broad in scope but is also more strategic. After each year, evaluate and adjust next year's goals based upon whether you accomplished this year's goals. Concentrate more on developing strong and tangible goals. In order to achieve this, limit your goals to five. Your goals must be:

- Challenging yet realistic
- Strong and specific
- Measurable
- Time-sensitive

50.3 Website

According to the HubSpot marketing statistics for 2019, 97% of consumers have searched online to find a local business. Even more compelling is the fact that 46% of all searches on Google are from potential buyers seeking information, and 88% of consumers will typically use the Internet to find a local business and visit them within 24 hours. For your practice, it's never been more critical to establish an online presence to attract leads and foster meaningful relations with potential patients. Establishing and maintaining an online presence begins with launching a strong website. Your website should be your anchor and referenced on all of your other social media sites. Hiring a consultant who can build a Wordpress site that integrates all your branding is the best investment you can make with your marketing budget. Some elements you should pay attention to while working with your consultant are as follows:

- The website should be mobile-responsive across multiple screen sizes and multiple browsers. It must offer an equally efficient user experience to people with different types of mobile devices.
- Highlight the features and procedures at the dermatology practice you offer which you want to grow and want people to be aware of.
- You have to have phone numbers, social media links, and forms.
- It has to be maintained on a weekly, if not monthly basis, to stay fresh and relevant.
- Categorize your site information in a sharp and logical manner, and create intuitive navigation, so that mobile users are able to find relevant information in as few clicks as possible. Have clear visual paths with succinct text presentations.
- Add a search button to your site to facilitate quick information access.
- Build a faster download speed for your site, considering the fact that many mobile users have limited time and patience. The mobile site should ideally load in four seconds or less.
- Must-have features include the ability for patients to book appointments online, access their charts/medical records, and potentially shop online.
- Optimize image files for mobile screen viewing.
- Size images so the reader does not need to scroll up or down to see a full image.
- Provide share buttons to encourage mobile users to make a phone call, send a mail directly from the web page, or access your social media pages.
- Post educational content, respond to comments and questions, share links to relevant websites, and post information about dermatology procedures and treatments.
- Remove duplicate data and add rich content and videos to help your Google ranking.
- Have the content SEO and SEM optimized with the help of a consultant.

A great website comes hand in hand with setting up your Google My Business (GMB) profile, customizing it, and gearing it toward online success for your health care marketing program. Dermatology practices that employ high-performance GMB growth tactics can rank at the top of Google's map pack, which is a rectangular box that displays nearby businesses in a searcher's area. As a result, the practice at the top of Google's map pack receives the lion's share of consumer clicks. Google's top map result has a 30% click-through rate (CTR), according to Smart Insights. Considering that thousands of people in your local area currently use search engines to find local businesses, that statistic is huge (see also Chapter 45).

50.4 Digital Media

As dermatologists, you should know how important photos, videos, and graphics are in gaining clients. Posting before-and-after photos and videos online may seem outdated, but it actually works, as it helps prospective patients create a connection with you and let you control the story that emphasizes how better a situation got after engaging in your services. Aside from the before-and-after photos or videos, a mixture of graphics and videos to create an informative animated video will most likely boost business by as much as three times with the help of SEO for medical practice marketing. The Internet provides a vast number of opportunities for free or inexpensive marketing, but that's not to say that traditional marketing strategies such as TV, print, and outdoor media are not required. The best marketing strategy to reach a wider customer base with minimum costs is one that balances both online and offline media. In a 2012 Google/Compete Hospital Study, almost 84% of patients were shown to use both online and offline media for health care research. Of those patients who used traditional media for research:

- 32% of patients used TV.
- 20% of patients used magazines.
- 18% of patients used newspapers.

Therefore, if implemented correctly, offline or traditional media can be just as powerful as online media. Online videos on channels like YouTube have proven to be very effective in marketing a medical practice. Some video production and promotion tips to maximize success are as follows:

Keep it short and sweet. Keeping videos between 1 to 5 minutes is generally recommended.

Health Insurance Portability and Accountability Act (HIPAA) still applies. Observe all HIPAA considerations and obtain signed releases (included different possibilities of use) from anyone who appears in, or whose stories appear in, your videos.

50.5 Search Engine Optimization

There are a lot myths floating around out there about what SEO actually is and how it can help you as a dermatologist. You may be questioning whether this is something your practice really needs and think that a high-quality website and active presence on social media is adequate to find and attract new patients. While these are certainly effective and necessary elements of a good online marketing campaign, they're only a piece of the puzzle, and without a strong presence on the search engines, you are practically invisible. A reliable search engine optimization strategy or SEO will get you that spot on Google's first page. But what is SEO? It is a conglomeration of strategies that help optimize your web pages to make them reach a high position in the search results of Google or other search engines. As you keep with the SEO strategy, your dermatology practice will soon become the one that people view, trust, and visit when they need your skin care solutions.

The best SEO campaigns for dermatology clinics should include both on-page and off-page elements.

- On-page SEO are the elements that you have the most direct control over and can easily update to meet search engine standards. These include mobile compatibility, load times, quality content, site navigation, and keyword usage. On-page SEO is something your Wordpress consultant can help you set up as you launch your website.

- Off-site SEO are the elements that you have less control over but are nevertheless an important part of SEO. These activities can show Google that you are an authoritative and important resource, but you need to put a lot of time and effort into implementing these strategies effectively. Some of these activities include creating linkable content, meaning amazing content, that other websites will naturally want to link to and share. Another off-site SEO strategy involves building relationships, for example, asking other sites to list your practice in their list of local businesses.

Something to remember, however, is that SEO is a fluid, dynamic set of practices and strategies, and things that worked amazingly well last year might not be all that helpful this time around. It can be difficult to stay fully up-to-date with all the changes in the search engines, so hiring a consultant on an as-needed basis may be beneficial to assess what needs to be tweaked on-page and off-site in order to stay relevant to the search engines.

50.6 Content

They say content is king and they say it for a reason. It's vital to know that great content will give you higher chances of getting promoted by Google online. Always publishing informative and useful content will give your website better chances at attaining higher rankings. Content can be a blog, link to a recent research article, or a visual like a picture of you using a new technology. Aside from helping in SEO, it will actually improve your credibility online. Your patients will get the sense of authority and expertise in your field and give them a chance to engage with you and grasp a bit of who you are. Aside from helping our business, let's not forget that, as physicians, it is our moral obligation to teach and share our knowledge. When we impart the knowledge, we have collected through our many years of training, or our recent research, it differentiates us from those who can't or won't. I teach my patients about the aging process, how lasers work, and the different properties of the fillers. This adds tremendous value to the provided service and bolsters the image of medical excellence.

50.7 Social Media

Social media is an important piece of the digital marketing puzzle and shouldn't be taken lightly. It is where you can attract more clients, since an average person spends at least 2 hours of their time on social media, and the best place to gain an Internet following. Aside from costing time, it's pretty much a free marketing tool where you can promote your blog, website, services, or even yourself. Your best bet is to set up all your social media platforms by engaging the services of a marketing consultant. Simply having social media pages is not adequate. You have to manage your online presence carefully, because it's the first impression many potential customers will have of your practice. Creating your social media marketing plan starts with understanding a bit about how the major social platforms work, and how they differ from one another:

- **Instagram:** Instagram is all about images. The key to Insta-marketing is catching people's attention as they scroll through their timeline. To stand out, keep it interesting and don't share the same type of content every time you post. Consider sharing before-and-after shots of procedures or treatments you offer, or some creative shots of your office. Use very high-quality photos. Since influencers control Instagram, having thousands, if not millions, of followers on Instagram, leverage this phenomenon by striking up a deal with one of them.
- **Twitter:** Twitter is where people go for the hot take. Twitter posts should be quick and quotable. Twitter is the also the original home of the hashtag so using them (in moderation!) can help direct people to your posts. Marketing on Twitter means being aware of—and taking advantage of—trending topics. Jumping into trending discussions, which have some relevance to your field, can get your posts more exposure.
- **Facebook:** If you only choose to focus on one social media platform, let it be Facebook. More than 2 billion people are active on Facebook on any given day, and the average user logs in about 8 times per day to scroll through their news feed. Lest you think the social platform has reached its peak, consider that 400 new users sign up every single day, both young and old. Digital marketing experts know that Facebook offers the most bang for your buck in terms of social advertising dollars. Paid Facebook ads (when done right) can provide a substantial boost in your social media engagement, driving leads right to your website and not just any leads either. Facebook ads are great at helping you reach a precisely targeted audience and you get to draw on their vast bank of data to help you do it (see also Chapter 46).

While each platform has its own unique attributes, there are some hard and fast rules to follow:
- Strike a balance between sharing things posted by others and posting your own original content. Sharing relevant articles, pictures, or posts from others can keep it from seeming overly promotional and can also help build valuable relationships with people and businesses in your social network.
- Keep it professional. Which means no political rants, polarizing statements, and off-color humor as these things just alienate potential customers and diminish your credibility as a professional in your field.

- Never, ever disparage a colleague, employee, vendor, patient, or, well, anyone. It's incredibly unprofessional so just don't do it. Handle disputes and issues in the real world, not on social media.
- Connect your social media accounts. Then, connect those to your website. Make sure that people can find you, and that they can easily hop from your social sites to your website.
- Be consistent and know your brand. Use the same logo, voice, and overall aesthetic for your website and all your social media pages.

Some housekeeping tips for using social media in your marketing strategy are as follows:
- Keep professional and personal online personas separate.
- Never "friend" or contact patients through personal social media.
- Avoid using text messaging for medical interactions even with established patients.
- Use email or other electronic communications only when there is an established patient–physician relationship and with patient consent.
- Encourage an office visit or an emergency room visit as the situation demands, when patients whom they do not know seek out clinical advice online.

50.8 Newsletter, Blog

Blogging can add fresh content to your website on a regular basis and also help with SEO. Consistently posting original content on your blog shows that you know your business and are happy to keep your patients empowered and engaged. You may provide information about general dermatology procedures, share skin care tips, announce discounts and deals and announce updates about your practice. You can promote your blog using social media and use it to engage with existing and potential patients. Another marketing strategy involves getting email subscriptions to send newsletters. Contrary to popular belief, email is still heavily used by all generations, even by millennials. Leverage this fact by sending out newsletters that feel personalized and that deliver results which will keep clients from unsubscribing. Newsletters are a way to communicate any new development happening in your practice, such as an event, a new laser procedure, or some breaking news about skin care. Keep newsletters rich in visuals and light on text, so the information can be quickly digested by the readers.

50.9 Reviews

Online reviews will increase your credibility and online presence as a dermatologist. Asking past clients to post honest and positive reviews on your website or social media accounts like Yelp will get more potential clients to recognize you online. This is vital since there is an increase in the number of online patients reading past reviews. Sharing your reviews online can also get you recognized but make sure you have your patient's consent to do so and then post it in on your blog, website, or social media page. Another way to encourage positive online reviews is by sending a follow-up email thanking your patients for their visit and encouraging them to review your practice. You can even consider offering free services and discounts to reward patients for posting reviews of your practice. In addition to enhancing your brand image and credibility, online reviews increase the online visibility of your practice.

Managing bad reviews, otherwise known as reputation management, is also a crucial aspect of your local search strategy. While it doesn't entirely negate a negative listing, responding to issues can help your reputation. Ideally, you want to provide excellent customer service from the start to avoid receiving negative reviews, but when you do get one, be sure to respond so that others who come to your listing know that you care. Ensure your response acknowledges the incident, apologizes, and refrains from being defensive. You also want to weed out reviews that aren't actually about your dermatology practice, as sometimes people post on the wrong listing by accident. You can prove that these listings don't belong on your listing and request that they are removed. A good-to-know fact is that if the information in a negative review is false, aimed at destroying your practice, or uses inappropriate language, you can have the review removed.

50.10 Offers and Discounts

Deals and discounts will always catch people's attention online and entice them to visit your practice over another. It creates a buzz to promote your services and gives you a chance to market your website and engage with your patients. Some ideas are seasonal discounts like offering a discount for dads before Father's Day or in anticipation of Valentine's day. You can create contests that will give your clients a chance to interact with you by posting photos or videos, and present an offer that the best ones may get a chance to win a gift card or a percentage off on their next visit. You can also offer free consultation for a period of time. The only drawback of offers and discounts is that you need to invest marketing, advertising time, and budget, as a lot of campaigning will go into getting your contest or promos some buzz. Social media, email, and e-commerce sites are places where you can post about your contest, deals, and promos.

50.11 Online Shop

It would be a rare and even odd event if after personally meeting your clients, you wouldn't recommend a skin care regimen that will cater to their skin type or skin problems. Instead of having your clients visit your clinic to buy skin products, you can set up an online store, sell your skincare products, and increase your profit. Although some physicians feel uncomfortable selling products to their patients due to the physician–patient relationship, the truth is most, if not all, of my patients want me to sell skin care products. The main two reasons are trust and convenience. They want to make sure they are using the right products and don't want to allocate more time and effort in searching elsewhere for products. Important elements to consider when selling products online is to cater to all types of skin types, and be able to offer a customized efficacious regimen at a reasonable price. Partnering with your favorite brands and selling them on your online shop is always a win-win for both parties. It's important to educate your staff on the skin care you offer, ingredients they contain, best way to apply them, and any potential interactions with other skin care products or medications. Patients may choose to purchase products online or in person, so in case you or other physicians are not available, everyone from the front desk to the medical assistant should be able to guide the patients on what they are purchasing and why.

50.12 Conclusion

Becoming a dermatologist and having a fulfilling practice is one of life's greatest pleasures and accomplishments. Hopefully, this chapter will provide you with ideas and suggestions that will make you better businessmen and businesswomen. Remember that the only constant is change and a marketing plan is what you make of it. There is no "one-size-fits-all" or "one-budget-is-the-answer" approach that guarantees success. The best strategies are tailored to the individual practice's needs, with a clear goal that is set from the beginning and supported by a strong physical and virtual presence.

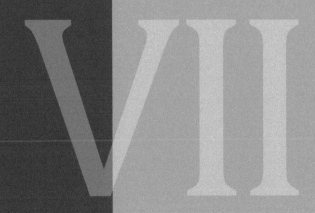

51 Growing Your Practice

Vince Bertucci MD, FRCPC; Alessia C. Bertucci B.Comm

Abstract

Growing a dermatology practice may appear to be a daunting task but, when approached systematically, is a highly achievable goal. By starting with a clearly defined practice purpose, and implementing changes through the lens of that purpose, a unique brand offering can be developed. Strategic growth may look different from one practice to another, and will be informed by a deep understanding of one's market segment, key performance indicators, analysis of strengths and weaknesses and individual business goals. Identifying the appropriate business levers and securing the necessary resources are two important pieces of a larger puzzle that will foster sustainable growth. In order to uncover the essential pieces that will support your practice's growth, it is necessary to look both internally and externally. Growth is rarely the product of one single solution, and therefore requires an in-depth understanding of what drives your practice.

Keywords: purpose, trust, brand loyalty, key performance indicators (KPIs), business model, competitive strategy, customer service, marketing

Top 10 Things You Need to Know

1. Create a solid foundation for growth by assigning the right staff and allotting adequate financial resources.
2. Know your "why": Define your "purpose" and let this permeate everything in your practice.
3. Define your market segment and cater to that group of patients.
4. Know your numbers: Measure relevant key performance indicators (KPIs) so that you can identify potential issues and measure the success of changes implemented.
5. Create a 5-star customer service experience in all aspects of the practice.
6. Deliver outstanding outcomes: Great results lie at the core of any practice. Only recommend treatments and procedures that will deliver excellent results and avoid those that will not be of benefit to the patient, even if the patient insists.
7. Build brand loyalty by showing patients that you care by according attention to detail in all aspects of their encounters with your practice.
8. Refine your patient schedule to allow adequate time to carry out full treatments, thus improving results, patient satisfaction, and word-of-mouth referrals.
9. Perform comprehensive consultations with customized and complete treatment plans.
10. Create a marketing plan that leverages your existing patient base with tactics such as email blasts, informational brochures, and video displays. Engage both existing and potential new patients through social media platforms.

51.1 Starting Out

Where does one start with a subject matter as broad as "Growing Your Practice," which is one that might easily occupy an entire book? Achieving growth in a practice is truly the sum of countless parts and one that requires attention to the foundations outlined in this book. As the topic is so broad, the mechanics of growing a practice can be somewhat daunting when first embarking on this journey. To make the task more approachable, the reader is encouraged to review the chapter, take an inventory of practice needs, select the most pertinent areas that need to be addressed, create an action plan, and then implement change in a step-wise manner.

51.2 Creating the Foundation for Growth

Even the best laid plans will fail if the infrastructure for growth isn't first put into place. Hire the right people and allocate adequate financial resources, so that you can execute your growth strategy. As dermatologists, we are busy attending to patients and often don't have the time or desire to take on administrative roles. A practice manager or clinic director who is well versed in change management and execution is critical to the growth strategy. Hiring a business consultant up front, with experience in dermatology practices, will help you crystalize your plans and guide you in your quest for growth. Speaking to colleagues you trust, ideally with similar practice settings but outside your immediate area, about how they went about growing their practice will broaden your horizons and help you avoid pitfalls. Once the right team is in place, plans can be framed and taken to fruition.

51.3 Define Your Practice Purpose and Ideals

People are influenced mostly by those they trust, admire, and believe care for them. Despite recognizing the importance of trust, few leaders give it the central focus it warrants.[1] If patients don't believe that you are acting in their best interest, you won't be successful in influencing them. Trust is built by being patient-focused. Communicating that we are patient-focused can be achieved in many ways, but perhaps most importantly through practice attitude and culture. Understanding who you are and the "purpose" or "why" of your practice will form the foundation of how everything in your practice is implemented and how your practice is viewed by others.[2] Defining your purpose precedes mission statements, strategies, and tactics. For example, if your purpose is to make people feel good about themselves, this will inform how you and your staff communicate with patients, look and feel of the office, your attitude when dealing with unhappy patients, and every other aspect of the practice. Starting with this exercise is very valuable in helping to build your practice brand and achieving both the desired culture within the practice and the patient-facing aspects of your practice. People are more likely to connect with your unique purpose than solely with a procedure or result that may equally be achieved by other practices. In his book, Jim Stengel describes five must-dos when building a brand[3]:

1. Discover an ideal or purpose in one of the fields of fundamental human values.
2. Build your business culture around your ideal.
3. Communicate your ideal to engage both your employees and customers.
4. Deliver a near-ideal customer experience.
5. Evaluate your progress and people against your ideal.

To help your practice team members discover their "why," you may wish to consider holding a team-building "purpose" workshop that allows staff members to identify, embody, and communicate their "why." This will result in improved staff satisfaction, better interactions with patients, and overall elevation of your practice brand.

51.4 Know Your Practice Type and Competitors

There are many dermatology practice models in today's market. When starting a practice, it's easy to fall into the trap of trying to cater to and attract overly broad segments of the market. The reality is that a practice is much more likely to be successful if it stays focused and in its "lane." To do so, it's important to identify both your practice type and market segment. Practices may be categorized in various ways, some of which include:

- Solo, group (dermatology only or multispecialty), academic, or third party corporate.

Market segments commonly include:

- Luxury, premium, midrange, and discount.

Once you define your target market and practice offering, it's much easier to focus on the patients who are most important to you. For example, if you decide to run a premium practice, you will concentrate on providing a higher level patient experience that pays attention to important details such as previsit preparation and information, in-office concierge-like service, and posttreatment follow-up to name a few. On the other hand, a discount practice is much more likely to focus on discounts, as the main driver of new patient acquisition and patient retention. The service levels and expectations in these models will necessarily be different and tailored to the patients that you choose to work with.

51.5 Ways to Grow Your Practice

Some of the basic ways to grow your practice are listed below.

- Become more efficient: This refers to being able to attend to more patients in the same amount of time or making sure that existing patients are aware of all your services, so that they can take advantage of them.
- Add new services or products: This might include new devices, skin care products, or procedures, to name a few.
- Hire new providers such as dermatologists or physician extenders.
- Add a new practice location: By expanding locations, the practice will be able to service more patients, thus increasing overall revenues.

Most practices would benefit from improved efficiencies. By understanding your growth goals and business model, it will be easier to decide which of the other growth options to pursue.

51.6 Physician Extenders

Practice extenders can take the form of assistants who help the dermatologist be more efficient, ensuring the latter only performs those tasks that s/he can uniquely do, thus offloading other tasks, and allowing the dermatologist to attend to more patients, consequently growing revenues. Depending on your practice model, you may also wish to add physician assistants (PAs) to carry out standard examinations, prescribe certain basic medications, and maybe even lengthen your days and hours of operation. Of course, you will need to consider whether adding PAs who provide independent patient care is right for you, as it changes the flavor of your practice from one where only physicians provide services to one where PAs also deliver patient care. The choice you make will depend on your practice philosophy and patient preferences in your area.

51.7 Know Your Numbers

It's not uncommon for practice owners to say that they have a "gut" feeling of how their practice is performing. However, the reality is that unless it's actually measured, it's not possible to precisely understand how the practice is performing, recognize areas in need of attention, and determine whether changes implemented are of value. It is only by tracking and measuring practice numbers that you can make informed choices and decisions with regard to every aspect of the practice, such as hiring, staff compensation, investing in equipment, marketing tactics, investment in physical space, and so on. These measures or metrics, often referred to as *key performance indicators* (KPIs), can be extensive and may seem daunting at first glance. Starting with the KPIs, which make the most sense for your practice and its strategic goals, and expanding as you become comfortable with the numbers is one way to manage all the data. Based on clinic-specific information on where your business currently stands and how you aim to grow in the future, you will be able to select the most relevant KPIs. For example, if you aim to increase top line revenues, looking at your average fee per patient is one possible avenue

to explore. Monitored closely over time, the average fee per patient will allow you to further understand how your patients invest their money, and tactics that can be implemented to allow patients to benefit from all your services, thus increasing the average fee per patient. If patients complain about long wait times in the office, measuring your on-time service performance will allow you to define the problem, implement change, and then reassess it to determine the success of the tactics.

Some of the KPIs to track are listed in the following table adaptation[4]:

Measure	Description
New patients	Number of new patients per health care provider per unit time (day, week, or month)
Patients per day	Total number of patients per practitioner per day
Average fee	Average fee received per visit to the practice
Lifetime value	Average total fees received per patient over lifetime with you
$ per hour	Average fees billed per practitioner (or per room, per device, etc.)
Utilization rate	Percentage of appointment time that is actually booked
Rebooking rate	Percentage of patients seen that have a future appointment booked
Conversion rate–phone calls	Percentage of phone call inquiries that book an appointment
Cancellations with no reschedule	Percentage of cancelled appointments that do not reschedule an appointment
No show rate	Percentage of appointments booked where the patient doesn't attend
Practice sales	Total practice sales over a defined period of time
Sales growth	Growth in practice sales over a defined period of time
Cross-selling	Percentage of patients booked for one service and also purchase another service
On-time service	Percentage of appointments seen within 5 minutes of the scheduled time

51.8 Service, Service, Service

It is said that people better remember how you make them feel than what you say. The same is true in dermatology practices. In fact, patients may have difficulty judging the quality of dermatologic care that you provide, but they are great judges of how they are treated by you and your staff.[5] The whole patient experience—from the time they first encounter your practice on the web or social media to their first email or phone call to the practice, to the time they walk into your office and are greeted by your reception staff, and to the manner in which they are treated by the dermatologist and assistants in the room—all of this and more determine how a patient feels about their experience and the impression formed of your practice. It is critical that each of these touchpoints is analyzed in detail and that the staff are trained to adhere to the practice culture, so as to provide an outstanding customer experience.

For example, training staff on answering phone inquiries is key. Having them answer the phone with the practice name and identifying themselves in a friendly, inviting manner helps potential patients make a connection and puts them at ease. After asking about and understanding the caller's concerns, having staff credential the office and the dermatologist instills confidence. Following it up with a credible and informed response to the issue raised, and finally, a call to action to book an appointment, will lead the caller to feel more confident about the practice and more likely result in booking a consultation with the dermatologist.

51.9 It's All about the Results

It goes without saying that delivering outstanding results is central to the patient experience. Great customer service without excellent results will eventually lead to poor word-of-mouth in the community and will invariably negatively impact the practice. Thus, keeping abreast of the latest treatments, techniques, and devices through continuing medical education in its many forms, so as to deliver excellent results, is at the core of all practices. Even the best marketing plans won't prevent a practice which delivers poor outcomes from sinking.

51.10 Show Patients that You Care

A simple follow-up phone call the day after a visit to find out if the patient has any further questions or to see how a procedure went shows that you care, especially after the first visit or after more complex procedures. For significant procedures, consider making yourself accessible to patients by providing an office extension that rings your mobile phone or an answering service where you can be reached after clinic hours. Surprisingly, patients rarely call but are very appreciative of your efforts to take care of them. For patients new to the practice, scheduling a return visit to assess treatment outcomes is very important in that it provides the opportunity to critically appraise your own work, thus improving your skills; it also allows you to follow-up with other skin-related health concerns the patient may have, thereby giving them the opportunity to benefit from your other services.

Finally, no discussion of service would be complete without stating that each office has its own unique flavor and it is considered favorable to let the office culture and staff personality shine through, so as to further entrench your unique brand.

In summary, implementing service measures that help to deliver positive patient experiences will result in loyalty to you, your practice, and your brand, spreading the word to friends, family, and coworkers.

51.11 Appointment Scheduling

Optimizing the booking schedule is critical in terms of achieving patient satisfaction, improving efficiencies, and growing the practice. This is an ongoing process that is tweaked based on the clinic flow as well as physician and patient requirements.

Case Study: Because we tended to run behind and sometimes didn't have time to fully address patient concerns during visits, we had a consultant come in to evaluate our booking schedule. After spending time observing in the office, the consultant advised us that there were a number of issues that needed to be addressed. First, our in-office wait times were too long, leading to patients experiencing dissatisfaction, sometimes resulting in patients leaving the office before being attended to. Second, appointment times were too short. It was pointed out that patients often came in wanting a particular service or procedure that they felt would address their needs but, after discussing their issue with the dermatologist or staff, it was determined that there were other issues that needed to be addressed, beyond what was originally envisioned. This created the unintended dilemma of forcing us to decide whether we would address the full gamut of issues, thus putting us behind in the schedule as time wasn't sufficiently allocated, or rebooking the patient at a separate time to deal with the other issues. We gathered from experience that when the latter route was chosen, patients often didn't return as their schedule didn't permit another visit or they lost interest.

After having a staff meeting to discuss the findings, it was decided that we would do several things to attempt to reduce wait times once the patient arrived in the office. First, we decided to lengthen appointment times to permit us to address more patient concerns at the time of their appointment, without having to bring them back on a separate date. Supplementary training of booking agents empowered them to more carefully inquire about patient goals on the phone prior to booking, allowing us to book times that better catered to patient needs; in general, this resulted in longer appointment times. While we were initially concerned that longer appointment times and fewer patients per day would translate into reduced revenues, we found that this wasn't at all the case. A number of positive outcomes were realized: wait times in the office were significantly reduced because more time was allocated for patient visits; we were able to perform more complete treatments beyond what was originally envisioned; and cross-selling was increased as we had more time to understand and discuss other concerns. The overall effect of the scheduling changes was to improve patient satisfaction with the office experience, improve patient results, and increase office revenues. Each practice is different but the take-home message is that identifying and understanding office issues and then implementing rational changes that can be tracked and measured often lead to practice growth and improved loyalty to your brand.

51.12 The Consultation

The consultation is arguably the part of the patient engagement process that has the highest potential to set your practice apart from others and help you grow your business. While many patients come into the office asking about a specific issue, we always ask patients if they'd like to take advantage of a full assessment and are open to being presented with a customized treatment plan with prioritized treatment options. Without fail, patients agree to this approach, even if they can't necessarily afford to proceed with all suggestions at the time of their visit. By taking an educational approach to the consultation, the patient acquires a deeper understanding of the issues at hand and the rationale for treatment and, perhaps most importantly, develops trust.

We have found that a professional, courteous approach in which the dermatologist calmly walks into the room, smiles, introduces him/herself and engages the patient with an anecdote or a talking point unrelated to the reason for the consultation is a great way to start off the visit. Putting patients at ease and not making them feel rushed goes a long way toward establishing a rapport. Sitting beside the patient, listening to their needs, and repeating a summary of their concerns to convey an understanding of their issues are some other strategies that help to show that you care, thus building confidence in and loyalty to the dermatologist and the practice. Since trust is critical, it is our office culture to only recommend treatments and procedures that will deliver great results and avoid suggesting those that will not be of benefit to the patient. The use of visual aids such as a tablet or computer with before-and-after photographs, ideally your own, to provide examples of patients with comparable issues, so as to explain treatment benefits and expected outcomes, will further help to build credibility and showcase the dermatologist's talents.

51.13 Marketing and Public Relations

In today's competitive environment, marketing and public relations (PR) are quite common in dermatology practices. Marketing can be broadly categorized as *internal* and *external*, with internal marketing referring to measures that are directed toward existing patients in the practice, while external measures are directed to individuals outside the practice. In a dermatology practice, internal marketing is considered the most effective and least costly.

Internal marketing starts with the look and feel of your office space, as it represents the brand that you choose to portray to your patients. An aesthetically pleasing, clean, organized office with calming music sets an inviting tone for visitors. Attention to amenities such as beverages and a selection of reading materials further enhances the experience.

Other helpful internal marketing tactics include having a video display in the waiting room and/or patient examination rooms with an educational presentation that both provides information about the skin and raises awareness about treatment options available in the practice for various concerns, both medical and cosmetic. Topics to consider covering include skin cancer statistics and information, sun protection tips, skin care pearls, skin disease information, before-and-after photos of procedures performed by the practice, highlights of video clips showcasing the dermatologist's expertise, and any other items that you deem appropriate for your target market. All of this can be easily accomplished using PowerPoint, Keynote, or similar presentation software.

Having brochures with procedures performed in the practice often raise awareness of solutions provided by the practice, especially since it has been our experience that patients are frequently unaware of all that the practice has to offer. In addition to specific procedural brochures, we have found that a brochure that is organized by "issue" and "solution" is a good way of providing a broad overview of services using a problem-oriented approach.

Further to this theme of patients being unaware of all that the practice has to offer, asking the patient for permission to discuss issues or solutions not raised by the patient will allow you to make the patient aware of other relevant treatment options that would be of benefit, perhaps even more so than what was originally requested. Patients frequently don't know the treatment that would best help them achieve their desired goal. Thus, if one only provides information about the specific treatment requested, suboptimal results will be achieved and the patient will be dissatisfied.

Increasing patient retention can also be aided with social media communication. Understanding your patients is important in being able to effectively communicate with them and ensure that you are utilizing the correct social platforms to create a dialogue with your target audience. For example, understanding the average age, gender, profession, and location of your existing patients will aid you in selecting the most effective marketing techniques (i.e., Instagram) to interact with your current patients.[6]

There exist multiple external marketing and PR tactics. Making yourself available to media and making the practice discoverable on social media is especially important as media mentions carry a lot of weight with respect to credentialing. Searching local media, pitching stories about the latest products, procedures, or treatment options, and sending thank you notes are all simple tactics that will help to raise the profile of your dermatology practice. Working with industry can be very helpful, provided that one maintains credibility by being truthful and showing integrity. Asking to become a spokesperson, media contact, speaker, or clinical trial investigator, or participating in product launches are but a few of the ways dermatologists can work with industry in a mutually beneficial manner.

Nowadays, external marketing often includes reaching out to current and potential patients through the Internet via a website and social media platforms. Practice websites not only provide a repository of detailed information about the practice such as products and services but also allow the practice to tell its story, credentialing dermatologists and other employees and, importantly, elucidating the practice purpose. Periodic updates when new products and services are offered, blogs, and other news items will help to keep the website fresh. Having the website optimized for mobile devices is a must, given that most searches now take place through mobile phones. Search engine optimization and keeping content up-to-date helps in garnering a higher ranking on search results. On the other hand, social media channels such as Instagram and Facebook keep patients engaged with shorter snippets of information that help build the practice brand and increase brand equity amongst patients.

Some established practices choose PR over advertising with the rationale that PR helps to build the brand. For example, by making potential patients aware of a unique quality or achievement of the practice such as a speaking engagement at an important meeting or a unique technique pioneered by the dermatologist, the patient may be more likely to develop trust and seek out services offered by the clinic. Spending money on advertising can be beneficial but, to make it most effective, it should be tied to the practice purpose and brand, so as to increase patient connection to the practice, thus increasing the likelihood of acquiring lifelong patients.

Ultimately, whichever marketing and PR tactic one chooses, the central message should always be one that keeps the practice purpose and brand at the top of mind.

51.14 Online Reviews

Increasingly, tech-savvy potential patients, especially those who don't know of the dermatologist by word-of-mouth, will seek information not only through the practice website but also online patient reviews. Online reviews are a useful tool as they are a form of earned media, which is often the most trusted source of promotion in the eyes of potential patients.[7] Building a positive online presence can be as simple as providing patients a card with a list of relevant online rating sites and encouraging them to rate you as they leave your office. While some negative reviews may be spurious, by checking your ratings regularly to look for trends, you'll be able to address complaints and implement changes in order to improve your practice. Furthermore, responding to reviews, positive and negative, while maintaining confidentiality will be a form of signal to potential patients that your practice is engaged and values feedback.

51.15 Conclusion

Growing your practice may seem like a daunting task but by approaching it systematically, it is highly achievable. A stepwise approach to growth involves creating a solid foundation with the right people and sufficient financial resources, defining your practice purpose, identifying and catering to your market segment, and understanding your performance by measuring KPIs. Paying attention to detail and creating a comprehensive 5-star customer experience in every aspect of the practice all the way, from the patient's first contact with the practice to their postvisit follow-up, will go far in helping a dermatology practice achieve its growth objectives.

References

[1] Horsager D. The Trust Edge: How Top Leaders Gain Faster Results, Deeper Relationships, and a Stronger Bottom Line. New York, NY: Free Press; 2012

[2] Sinek S. Start with Why: How Great Leaders Inspire Everyone to Take Action. New York, NY: Penguin Group; 2009

[3] Stengel J. Grow: How Ideals Power Growth and Profit at the World's Greatest Companies. New York, NY: Random House; 2011

[4] Clinic Mastery. Available at: https://www.clinicmastery.com/numbers/. Published 2017. Accessed April 20, 2019

[5] The Coker Group. Starting and Marketing a Dermatology Practice. Schaumburg, Illinois: American Academy of Dermatology; n.d.

[6] Practice Builders. Available at: https://www.practicebuilders.com/blog/top-25-ways-to-attract-more-patients-to-your-medical-practice/. Published 2018. Accessed April 20, 2019

[7] R1 Revenue Cycle Management. Available at: http://www.r1rcm.com/blog-posts/5-ways-to-increase-patient-volume-and-grow-your-medical-practice. Published 2016. Accessed April 20, 2019

52 Mohs: Outsource or Keep In-House

Allison Hanlon MD, PhD

Abstract

Mohs micrographic surgery is the preferred skin cancer treatment for tumors located in anatomically sensitive areas. Thoughtful consideration of the practice's resources and needs is crucial prior to expanding into Mohs micrographic surgery.

Patient population, personnel training, clinic space and cost all need to factor into whether Mohs services is an area for practice growth.

Keywords: Mohs micrographic surgery, skin cancer, CLIA

Top 10 Things You Need to Know

1. Mohs micrographic surgery is the preferred treatment for skin cancers in anatomically sensitive areas for complete evaluation of the surgical margin.
2. The American Board of Dermatology has approved a subspecialty certification in micrographic dermatologic surgery.
3. The ideal clinical space is patient-focused and efficient for staff. The space needs to include a Mohs micrographic surgery laboratory, procedural waiting room, and surgical rooms.
4. Before any buildout or room conversion, confirm that the proposal meets the local codes.
5. Capital investment in equipment is significant for clinical and laboratory space.
6. A clinical laboratory improvement amendments (CLIA) certification for high complexity is necessary to perform Mohs micrographic surgery.
7. The laboratory staff training includes Mohs micrographic processing of tissue, procedures for lab maintenance, and CLIA certification.
8. The physician performing Mohs micrographic surgery will need malpractice insurance to include more complex surgical procedures.
9. The clinical staff skills include assisting in surgical procedures, management of surgical patients, and multitasking.
10. State laws regulate the medical assistant, licensed practical nurse, and registered nurse duties. Verifying the state regulations is important before defining clinical staff roles.

52.1 Introduction

Mohs micrographic surgery is the preferred skin cancer treatment for tumors located in anatomically sensitive areas. First developed by Frederic Mohs, MD, in the 1930s, Mohs micrographic surgery (MMS) involves the physician functioning as both surgeon and pathologist. The physician removes the skin cancer as a thin disc and examines the frozen processed specimen to map out areas of tumor involvement. The precise mapping allows for removal of positive tumor margins in the corresponding anatomic site while sparing healthy tissue. The number of Mohs micrographic procedures has grown with increasing skin cancer incidence. The decision to incorporate MMS in one's clinical practice depends on multiple decision points.

Dermatology residents are introduced to MMS as part of the Accreditation Council for Graduate Medical Education (ACGME) dermatology curriculum. The residency exposure can vary depending upon the training site. The American Society for Mohs Surgery (ASMS) provides continuing medical education courses postresidency for Mohs micrographic surgery and surgical reconstruction training. Formal training in cutaneous oncology, MMS, and surgical reconstruction is available through the ACGME Micrographic Surgery and Dermatologic Oncology Fellowship. In the 1- to 2-year fellowship, physicians are trained on the treatment and management of skin cancer and cutaneous surgical reconstruction. In October 2018, the American Board of Dermatology approved the creation of a subspecialty certification in micrographic dermatologic surgery. How board certification will impact reimbursement and practice scope is not known at this time.

Early Mohs micrographic surgery practices were consult based where patients were referred for skin cancer treatment. Few practices have maintained this model. The incorporation of MMS within a general dermatology practice is on account of increased patient demand coupled with physician training during residency and fellowship. Large private practices, multispecialty groups, and academic centers often have MMS as part of the services offered. For solo practitioners or small group practices, when to incorporate MMS in the practice depends on multiple factors. Are the physician members trained in MMS? Does the practice have the patient volume to support a Mohs surgeon? Is the clinical space able to contain a Mohs unit? Do you want to hire additional technical and support staff? Do you want to incorporate more complex procedures in the practice? We will review here some of the decision points to consider prior to incorporating MMS within a practice and the steps to do so.

52.2 Clinical Volume

The clinical volume to support a full-time Mohs surgeon is thought to be three full-time general dermatologists. Before expanding to include Mohs surgery, it makes sense to know if the practice has the clinical demand. If the clinical volume does not support a full-time Mohs surgeon, a part-time hire can be considered, but the return on the surgical buildout and space needs to be considered. Building referral patterns with local plastics, oculoplastics, otolaryngologists, dermatology, and primary care providers can increase Mohs referrals.

It is also important to understand your payer mix. Some commercial insurance plans may not pay adequately per case to cover overhead. In some areas, Medicare will not cover beyond five stages. Understanding your payer mix will also help you calculate overhead and understand the minimum number of cases you will require to perform in order to keep the Mohs unit running successfully. If you decide to outsource Mohs, understand what these implications are expensive.

52.3 Clinical Space

The ideal clinical space for MMS is patient-focused and efficient for staff. The space needs to include a laboratory, surgical rooms, and a patient waiting room. Room planning should be functional so that the physician can efficiently attend to patients with staff nearby. A large, spread out space does not allow for effective communication amongst the clinical team and staff can get "lost" easily. Before any buildout or room conversion, confirm the proposal meets local codes.

The laboratory is where tissue processing takes place. The laboratory is located near the surgical space in a direct route from the patient rooms. The laboratory should not be within the path where patients walk between surgical rooms, waiting room, or check-in desk. Direct tissue transport is important for efficiency. Also, most patients prefer not seeing tissue being transported. Depending upon the laboratory size, physicians can perform slide review within the space, allowing direct communication with regard to slide quality. If the laboratory space is small, slides can be reviewed in another location, but time is added for slide transport. The laboratory space needs to be adequately large to include a cryostat, linear stainer, fire cabinet for solution storage, and sink for stainer drainage.

During tissue processing, patients can stay in the procedure room or a nearby waiting room. If patients stay within the surgical room, the space cannot be used to treat another patient. The benefit of keeping the patient in the room is no room turnover time, but the short turnover time does not equate to keeping the procedure room occupied by one patient. A patient waiting area near the nursing staff is ideal for patients to stand by between stages. The waiting room design should include space for a family member to accompany the patient. Refreshments and comfortable seating enhances the patient experience. Keeping the Mohs patients separate from the general dermatology or cosmetic patients is considered best. Most patients do not want to see other patients with bandages in place or bleeding, if that occurs.

The procedure rooms will need adequate lighting, a surgical table, electrosurgical unit, storage space, and sink. If overhead surgical lights are required, supportive beams may be needed to suspend the light safely. The room space needs to accommodate a fully expanded surgical table with room for the physician and staff to easily walk around the patient. Electrosurgical units can range in complexity with some having attached vacuums. The cost varies and often depends on the surgeon's preference; including a vacuum within the system adds to expenses but decreases the smoke plume.

52.4 Staffing

The staffing required for Mohs micrographic surgery includes a physician, laboratory staff, and clinical staffing. I recommend the physician should have completed an ACGME Micrographic Surgery and Dermatologic Oncology Fellowship. While a fellowship is not required to perform MMS at this time, the training includes 1 to 2 years of training in MMS, reconstruction, and cutaneous oncology.

A histotech manages the laboratory and processes the tissue for histology review. The histotech can possess training ranging from a graduate of an accredited histology program and courses through the American Society for Mohs Histotechnology to in-house training. The histotechnician's salary can vary based on training. Slide quality is very important for patient safety and outcomes. A physician cannot accurately evaluate poor-quality slides resulting in time delays for recuts or additional tissue layers. The time delays impact efficiency and patient care. A competent histotech produces consistent, high-quality slides, and is worth the salary.

Clinical staff includes medical assistants (MA), licensed practical nurses (LPN), and/or registered nurses (RN). State laws define the MA, LPN, and RN duties. Verifying the state regulations is important before deciding clinical staffing and duties. Multiple staffing models are possible, but clinical volume and complexity will determine the nursing staff number. MMS requires personnel who can assist in surgical procedures, multitask, and work as a team.

52.5 Certification

CLIA was established by the federal government to establish quality standards for laboratory testing. A CLIA certificate can be obtained directly through your local state CLIA office or through an accreditation agency that certifies the laboratory in place of the state. CLIA has different certificates based on the tests performed. There are three levels of complexity: waived, moderate, and high; Mohs micrographic surgery is considered to belong to the high level of complexity.

To maintain CLIA certification for Mohs micrographic surgery the following is required:

- Create a laboratory procedure manual for each test and equipment used.
- Establish a quality assessment program for all laboratory tests performed. Standard operating procedures for quality control of patient specimens, personnel training, and competency. Establish safety policies and procedures.

CLIA requires that anyone performing a high-complexity test possess at least an associate degree in laboratory science or medical laboratory technology, or at least 60 semester hours of higher education, including at least 24 semester hours that are science-based. If your practice has a medical assistant or histotechnologist grossing tissue or performing any high complexity testing, they are mandated to meet those requirements. Maintaining a laboratory procedure manual, and quality assessment (QA) and quality control (QC) logs are important for CLIA requirements. CLIA representatives review the documents during inspections. The American Academy of Dermatology and the American Society for Mohs Histotechnology are resources for log examples.

52.6 Conclusion

The decision to incorporate MMS within a general dermatology practice depends upon the clinical need, staffing, and space. Expanding services to include MMS allows for continuity of patient care within one practice and an additional source of revenue. Multiple decision points are needed to develop an efficient and patient-friendly clinical space, trained staff, and certification maintenance.

Suggested Readings

AAD Clinical Laboratory Improvement Amendments for Dermatology Manual. Publisher American Academy of Dermatology

American Society for Mohs Histotechnology (ASMH). Available at: http://www.mohstech.org. Accessed November 13, 2019

Manual of Frozen Section Processing for Mohs Micrographic Surgery.Publisher American College of Mohs Surgery

53 The Ground Rules of Teaching in a Private Practice

Lauren Taglia MD, PhD

Abstract

Outpatient practice in the field of dermatology provides an excellent opportunity for teaching given its visual nature and patient volume. This chapter explores the potential obstacles as well as identifies strategies for educating in the private practice setting. The methodologies provide a practical guide for establishing a successful teaching program.

Keywords: mentoring, private practice teaching, education at bedside

Top 10 Things You Need to Know

1. The private practice dermatologist has a unique and valuable perspective to share.
2. Visual aspects of dermatology are uniquely applicable to bedside teaching and modeling.
3. The large volume of clinical cases observed in private practice, as well as the relatively low cost and equipment required to assess the skin, provide infinite teaching opportunities.
4. Lack of access to dermatologists in the US presents an opportunity to partner with primary care physicians to improve referrals and melanoma detection.
5. Teaching in private practice presents an opportunity to mentor future generations and directly impact the communities served.
6. Potential obstacles to teaching in a private practice include limited dedicated training time, lack of experience in teaching, and potential financial impact of replacing clinical work with training sessions.
7. Effective teaching requires planning and realistic goal setting to be successful for both the teacher and the learner.
8. Strategies to enhance bedside teaching include asking questions, identifying general rules, and providing feedback to learners.
9. The special relationship between teacher and learner provides a source of personal and professional gratification apart from patient care.
10. Developing effective training goals and teaching plans require continuing education of current skills and practices which further the provider's opportunities for career fulfillment and satisfaction.

53.1 Introduction

After many years of hard work, dedication, Kodachrome sessions, and days spent hunched over the microscope reviewing slides, you successfully completed residency. After passing the boards, you set your sights on the ultimate goal driving you all these years: *actually practicing medicine.* After clearing the final board exam hurdle, you still have some important choices to make. Will you choose to focus on a subspecialty such as surgery or pediatric dermatology? Where will you choose to start your career geographically? Perhaps the biggest of all early career decisions is whether to practice in an academic or private practice setting. Studies of career surveys find those interested in an academic career achieve professional satisfaction related to teaching, research, and scientific writing.[1] For others, the choice to join a private practice offers the opportunity for greater control in decision-making, greater income potential, and a lack of institutional requirements. While, at first blush, the choice to embark on a career in an academic setting or private practice seems to be a decision between two extremes, there are significant shared goals for both settings. Those goals include excellent patient care, clinical challenge, and continuous professional growth.

53.1.1 Challenges that Prevent Private Practitioners from Teaching

Continuous professional growth requires a lifelong devotion to learning but no one takes this journey alone. Success as a dermatologist is dependent on the effort and effectiveness of teachers and mentors, and participation in teacher/learner relationships is part of the social contract of being a member of the medical community. While many dermatologists can quickly recall the teachers and mentors who have had the most impact on their lives, it is all too easy to forget that once you are a fully practicing physician, you share in the responsibility to teach others. The task of teaching can be daunting for a variety of reasons. See below a list of challenges that are especially relevant in the private practice setting.

- Lack of experience in teaching or lack of confidence in ability to teach.
- Lack of protected time to prepare and educate.
- Potential for running behind in clinic due to time required to teach.
- Potential impact on income if time is allotted for teaching versus attending to more patients.
- Patient preference to not have other providers involved in the clinic visit.

53.1.2 Benefits of Teaching

In spite of these challenges, the decision to commit to teaching in private practice should emerge from the desire to give back to learners as prior teachers have provided you with. The Hippocratic oath states it is the role of the physician "to not only respect the scientific gains in those physicians whose steps I walk, and gladly share such knowledge as is mine with those who are to follow." Once a private practice dermatologist has committed to actively teaching in his or her clinic, there are multiple benefits he or she will realize. Such benefits will improve the personal career of the teacher and the overall effectiveness of the practice, and therefore should not be limited to just the academic clinic.

- Teaching is an opportunity to continue to learn through both preparation of training and feedback from learners. "To teach is to learn twice."
- Dermatology's visual nature and private practice's large patient volume provide excellent opportunities for teaching at the bedside.
- Teaching provides the opportunity for feedback and collaboration with learners and therein lies the potential for immediate impact on quality of patient care.
- The special relationship created between teacher and student provides a potential source of personal and professional gratification unique from clinical work.

You are coming around to the idea that teaching is a necessary and beneficial element of a healthy private practice clinic, but you are still unsure if you will be able to commit to such a large undertaking. There is hope for you, the overburdened private practice dermatologist. A recent comprehensive review of education in the general medicine ambulatory setting uncovered important elements for effective teaching. First, the behavior of teachers strongly influenced the outcome and perceived success of the experience. Teachers who were considered effective showed interest, asked questions, defined goals, demonstrated competence, and importantly, spent time with the learner. Surprisingly, the environmental variables such as case load, pace of workload, space, and structured time for teaching all had little impact on the overall rating on teacher effectiveness. The key point is that effectiveness of teaching is driven by the learners' perceptions of what is effective and not reliant on rigid academic structure. Another key finding is that role modeling greatly influenced learners. For example, in one study, there were similarities in what teachers wanted to share with their students, what these teachers most valued about their own mentors, and what the students wanted to emulate following their rotation. Therefore, the goal of teaching in the private dermatology clinic should not only create an opportunity for learning that is both effective and rewarding for both the teacher and the learner but also draw from the ongoing goals and everyday operations of the practice.

53.1.3 Strategic Questions and Opportunities

So, you have made the decision that teaching is a valuable exercise and you want to take on the challenge in your own practice. Where do you begin? Success will emerge from a solid strategy. The bullet points below capture some strategic questions and opportunities private practice clinicians should consider.

- Define realistic goals and set a plan: Once time is set aside for preparation and delivery of teaching, it will make the process more enjoyable for both the learner and the teacher.
- Take advantage of available opportunities to teach including partnering with full-time faculty at local medical centers, joining university faculty as a part-time teacher, or reaching out to colleagues in other private practice clinics to establish shared sessions

- Determine the audience: Would you like to teach medical students, residents in dermatology or primary practice, primary care physicians, or advanced practitioners? Or would you prefer to teach to nonmedical individuals such as clinic staff or patients?
- Consider opportunities in the community: Churches, small interest groups, and local businesses provide teaching opportunities and a potential for name recognition and patient referral. This is especially important for early career physicians.
- Look for teaching opportunities with colleagues during society meetings. Such opportunities not only offer unique experiences for greater learning but also relationship-building within the field.

53.2 Methodology for Establishing a Teaching Program

53.2.1 Step One: Preparation

To be successful, it is important to first set the plan for the teaching experience. First, consider the five "w's" of your goal: who, when, where, what, and why.

- **Who:** Is your goal to teach to reach early learners such as medical students or would you prefer a more seasoned professional like a resident in either dermatology or outside the field? Identifying the group you are most excited to reach will drive required material and likely predict a greater opportunity for success.
- **When:** Are there days in the week, month, or year that more easily lend themselves to teaching? Some things to consider may be natural slow times in clinic such as early in the year when patients have not yet reached their deductible and may be less likely to seek care.
- **Where:** Do you prefer to teach in clinic with the learners at bedside or do you prefer to reach a broader audience by participating in teaching opportunities in the community (i.e., educational sessions held in local churches or small businesses)?
- **What:** Are there specific conditions you wish to teach, such as educating primary care physicians on the differential diagnosis of groin rashes? Are there broader objectives you

wish to cover, such as teaching junior clinical staff the components of the total body skin examination?
- **Why:** What motivates you as the teacher? Do you wish to become involved in your local health care community, stay current with literature and practices, and establish rapport with students? Defining the "why" of anything we do makes the experience more memorable and rewarding.

Once these questions have been answered, the teacher should define the specific role of the learner in the desired training. For example, the teacher may choose to sit down with the learner prior to the start of clinic and set up the expectations for the experience. Points to discuss may include number of patients the learner should attend to, what the learner may encounter during the clinical visits, how to consult with the teacher and patient during the training visit, and what, if any, conditions the learner might like to focus more time on.

53.2.2 Step Two: Teaching during the Visit

There are a few key elements to teaching during the visit that allow for more meaningful experiences for the learner. First, it is important for the teacher to ask questions. By asking questions, the teacher encourages active participation of the learner and identifies strengths and shortcomings in understanding. The teacher may choose to ask questions after the clinical visit or even prior to seeing the patient to better "prime" the learner. It is also important to allow adequate time for the learner to answer questions, so choosing *when* to ask is equally as important as *what* to ask.

The teacher may want to identify a general rule to summarize important teaching points most appropriate to the clinical experience. The general rule should be brief, contain both the patient's concern and learner's need, as well as emphasize a useful principle. The teacher may ask themselves this one simple question to identify an important general rule, "what do I want the learner to take away from this patient's visit"? When there is insufficient time to address all relevant issues related to a patient case, a useful technique for teaching in the clinic is modeling. The teacher can simply think out loud by sharing clinical clues and insights as well as pointing out considerations and dilemmas when deciding on diagnosis and plan for care. In addition, modeling offers a unique technique for teachers to demonstrate the importance of asking questions while demonstrating compassionate care to both the learner and patient. This can be especially useful in the busy private practice setting.

53.2.3 Step Three: Teaching after the Visit

It is important at the end of the experience to provide feedback to the learner. Effective feedback should include specific examples directly observed by the teacher and should be nonjudgmental in nature. A learning environment, one that is supportive and nonthreatening, will facilitate healthy relationships between the learner and teacher. In the private practice setting, the teacher may wish to use time at the end of the busy clinic day to review general rules encountered as well as take time to answer any questions not addressed earlier.

Private practice dermatologists can avail of a unique opportunity to not only provide excellent care to patients but also influence learners at any stage in their career. By developing goals and setting a thoughtful plan, the rewards of teaching provide further opportunity for career fulfillment and satisfaction.

Suggested Readings

Brodell RT. The role of the part-time physician-teacher in dermatology. Arch Dermatol 1996;132(7):758–760

Mayer JE, Swetter SM, Fu T, Geller AC. Screening, early detection, education, and trends for melanoma: current status (2007–2013) and future directions: Part I. Epidemiology, high-risk groups, clinical strategies, and diagnostic technology. J Am Acad Dermatol 2014;71(4):599.e1–599.e12, quiz 610, 599.e12

McCleskey PE. Commentary: to improve melanoma detection, help teach our colleagues. J Am Acad Dermatol 2015;73(6):966–967

McGee SR, Irby DM. Teaching in the outpatient clinic. Practical tips. J Gen Intern Med 1997;12(2, Suppl 2): S34–S40

Tierney EP, Hanke CW, Kimball AB. Career trajectory and job satisfaction trends in Mohs micrographic surgeons. Dermatol Surg 2011;37(9):1229–1238

54 Staying Active Nationally in the Years after Residency

Susan H. Weinkle MD

Abstract

This chapter addresses ways to stay active in dermatology nationally in the years after residency. There are ten top things you need to know in order to accomplish this goal. First, there is the question of why you would want to do this. Being involved nationally can add an entire broader professional experience. Leadership is the first step to building this profile. Teaching is a way to give back and share your passion and expertise. Clinical research allows you the opportunity to be part of growing the specialty. Advisory boards give you the interactions with colleagues. Becoming a volunteer faculty member is another way to give back. Publishing is certainly a way to establish expertise. Advocacy involvement can help to assure the needs of our specialty. Charity is giving back financially and can inspire others. Mentoring is another way to share your skills. International involvement provides a broader global perspective. Most importantly, staying active nationally can help you to continue to grow both personally and professionally.

Keywords: leadership, teaching, clinical research, advisory boards, publishing, mentoring

Top 10 Things You Need to Know

1. Leadership opportunities abound in your local community and on the national stage. Any leadership role builds your profile and opens new opportunities for professional advancement.
2. Teaching allows you to sharpen your communication skills and expand your own knowledge, whether speaking to civic groups, training residents, or presenting on a national stage. These skills will prove to be invaluable as you advance on both local and national levels.
3. Clinical research offers the opportunity to stay informed about emerging therapeutics with flexible options for involvement. Those possessing early clinical experience of a novel intervention are the first to be called upon to lecture or comment.
4. Consulting/advisory boards let you learn about new products or interventions.
5. Volunteer faculty positions allow you to give back, hone your teaching skills, and stay up-to-date on new advancements.
6. Publishing is the primary way to establish expertise. In fact, it is rare to be called upon to lecture on a topic you have never published on. Also, consider opportunities to collaborate with medical or lay media outlets as an expert source to further establish your acumen.
7. Advocacy opportunities range from the local to the national scale and allow you to support issues you are passionate about. Effective advocacy involves networking and outreach that keep you active in the specialty.
8. Charitable contributions, like advocacy opportunities, allow for networking and the chance to be informed about key issues affecting the specialty and the public.
9. Mentoring is as much about gaining knowledge and insight as it is about sharing it. Communication and interpersonal skills honed as a one-on-one mentor will serve you well on a larger stage.
10. International involvement affords the opportunity to learn about advancements in other parts of the world, meet colleagues from other countries, and elevate your status in the US.

54.1 Introduction

Early in my career, I was asked by Lyn Drake, MD, to chair a surgical session at the American Academy of Dermatology (AAD). I was honored and excited. I worked really on that session, and we were successful. The course had very good reviews and since that time, I've had the opportunity to direct a course at the AAD every year for more than 25 years. It was a great chance that I availed of because someone opened the door to me with an opportunity, and I focused on producing the desired result.

To stay active on the national level postresidency comes down to those two key elements: opportunity and delivery. However, opportunities do not always fall in your lap. The dermatologist must seek opportunities, all the while developing the skills required to be successful.

There are numerous avenues for finding opportunities as well as honing talents and skills. The top 10 opportunities are in some ways interrelated, and they all offer a degree of flexibility to match your particular interests and availability. It is essential, therefore, to start by identifying your passion. Where have you specialized your practice and what is your expertise? To benefit most from your activities, find your passion and focus on opportunities that align with it. If you've never prescribed a biologic, don't pursue opportunities in biologics. Conversely, if you don't even inject botulinum toxin, steer clear of programs in aesthetics.

54.2 Why Be Active Nationally?

Many dermatologists will have rewarding careers, serving their local patient base and being active contributors to their local communities. They will be successful and satisfied, focusing efforts close to home. However, some dermatologists will be drawn to be active nationally.

Why? A national profile creates opportunities to learn, lead, and serve. There is no shortage of opportunities or benefits. In fact, many dermatologists find that each opportunity may open the door to additional or different opportunities.

A national profile can benefit your practice and create opportunities for increased revenue streams. More importantly, it can enrich your professional experience and enable you to optimize the care provided to patients.

54.3 Leadership

Leadership is, in fact, the first step to building a national profile. Some may mistakenly conceive of leadership positions as the "reward" for attaining a higher profile. The reality is that leadership is the foundation upon which a high-profile career is built. Leadership opportunities exist at the local, state, and national levels. Dermatologists at any stage of their career can volunteer for committee work.

Reach out to state, regional, or national dermatology societies or organizations, as well as general medical organizations, such as your state medical society. These groups are continuously seeking individuals willing to serve on and lead committees. The time and work required may vary by committee, season, or year. Find opportunities that match your interests and your available time.

Each leadership position prepares you to take on additional positions, if you desire. It gives you experience and confidence. In addition, society service is an ideal opportunity to network with others inside and outside of dermatology who can serve as valuable resources, support, and conduits to future opportunities.

54.4 Teaching

Doctors have always been teachers; it's as if we are wired to want to share the knowledge we acquire, so that others can better serve their patients. Give a lecture locally, feel comfortable with teaching, and then lecture at larger meetings and presentations. Gradually, you can go higher up this ladder to become director of courses or even of conferences.

Establish your areas of expertise and passion. Reach out to let others know you are interested in a topic and presenting on it.

54.5 Clinical Research

There's no denying that clinical research can be complex and time-consuming, but it can also be enjoyable and immensely rewarding. Opportunities vary, as does the complexity of each trial. An open-label, postmarketing trial of a topical cream will be less intensive than a double-blind, phase 3 trial of an investigational agent. Participating in clinical trials may require, at least, modest investments in physical changes or upgrades to your office and possibly dedicated staff to assist in trial management.

In the field of aesthetics, involvement in trials may provide you with access to new devices, fillers, or other treatments before the majority of your peers are even aware of them. This benefits you, your patients, and also makes you "in the know."

Investigators are frequently called on to attend advisory board meetings, and present on study results locally, nationally, or even globally. You may be tapped by national newspapers or magazines to discuss a new or emerging drug.

Talk to peers who pursue clinical research to explore the opportunity and be able to fully understand the requirements and commitment. They can provide you with insights and possibly make the introductions to help you get started.

54.6 Consulting and Advisory Boards

The degree to which a dermatologist gets involved in consulting and advisory boards can be variable. To get invited back, ensure that your participation is valuable both to the sponsor and to you. The organizers expect your active participation. Come prepared and conduct research in advance of the meeting, if needed. Be candid—your expertise and opinion are assets in this setting, and the sponsor is asking for your contribution. It is important to listen and always be open to learning from those around you.

The best experiences will come when you commit to opportunities that align with your professional passions. If the opportunity isn't a good fit, pass, and let someone else serve. Industry partners will appreciate your honesty and courtesy, which will serve you well in the future.

54.7 Volunteer Faculty

Most dermatologists serve as volunteer faculty, as they should. It's a great way to give back and support the next generation of dermatologists. Interacting with dermatologists in training may help you learn about new developments, and your affiliation with the university may lead to opportunities via the institution.

54.8 Publishing and Media

Being published is a key way to establish expertise. When your name appears on a study in a peer-reviewed journal, your peers know that you are an expert on a topic.

It may also be beneficial to cultivate opportunities in the national medical or lay media. Being quoted in publications geared to other medical professionals or consumers can highlight your expertise.

54.9 Advocacy

Advocacy can take many forms. Organizations like the AAD organize fly-ins that bring physicians to Washington, DC, to meet with Congressional representatives. This is a very effective approach, but it's just one of many. Advocacy efforts can include making phone calls, writing letters, and organizing others to do the same.

Sometimes, the opportunity to advocate between specialties is overlooked. It can be very rewarding to work with other core specialties over the years and develop mutually beneficial professional and personal relationships in this way.

54.10 Charity

It's really important to be recognized as giving back. In addition to mentoring, research, and teaching, you can give back financially. Supporting professional societies or their missions is a way to demonstrate your dedication to the specialty. Donors are often the first to be informed about issues facing the organization, and they may be called upon to assist in leadership on key initiatives. Beyond personal financial donations, consider donating time, leading a fundraising drive. It's a great opportunity to reconnect with colleagues and network.

54.11 Mentoring

Mentoring is another form of giving back and sharing your skills with others. Opportunities for mentoring abound. Consider formal opportunities, such as through the Women's Dermatology Society mentoring program or The American Society for Dermatologic Surgery resident preceptorship program. Informal mentorships are great too. You may learn as much as you share. And while you, as the mentor, may find yourself directing your mentee to new opportunities, over time, you may find that your mentee is inviting you to panels, papers, and more.

54.12 International Involvement

International involvement provides a broader global perspective on our profession and can frequently put you ahead of the curve in terms of knowing where our specialty is going.

Traveling to international meetings allows you to learn about so many things that we don't have here in the United States.

It also enables you to connect with numerous professionals internationally with whom you may have the opportunity to work with on clinical trials throughout the years.

54.13 Keep Growing and Enjoying Practice

As you identify your focus and work within it to build a national profile, be flexible and recognize that your focus may shift or expand. Allow for evolution within your skill set and your experience and expertise will evolve.

Staying active nationally is less about "being seen" and more about growth and professional and personal expansion beyond day-to-day care of patients. Of the many opportunities available, focus on the ones you find most rewarding. The most meaningful opportunities help you enhance your ability to care for your patients.

As the medical community increasingly addresses the problem of burnout, you will find involvement outside the four walls of your practice actually helps you enjoy practice more. I feel I have a better balance on my professional life which helps prevent boredom and burnout.

Staying active and involved outside your practice broadens your palate. It's often said, "you get what you give 10-fold over." You have to give time, energy, money, commitment, but you get what you give 10-fold over.

Ultimately, my personal motivation has been the opportunity to develop invaluable lasting friendships and supportive colleagues.

Dos and Don'ts

- Do not over commit. Know your limitations and avoid taking on responsibilities you simply cannot handle at the moment. If you'd like to be considered at a later date, when your schedule permits, feel free to say so.
- Be candid. If an opportunity arises but you have reservations, ask for clarification before you decline. Conversely, if something simply is not of interest, say so.
- Be true to yourself in the moment. Give yourself some time to grow and focus on what is important at each stage in your life and career. Your interests and availability may change. This is not only acceptable but beneficial.
- Be on time. If everyone agrees to meet or to be on a call at a certain date and time, be punctual. It's not fair to your colleagues who have also adjusted their busy schedules. Emergencies will arise, but be sure to communicate as quickly as possible if you absolutely must cancel or delay.
- Be reliable and follow through. If you say you will do something, do it.
- Do not feel you must say "yes" to every opportunity, especially if you know you cannot deliver. As you become more recognized and your expertise is established, additional opportunities will follow.
- Get started. Once you get your toe in the water, and you begin to establish yourself and earn respect from your peers, the rest will follow.
- Express gratitude for meaningful opportunities. Consider an old-fashioned handwritten note, which never goes out of fashion.
- Pay it forward. Support peers and share appropriate opportunities with others who are qualified.

55 Getting Involved in Advocacy

Byron K. Ho MD, Nikki D.Y. Tang MD, Anthony M. Rossi MD, FAAD

Abstract

Advocacy has many facets: increasing dermatologists' participation, from grassroots local efforts to legislative lobbying, is vital for the betterment of patients, physicians, and the future of the specialty. Issues such as access to care, prescription drug pricing, truth in advertising, and scope of practice affect dermatology in major ways. As physicians and members of the House of Medicine, we must devote time, effort, and spending to advocate for our field.

Keywords: advocacy, federal legislation, state legislation, patient advocate, health policy

Top 10 Things You Need to Know

1. Medical advocacy can be considered any effort to improve patient care or medical practice.
2. Dermatologists act as patient advocates every day by helping them get the care and treatment they need.
3. Quality and practice improvement projects can help us optimize patient care.
4. Physician advocacy groups, such as the American Academy of Dermatology or American Society for Dermatologic Surgery, have multiple resources to help improve care.
5. Patients' health is affected by social and economic factors, so advocacy can also take place outside of medicine beyond the clinic and hospital.
6. Community activism and engagement allows dermatologists to support local organizations that help their patients.
7. Health policy framing and reform are occurring irrespective of the participation of physicians.
8. There are many steps for a bill to become a law and physicians make an impact at each stage.
9. Legislative advocacy has tremendous potential to effect change and helps protect patient and physician interests.
10. Advocacy is a broad term that includes myriad activities which benefit our patients and is believed to be the first step to get involved.

55.1 Introduction

Many physicians and dermatologists can think of, at least, a few ways that they can improve either their practice, health system, or community at large to positively affect patient care and the practice of medicine. Implementation of those changes, however, can seem insurmountable. Advocacy is the process of identifying these areas of potential change and working to develop ideas into actions, which will drive real transformation.

As physician advocate, dermatologists have the potential to effect positive changes for both our patients and our field as a whole. It may feel both challenging and unappealing to engage in "politics," but advocacy can happen at a grassroots level as well as an organizational one. Engagement is less intimidating by targeting what to advocate for, organizing goals or initiatives, and formulating a strategy composed of discrete and actionable items.

Advocacy can be categorized by both type and level. Types of advocacy include health advocacy and legislative advocacy. Dermatologists can engage in these types of advocacy at different levels of civil society and government. Many of us are already participating in medical advocacy and may not even know it. In doing so, we are shaping the future of health care.

55.2 Why Advocate?

With the majority of physicians dedicated to traditional patient care, it is natural that we might be interested in working outside of the clinic to improve our patients' well-being. Our patients' health and our own abilities to deliver care are all impacted by patient, practice, and community factors. Some of these can be addressed in the clinic, but many require broader community activism and public policy initiatives for change. Thus, advocacy in medicine encompasses any effort to positively affect patient care or medical practice. This can include advocacy in areas that are not strictly within the health care sphere. Indeed, some writers expand the concept of physicians as advocates to include the promotion of health and well-being and reduction of suffering via any social, economic, educational, or political change.[1]

There are multiple social and economic determinants of health. In trying to care for our patients, we regularly attend to them in practice. A patient's economic status, health literacy, insurance status, social supports, transportation barriers, employment constraints, childcare needs, and many other aspects of their life all affect their health and ability to obtain medical treatment. In turn, these factors are further influenced by wider societal structures. For example, insurance status and insurance policies affect patients' access to specialists and also the medications we can prescribe. Medication price burden, access to medications, and pharmaceutical price tiers affect adherence and disease control. Health literacy and beliefs factor daily into patient counseling and are also influenced by patients' cultures, educational backgrounds, and communities. Barriers to health care access can significantly impact disease severity or even prognosis; one example would include delayed melanoma diagnoses. Becoming engaged in advocacy allows us to address these systemic issues, and thereby improve our patients' health as well as our own success in treating them. This is a belief that many physicians share; in 2004, a survey found that 90% of physicians felt physician advocacy was important.[2]

Furthermore, health care policy is being framed irrespective of the participation of dermatologists. As frontline providers, physicians are uniquely positioned to help inform public initiatives but, at the same time, are highly vulnerable to their implications. We are major stakeholders in almost any public policy change, especially with regard to health care policy. One obvious example is the Affordable Care Act, which has been controversial and subject to attack since its passing. However, all proposed federal regulatory models have major implications for our patient populations, compensation, and practice environments. Beyond

the realm of health policy, related fields such as education reform or tax policy can have lasting impacts on socioeconomic determinants of health via inequities. Even immigration policy can affect the demographics of our patient population, staff, and future physicians. Being involved in drafting public policy helps ensure that physician interests and patient interests are represented.

Encouragingly, dermatologists have successfully advocated for our patients and our field. The Affordable Care Act of 2008 contained a provision heavily taxing the tanning bed industry. This is credited with the closure of over 10,000 tanning salons and has contributed to the 50% reduction in tanning salon use among high school students between 2009 and 2015.[3] Many states also ban the use of tanning beds by minors under the age of 18 due to initiatives championed by dermatologist advocacy groups at the local and state level. Dermatologist advocacy initiatives have also played a major role in shaping compensation schedules and billing recommendations from both the Centers for Medicare and Medicaid and Services as well as large commercial insurance carriers.

Dermatologists advocate for patients every day in their clinical practice. Unfortunately, this means that we face barriers to care daily that require individual patient advocacy. Becoming engaged with our communities can help us create more equitable, efficient, and effective health systems.

Although engagement can take many forms, most physician advocacy activity primarily falls within either health advocacy or legislative advocacy. Health advocacy refers to any advocacy activity that relates specifically to the improvement and accessibility of health care. Legislative advocacy refers specifically to the use of state or federal legislation to effect policy change. While there may be overlap, as in health groups working on the Affordable Care Act of 2008, it is useful to think about them separately.

55.3 Health Advocacy

Many physicians are familiar with health advocacy and have participated in at least one health advocacy activity at some point in their careers. Advocating for our individual patients is a universal experience and example of health advocacy. Supporting physician groups and other nongovernmental organizations are other ways to promote patients' health.

55.4 Patient Advocacy

Physicians as patient advocates is likely a familiar concept. Every day in clinical practice we advocate for our patients by elucidating their goals, prescribing medications regimens that they can afford and follow, or referring them to appropriate specialists and services. Submitting prior authorizations and appealing denials are an important component of patient advocacy. Many writers and medical ethicists have analyzed how physicians are patient advocates. These include providing informed consent, protecting patient autonomy, facilitating surrogate decision-making, and ensuring access to health care resources.[4]

But patient advocacy in the clinical setting can be taken a step further in the form of care and quality improvement projects. Improving our local health systems lets us make daily patient care better for both patients and ourselves. There are a multitude of potential initiatives. To help us address socioeconomic barriers, we might create or expand access to social workers and care coordinators. To help us treat the psychosocial impact of disease, we might partner with patient support groups to provide their contact information and educational resources. If you notice a recurring problem in your clinical environment (e.g., timely biopsy result notification, pathology processing, clinic flow, or clinic wait times) perhaps you may be motivated to undertake a quality improvement project.

The possibilities for improvement can seem endless but all it takes is a single moment to identify an issue that can be addressed. Any single effort to advance patient care, no matter how small, is a step in the right direction.

55.4.1 Physician Advocacy Groups

There are many physician advocacy groups with differing scopes and specialty niches. Joining your local state dermatologic and physician societies, American Academy of Dermatology (AAD), American Society for Dermatologic Surgery Association (ASDSA), and American Medical Association (AMA) are excellent places to start. These societies often have ongoing advocacy and service projects and many seek volunteers (▶ Table 55.1). Each society has both state and legislative advocacy efforts. These can include patient-directed advocacy, such as skin cancer screenings, as well as

Table 55.1 Physician advocacy group advocacy and volunteer opportunities

American Academy of Dermatology[a]	• AccessDerm • Camp Discovery • Health Volunteers Overseas Native American Health Services Resident Rotation • Resident International Grant • Shade Structure Program • Skin Cancer for Developing Countries Grant SPOTme Skin Cancer Screening Program • SPOT Skin Cancer Academic Dermatology Leadership Program • Diversity Mentorship Program
American Society for Dermatologic Society Association[b]	• Choose Skin Health • Skin Cancer Is Color Blind • SPF for All • Stylists Against Skin Cancer • Sun Safe Soccer • Sun Safe Surfing
American Medical Association[c]	• Liability & Risk in Digital Health Innovation • FDA Issues • Target:BP™ • Reversing the Opioid Epidemic

[a]Updated as of January 20, 2019 at www.aad.org/members/volunteer.
[b]Updated as of January 20, 2019 at www.asds.net/Medical-Professionals/Public-Service-Programs.
[c]Updated as of January 20, 2019 at www.ama-assn.org/advocacy/physician-advocacy/national-advocacy

legislative efforts, such as lobbying days on Capitol Hill (see below).

The AAD and ASDSA have several volunteer opportunities for dermatologists listed on their websites at www.aad.org/members/volunteer and www.asds.net/ASDSA-Advocacy. These include a teledermatology program to expand access to underserved areas, summer camp for children with dermatologic diseases, free skin cancer screening program, and much more. In addition to these service opportunities, you can also volunteer to mentor medical students and young dermatologists. Joining the AAD also opens up the opportunity to apply for and join its numerous committees, positioning you as a leader in our field.

The AMA also undertakes many advocacy initiatives. While they aim to represent all physicians, many directly affect dermatology. Efforts such as its Truth In Advertising Campaign and Scope of

Practice Partnership directly affect dermatology and our patients.

55.4.2 Local Charities and Organizations

There are thousands of local, state, and national nongovernmental organizations that are interested in promoting human well-being and improving our society. Partnering with them can be a simple way to align and integrate your practice with and into your community. For example, one could hold skin cancer screenings with local melanoma and skin cancer awareness groups. One could also establish one's clinic as a food or clothing drive drop-off site. There are multiple nonprofit organizations dedicated to dermatologic disease, melanoma, and skin cancer awareness and prevention that are easy to partner with (▶Table 55.2).

Our civic engagement, as physicians, also need not be restricted to health care initiatives. Building stronger communities and empowering civil society also advances the goals of health and wellness. This could include supporting local schools, shelters, community centers, or religious organizations. Engaging with these organizations not only strengthens our social fabric, but also reinforces physicians' roles as community leaders.

55.5 Legislative Advocacy

Legislation can have enormous ramifications upon patient care and our professional lives. For this reason, many important health policy discussions occur in the sphere of legislative action. The idea of joining legislative initiatives may feel intimidating because the legislative process can be long, cumbersome, and confusing. First understanding how legislation is created can make it far less daunting to get involved.

55.5.1 Legislative Structure

The federal government comprises the executive, legislative, and judicial branches. The legislative branch, or Congress, passes bills for signature and enforcement by the executive branch. The judicial branch is largely tasked with settling disputes regarding the constitutionality of legislation. The process to create federal legislation is discussed below, but the process for most state legislation is fairly similar.

Congress has two chambers: The House of Representatives and the Senate. The House currently has 435 members with state representation determined roughly by population. Representatives are elected to 2-year terms. The Senate has 100 members, two from each state. Senators serve 6-year terms with reelections taking place every other year for one-third of the senators in a staggered fashion.

For a particular bill to pass, it must pass independently in both the House and Senate (▶Fig. 55.1). The bills may be modified or amended in the process. The two bills are then reconciled with each other and sent back to the chambers for a final vote. If the reconciled bill is approved by both chambers, then the President can either sign or veto the bill. A presidential veto can be overridden with a two-thirds vote in both the House and Senate.

Each chamber of Congress has multiple committees with differing purviews for related legislation. Each committee is chaired by a senior

Table 55.2 Dermatologic nonprofit organizations

Nonprofit organization	Website
The Skin Cancer Foundation	skincancer.org
American Melanoma Foundation	myamf.org
National Council on Skin Cancer Prevention	Skincancerprevention.org
Children's Skin Disease Foundation	csdf.org
National Alopecia Areata Foundation	naaf.org
National Eczema Association	nationaleczema.org
The Foundation for Ichthyosis & Related Skin Types	firstskinfoundation.org
The National Psoriasis Foundation	psoriasis.org
The National Rosacea Society	rosacea.org
American Vitiligo Research Foundation	avrf.org
Scleroderma Research Foundation	srfcure.org
Lupus Foundation of America	lupus.org
American Skin Association	americanskin.org

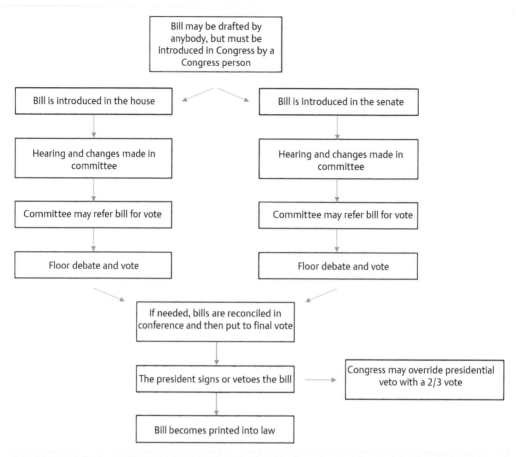

Fig. 55.1 The federal legislative process. Anybody may draft a bill to be considered in Congress, but the bill must be introduced by a Congressperson. Versions of the bill progress through each chamber. If approved by majority vote in each chamber, then the two bills are reconciled and a final vote is taken prior to going to the President for signature or veto. A veto may be overridden by a two-thirds vote in each chamber.

Congressperson from the political party that has a majority. This grants the majority party in each chamber tremendous power over Congress' legislative agenda.

With regard to health care, the relevant House of Representatives committees include Energy and Commerce, Ways and Means, Budget, and House Appropriations. The Energy and Commerce Committee has a Health Subcommittee and also has oversight of Medicare Part B. The Ways and Means Committee is involved with taxation but also has a Health Subcommittee that oversees Medicare Part A, Medicare Part B, and parts of the IRS, which is involved with health care costs. The Budget Committee and House Appropriations Committee

have control over federal spending and allocations to particular government programs. Medicare Part A covers inpatient, nursing facility, hospice, and home health care. Medicare Part B covers ambulatory and psychiatric services, durable medical equipment, and some prescription drug costs.

In the Senate, the relevant health care committees are the Senate Finance Committee and Health, Education, Labor, and Pensions (HELP) Committee. The Senate Finance Committee oversees Medicare, Medicaid, and State Children's Health Insurance program. It also oversees some health programs that are financed by specific taxes or funds. The HELP Committee oversees public health projects and health insurance carriers. It also oversees most of the Department of Health and Human Services including the Food and Drug Administration, Centers for Disease Control and Prevention, and National Institutes of Health.

Congresspersons also organize into caucuses to promote specific interests and goals. The bipartisan Skin Cancer Caucus was established in 2013 with support from the American College of Mohs Surgery and the AAD. The members of this Congress work to support legislation that raises skin cancer awareness and increases access to skin cancer treatment.[5]

55.5.2 Lobbying

Essentially every major industry and professional organization keeps in regular contact with Senators and Representatives on their relevant committees to promote their priorities. This is no different for physician groups and dermatologic societies. Even while the political climate, partisan politics, and balance of power may change annually, consistent lobbying efforts help ensure that legislation is crafted with physician input for the benefit of both patients and providers.

Many professional groups and their lobbyists will also strategically target members of Congress to influence a bill's contents and its chances of passing. This strategy might take into account a member's committee membership, party, and/or political vulnerability. Lobbying can take the form of petitions, letter writing, ads, campaign contributions, and direct contact with Congress members and their aides.

For example, members of the AAD and ASDSA make regular trips to Washington D.C. (AAD Legislative Conference and ASDSA Virtual Fly-In) in an effort to meet with Congress members and educate them on patient and physician needs.[6] Influencing the legislative process can therefore be as indirect as supporting our professional societies to as direct as working closely with Congress members to draft bills.

55.5.3 What You Can Do

One simple way to influence legislation is to write to your elected representatives. Many physician societies such as the AMA, AAD, and ASDSA organize letter writing campaigns in support or against legislative items. These societies also keep members abreast of legislative efforts and concerns with email notifications and prompts to contact state and local representatives. They also have pretemplated letters that make this even easier and less cumbersome. The AAD, for example, lists your state and federal representatives to whom you can then edit and send email templated letters regarding ongoing legislative efforts ▶ (Table 55.3).

Voting is another simple way to advocate. Voter turnout is historically the highest in presidential and midterm election years, but there are important measures on your local ballot every year. Local elections and ballot questions can have major implications on your community and patients. Familiarity with candidates for local office can help you understand how to vote in alignment with your health advocacy priorities.

Some physicians will even feel motivated to work on political campaigns for candidates that inspire them. In backing candidates that might

Table 55.3 Physician advocacy group lobbying efforts

American Academy of Dermatology[a]	Tell Congress to Maintain the Tanning Tax
	Support Skin Cancer Awareness in Congress
	Support Transparency in Medical Advertising
	Increase Transparency in Pharmaceutical Costs
American Society for Dermatologic Society Association[b]	SUNucate/Reducing the Risk of Skin Cancer and Excessive UV Exposure in Children Act
	Safe Laser and Energy-based Device Act
	Truth in Advertising and Scope of Practice
American Medical Association[c]	Administrative Simplification Advocacy
	AMA Vision on Health Care Reform
	Advocating for Diabetes Prevention
	Save Graduate Medical Education
	Join the Campaign to Promote Transparency in Drug Prices

[a]Updated as of January 20, 2019 at www.aad.org/advocacy.
[b]Updated as of January 20, 2019 at www.asds.net/ASDSA-Advocacy/Advocacy-Activities/Model-Legislation.
[c]Updated as of January 20, 2019 at www.ama-assn.org/advocacy/physician-advocacy/national-advocacy

promote human health and wellness, we can also advocate for patients. Campaign volunteering activities might include participating in telephone bank calls, canvassing, or voter registration drives.

55.6 Conclusion

Advocacy for the practicing dermatologist can take many forms. Most of the advocacy we are a part of occurs every day with our patients. However, there are many ways to get involved outside of the clinic and hospital. You can start an improvement project in your clinic, volunteer at a local school, contact your representatives, and be engaged members of your local, state, and national professional organizations. These actions not only help our patients and communities at large but also our own profession. Health care is constantly changing; if dermatologists are at the table making our voices heard, we can help guide change to the benefit of patients and providers alike.

References

[1] Luft LM. The essential role of physician as advocate: how and why we pass it on. Can Med Educ J 2017;8(3):e109–e116

[2] Gruen RL, et al. Public roles of US physicians: community participation, political involvement, and collective advocacy. JAMA 2006;296(20):2467–2475

[3] Ryan E. The "Tanning Tax" is a Public Health Success Story. Available at: www.healthaffairs.org. Published 2017. Accessed January 20, 2019

[4] Schwartz L. Is there an advocate in the house? The role of health care professionals in patient advocacy. J Med Ethics 2002;28:37–40

[5] Dermatology Times. Congress Forms Caucus on Skin Cancer. Available at: www.dermatology-times.com. Published 2012. Accessed January 20, 2019

[6] Olbricht S. Tis The Season for Getting Involved! Available at: www.aad.org. Published 2018. Accessed January 20, 2019

Index

Note: Page numbers set in **bold** or *italic* indicate headings or figures, respectively.

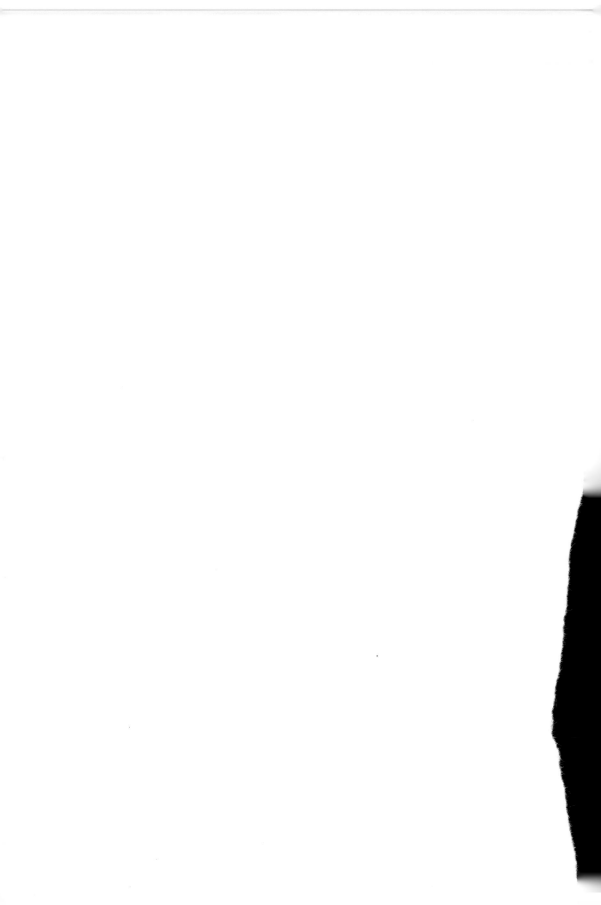